# THE WASHINGTON MANUAL® OF DERMATOLOGY DIAGNOSTICS

**Second Edition**

## M. Laurin Council, MD, MBA
Professor of Dermatology
Department of Medicine
Washington University School of Medicine
St. Louis, Missouri

## Lynn Cornelius, MD
Professor and Chief, Dermatology
Department of Medicine
Washington University School of Medicine
St. Louis, Missouri

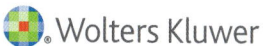

Philadelphia • Baltimore • New York • London
Buenos Aires • Hong Kong • Sydney • Tokyo

*Acquisitions Editor*: James Sherman
*Development Editor*: Eric McDermott
*Editorial Coordinator*: Chester Anthony Gonzalez
*Editorial Assistant*: Kristen Kardoley
*Marketing Manager*: Kirsten Watrud
*Production Project Manager*: Kirstin Johnson
*Manager, Graphic Arts & Design*: Stephen Druding
*Manufacturing Coordinator*: Lisa Bowling
*Prepress Vendor*: Straive

2nd edition

Copyright © 2026 Department of Medicine, Washington University School of Medicine

Copyright © 2016 by Department of Medicine, Washington University School of Medicine. All rights reserved. This book is protected by copyright. No part of this book may be reproduced or transmitted in any form or by any means, including as photocopies or scanned-in or other electronic copies, or utilized by any information storage and retrieval system without written permission from the copyright owner, except for brief quotations embodied in critical articles and reviews. Materials appearing in this book prepared by individuals as part of their official duties as U.S. government employees are not covered by the above-mentioned copyright. To request permission, please contact Wolters Kluwer at Two Commerce Square, 2001 Market Street, Philadelphia, PA 19103, via email at permissions@lww.com, or via our website at shop.lww.com (products and services).

9 8 7 6 5 4 3 2 1

Printed in Mexico

---

**Cataloging in Publication Data available on request from Publisher**

ISBN: 978-1-9752-3803-2

---

This work is provided "as is," and the publisher disclaims any and all warranties, express or implied, including any warranties as to accuracy, comprehensiveness, or currency of the content of this work.

This work is no substitute for individual patient assessment based upon healthcare professionals' examination of each patient and consideration of, among other things, age, weight, gender, current or prior medical conditions, medication history, laboratory data and other factors unique to the patient. The publisher does not provide medical advice or guidance and this work is merely a reference tool. Healthcare professionals, and not the publisher, are solely responsible for the use of this work including all medical judgments and for any resulting diagnosis and treatments.

Given continuous, rapid advances in medical science and health information, independent professional verification of medical diagnoses, indications, appropriate pharmaceutical selections and dosages, and treatment options should be made and healthcare professionals should consult a variety of sources. When prescribing medication, healthcare professionals are advised to consult the product information sheet (the manufacturer's package insert) accompanying each drug to verify, among other things, conditions of use, warnings and side effects and identify any changes in dosage schedule or contraindications, particularly if the medication to be administered is new, infrequently used or has a narrow therapeutic range. To the maximum extent permitted under applicable law, no responsibility is assumed by the publisher for any injury and/or damage to persons or property, as a matter of products liability, negligence law or otherwise, or from any reference to or use by any person of this work.

shop.lww.com

*To Arthur Eisen, MD, our mentor and friend.*

# Contributors

**Damien Abreu, MD, PhD**
Chief Resident
Division of Dermatology
Department of Medicine
Washington University School of Medicine
St. Louis, Missouri

**Joel Adu-Brimpong, MHI**
MD/MBA Candidate
School of Medicine & Graduate School of Business
Stanford University
Stanford, California

**Milan Anadkat, MD**
Professor
Division of Dermatology
Department of Medicine
Washington University School of Medicine
St. Louis, Missouri

**Susan Bayliss, MD**
Professor Emeritus of Dermatology
Department of Internal Medicine
Department of Pediatrics
Washington University School of Medicine
St. Louis, Missouri

**Cynthia Chen, BS**
Medical Student
Division of Dermatology
Department of Medicine
Washington University School of Medicine
St. Louis, Missouri

**David Chen, MD, PhD**
Assistant Professor
Department of Medicine
Washington University School of Medicine
St. Louis, Missouri

**Emily Cole, MD, MPH**
Assistant Professor
Division of Dermatology
Department of Medicine
Washington University School of Medicine
St. Louis, Missouri

**Lynn Cornelius, MD**
Professor and Chief, Dermatology
Department of Medicine
Washington University School of Medicine
St. Louis, Missouri

**M. Laurin Council, MD, MBA**
Professor of Dermatology
Department of Medicine
Washington University School of Medicine
St. Louis, Missouri

**Yuliya Kozina, BSc**
Student
Department of Medicine
Washington University School of Medicine
St. Louis, Missouri

**Ali Malik, MD**
Resident Physician
Division of Dermatology
Department of Medicine
Washington University School of Medicine
St. Louis, Missouri

**Caroline Mann, MD**
Dermatologist
Department of Internal Medicine
Washington University School of Medicine
St. Louis, Missouri

**Rabia Mayer, MD, PhD**
Assistant Professor of Dermatology
Department of Medicine
Washington University School of Medicine
St. Louis, Missouri

**Aubriana M. McEvoy, MD, MS**
Physician
Division of Dermatology
Department of Medicine
Washington University School of Medicine
St. Louis, Missouri

**Basia Michalski-McNeely, MD**
Assistant Professor
Department of Medicine
Washington University School of Medicine
St. Louis, Missouri

**Amy Musiek, MD**
Professor Medicine
Division of Dermatology
Department of Medicine
Washington University School of Medicine
St. Louis, Missouri

**Muithi Mwanthi, MD, PhD**
Assistant Professor
Division of Dermatology
Department of Medicine
Washington University School of Medicine
St. Louis, Missouri

**Spencer Ng, MD, PhD**
Assistant Professor
Division of Dermatology
Department of Medicine
Department of Pathology/Immunology
Washington University School of Medicine
St. Louis, Missouri

**Morgan Nguyen, MD**
Resident Physician
Division of Dermatology
Washington University School of Medicine
St Louis, Missouri

**Jennifer Pugh, MD**
Resident Physician
Division of Dermatology
Department of Medicine
Washington University School of Medicine
St. Louis, Missouri

**Sunaina Rengarajan, MD, PhD**
Instructor of Dermatology
Department of Medicine
Washington University School of Medicine
St. Louis, Missouri

**Aaron Russell, MD**
Assistant Professor
Division of Dermatology
Department of Internal Medicine
Department of Pathology & Immunology
Washington University School of Medicine
St. Louis, Missouri

**Liza Siegel, MD**
Assistant Professor of Dermatology
Department of Internal Medicine
Washington University School of Medicine
St. Louis, Missouri

**Carly Stevens, MD**
Resident Physician
Department of Internal Medicine
Tulane University
New Orleans, Louisiana

**M. Slade Stratton, MD**
Assistant Professor
Division of Dermatology
Department of Medicine
Washington University School of Medicine
St. Louis, Missouri

# Preface

Dermatology has entered an exciting era. Novel targeted therapies are emerging for severe forms of common conditions, such as hidradenitis suppurativa and alopecia areata. Advances have been made in the treatment of deadly skin cancers, such as Merkel cell carcinoma and melanoma, extending the lives of our patients by years to decades. On the cosmetic side, energy-based devices and injectables have evolved to reverse the signs of aging. Now, more than ever, we are gaining greater insight into the science behind skin conditions and developing targeted therapeutic modalities.

Whether you are a medical student aspiring to become a dermatologist, an intern rotating through hospital wards, a primary care physician treating patients with skin concerns, or a specialist aiming to garner a greater understanding of dermatology, we hope that you will find this book to be a valuable resource. The *Washington Manual of Dermatology Diagnostics* covers the fundamentals of the study of the skin, hair, and nails. Now in its second edition, this text provides an overview of the most important aspects of the study of dermatology. Basics, such as terminology used when describing skin lesion morphology and important steps of the skin examination, are covered in the first chapter. The structural importance of the skin and normal skin function are described in Chapter 2.

Chapters 3 to 10 describe the most common skin conditions, which one will encounter in medicine. The next few chapters elaborate on subspecialties of dermatology: dermatologic surgery, aesthetic dermatology, pediatric dermatology, and geriatric dermatology, respectively. Given a need to understand how different conditions manifest in those with different skin types, this edition includes a chapter on dermatology in skin of color. This book also covers the importance of sun safety (Chapter 16) and includes a chapter on common therapies used in dermatology (Chapter 17). We trust that you will find the information contained in this edition helpful in the care of your patients.

This manual would not be possible without the dedicated authors of Washington University. We thank you for the countless hours of reviewing the literature and succinctly summarizing the most pertinent facts for this text, and we thank you for contributing classic examples of conditions from your image collections. Finally, and most importantly, we would like to thank the patients of our clinics and hospitals, for allowing us the opportunity to learn from you and allowing us to share what we have learned with others.

*M. Laurin Council, MD, MBA*

# Contents

**Contributors** iv
**Preface** vi

**1 The Skin Examination** 1
M. Laurin Council, MD, MBA

**2 Basic Science of the Skin** 10
Jennifer Pugh, MD and Joel Adu-Brimpong, MHI

**3 Inflammatory Disorders** 24
Amy Musiek, MD

**4 Infections and Infestations** 58
Rabia Mayer, MD, PhD

**5 Reactive Disorders and Drug Eruptions** 95
Yuliya Kozina, BSc and Milan Anadkat, MD

**6 Disorders of Pigmentation** 125
Cynthia Chen, BS, Caroline Mann, MD, and Sunaina Rengarajan, MD, PhD

**7 Benign Skin Lesions** 146
Aaron Russell, MD and M. Laurin Council, MD, MBA

**8 Malignant Skin Lesions** 157
Aubriana M. McEvoy, MD, MS, Ali Malik, MD, David Chen, MD, PhD, Amy Musiek, MD, and Lynn Cornelius, MD

**9 Disorders of the Hair and Nails** 183
Caroline Mann, MD and Aaron Russell, MD

**10 Cutaneous Manifestations of Systemic Disease** 201
Amy Musiek, MD

**11 Dermatologic Surgery** 215
Ali Malik, MD, Aubriana M. McEvoy, MD, MS, and M. Slade Stratton, MD

**12 Aesthetic Dermatology** 233
Morgan Nguyen, MD, Ali Malik, MD, and Basia Michalski-McNeely, MD

**13 Skin of Color Dermatology** 251
Muithi Mwanthi, MD, PhD and Damien Abreu, MD, PhD

**14 Pediatric Dermatology** 291
Carly Stevens, MD, Liza Siegel, MD, and Susan Bayliss, MD

**15 Geriatric Dermatology** 316
Spencer Ng, MD, PhD

**16 Sun Safety** 333
M. Laurin Council, MD, MBA

**17 Dermatologic Therapies** 340
Emily Cole, MD, MPH

**Index** 363

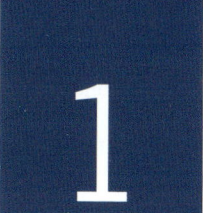

# The Skin Examination

M. Laurin Council, MD, MBA

Unlike other medical disciples, dermatology is a predominantly visual field. By directly observing and palpating the skin, one can obtain vital information, which can lead to the correct diagnosis and treatment. Pointed questions and, occasionally, ancillary tests are also useful to this regard. This chapter covers the nuances of examination of the skin.

## 1. Dermatologic History

- History of present illness
  - In most medical specialties, a thorough history is obtained first from the patient followed by a physical examination. In dermatology, the physical examination is essential to achieving a diagnosis, so it is best to obtain the medical history before, during, and after physical examination. Key questions to ask include the following:
    - "How long?"
    - "Does it hurt or itch?"
    - "What treatments have you tried?"
    - "Have you had any other symptoms?"
- Past medical history
  - Obtaining a focused past medical history is also essential to the dermatologic examination. Questions that are helpful to ask include, "Have you had similar rashes before?" This may assist in the diagnosis, and if previous treatments have been employed, they may assist in treatment as well. Prior to prescribing any systemic medications, other illnesses should be documented.

## 2. Indications for Total-Body Skin Examination

- In 2023, the U.S. Preventive Services Task Force (USPSTF) reported insufficient evidence for or against screening for skin cancer in asymptomatic adults and adolescents.[1] It is important to note that USPSTF comment is limited to *asymptomatic* individuals and that the American Academy of Dermatology encourages patients at higher risk of developing skin cancer to see a board-certified dermatologist.[2]
  - Patients with history of extensive sun exposure or sunburn
  - Patients with fair skin over age 65
  - Patients with clinically atypical nevi
  - Patients with more than 50 nevi
- In 2018, the USPSTF gave a grade "B" recommendation to the practice of counseling fair-skinned children, adolescents, and young adults ages 6 months to 24 years about reducing their risk of skin cancer. They concluded that "insufficient" evidence existed for similar counseling for adults.[3]

---

*The authors would like to acknowledge the first edition authors* Rebecca Chibnall, Susan Bayliss, and Arthur Eisen.

- Our recommendations are that any fair-skinned individual who has had considerable sun exposure during the early periods of his or her life needs to be examined at least yearly. Individuals who have numerous nevi should also be examined annually. Additionally, patients with a family history of melanoma in a first-degree relative also warrant an annual skin examination. Patients should be instructed in the ABCDEs of melanoma, which are as follows:
  - A—Asymmetry
  - B—Border irregularity
  - C—Color variation
  - D—Diameter greater than 6 mm (the size of a pencil eraser)
  - E—Evolution

## 3. Examination Tools

- Potassium hydroxide mount (Fig. 1-1)
  - This technique is useful for diagnosing dermatophyte infections and can be easily employed in any clinic equipped with a microscope. The following steps will ensure an adequate and clinically helpful sample:
    - Hold a microscope slide perpendicular to the skin just inferior to the area identified for scraping. Using a 15-blade scalpel, vigorously scrape the scale from the edge of the lesion onto the slide.
    - Apply a cover slip to the portion of the slide with scale pieces. Place 1 to 2 drops of 20% KOH with dimethyl sulfoxide (DMSO) beneath the coverslip so that the entire field is covered.
    - Blot excess KOH with a paper towel. This allows the scale to be evenly distributed and prevents KOH from coming into contact with the microscope objective.
    - Scan the slide at low power (10×) searching for fungal elements, which appear as refractile, large, branching hyphae that cross cell membranes.
    - Higher-power examination of a suspicious area (40×) confirms the diagnosis.
  - This technique may also be used for diagnosis of scabies. Vigorous scraping of suspected burrows or papules should be performed to maximize the ability to find the mite.
- Culture
  - Occasionally, lesions will present with crust, purulent drainage, or ulceration. If infection is suspected, a culture swab may be taken to identify the causative organism. If crust is present, it should be removed and the exudate below swabbed for aerobic culture. Fungal cultures may also be performed in this way; however, if a deeper tissue infection is suspected, a tissue biopsy and culture will have greater yield.
  - Cultures or polymerase chain reaction may also be performed for viruses such as herpes simplex and varicella-zoster. Viral transport medium must be used, and vesicles should be deroofed or crust removed. The serum at the base should be vigorously swabbed to give the highest possible yield. Polymerase chain reaction results can be available relatively quickly, whereas culture results generally take 7 to 10 days.
- Dermatoscopy and other imaging tools
  - A dermatoscope is a noninvasive tool which can be used during the skin examination for a more in-depth look at skin lesions.
  - In dermoscopy, light and magnification are used on individual lesions to look for patterns and aid in diagnosis. Should a lesion remain suspicious even at a closer look, the gold standard is to remove the lesion for histopathological evaluation.

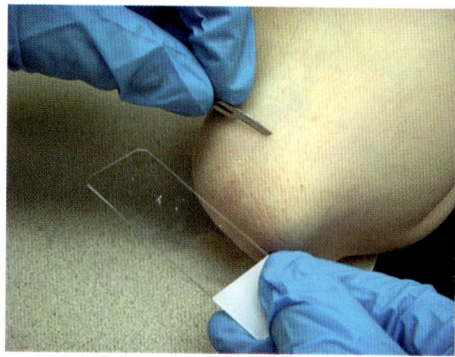

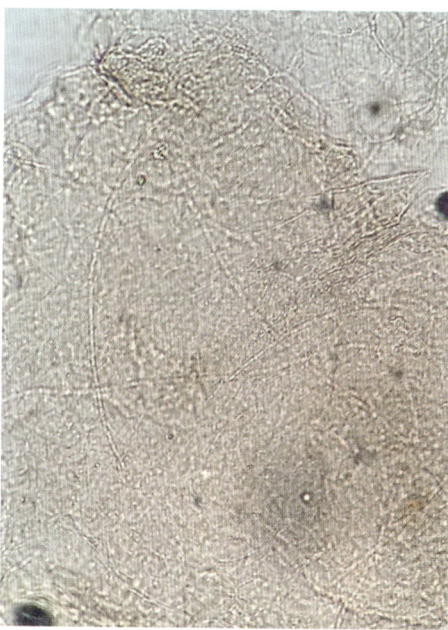

**Figure 1-1. A.** Skin scraping for a potassium hydroxide preparation. **B.** Positive prep for hyphae and yeast forms. (Courtesy of David Sheinbein.)

- Other imaging tools such as reflectance confocal microscopy, optical coherence tomography, and high-frequency ultrasound are used, although use is typically limited to research studies.
- Biopsy
  - The gold standard for precise diagnosis of many skin conditions remains tissue biopsy. The two most employed techniques are shave biopsy (Fig. 1-2) and punch biopsy (Fig. 1-3). Both are relatively simple and noninvasive procedures that can

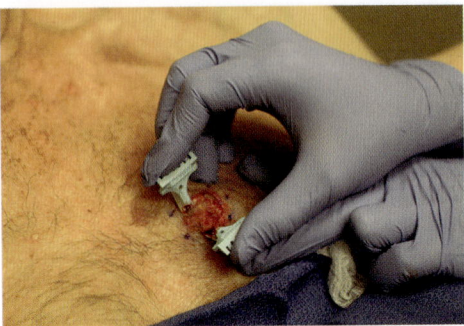

**Figure 1-2.** The shave biopsy technique. (Courtesy of M. Laurin Council, MD.)

be quickly performed in an outpatient setting. Shave biopsies are best utilized for lesions concerning for neoplasms such as nonmelanoma skin cancers or atypical moles. Care should be taken to entirely remove pigmented lesions through shave biopsy so as to not encounter sampling error. Punch biopsies are best employed for rashes or other inflammatory skin processes. The best site for a punch biopsy depends on the patient's rash. For ulcerated or necrotic lesions, the leading edge of the rash, especially if there is erythema, will give the highest yield. For primary blistering disorders, biopsy should be performed at the edge of the blister to include some intact skin as well. Steps taken for biopsy should be as follows:

- Identify and mark the site of biopsy. Obtain informed consent from the patient. Set up all supplies including properly labeled specimen cups.
- Cleanse the area, and then using a small-gauge (the author recommends 30-gauge) needle, infiltrate the area with 1% lidocaine with epinephrine 1:100,000 or similar local anesthetic so that a wheal is formed.
- For shave biopsy, a scalpel is used parallel to the skin or in a "scooping" fashion to remove the suspicious lesion. For punch biopsy, a firm twisting motion is employed perpendicular to the skin until the desired depth is achieved. The portion of tissue removed with the punch tool can then be gently lifted with forceps and snipped with scissors at the base.
- Tissue specimens should then be handled with care with forceps and placed in appropriately labeled specimen cups containing formalin.

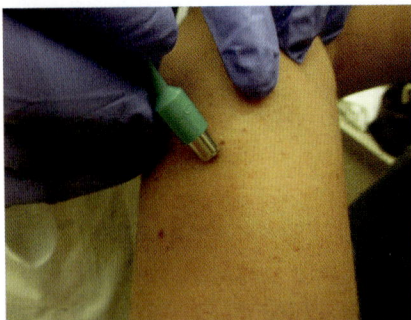

**Figure 1-3.** The punch biopsy technique. (Courtesy of M. Laurin Council, MD.)

- Hemostasis in shave biopsy can be achieved with electrocautery, firm pressure, or a 20% aluminum chloride solution. Hemostasis in punch biopsy can be achieved with the means above, but more commonly one or two simple interrupted sutures are placed.

## 4. Morphology of Skin Lesions

- In dermatology, terms used to describe specific lesions or patterns of lesions are standardized. Primary lesions are covered in Table 1-1. Secondary lesions, or lesions that appear because of an underlying or exogenous process, are demonstrated in Table 1-2. Table 1-3 describes various patterns of dermatologic lesions.

| TABLE 1-1 | Primary Lesions | |
|---|---|---|
| Macule | • Nonpalpable<br>• <1 cm in diameter | |
| Patch | • Nonpalpable<br>• >1 cm in diameter | |
| Papule | • Palpable<br>• <1 cm in diameter | |
| Plaque | • Palpable<br>• >1 cm in diameter | |

(*continued*)

| TABLE 1-1 | Primary Lesions (*continued*) | |
|---|---|---|
| Nodule | • Palpable, but deeper than a papule<br>• Often >1 cm in diameter | 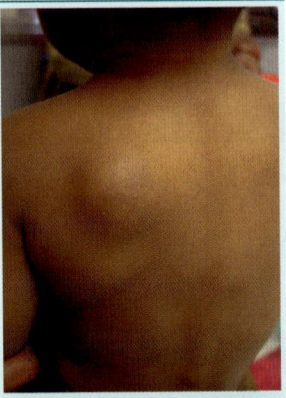 |
| Vesicle | • Palpable and filled with fluid<br>• <1 cm in diameter | 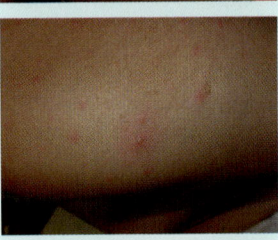 |
| Pustule | • Palpable and filled with purulent fluid<br>• <1 cm in diameter | 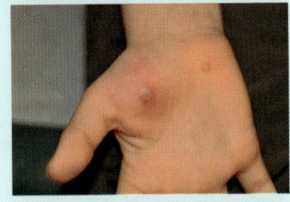 |
| Bullae | • Palpable and filled with fluid<br>• >1 cm in diameter | 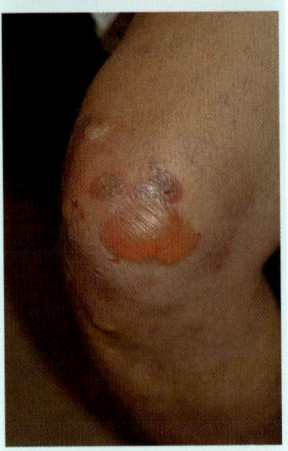 |

| TABLE 1-2 | Secondary Lesions | |
|---|---|---|
| Scale | • Keratin accumulation from the stratum corneum (outermost layer of skin) | |
| Crust | • Dried exudate or transudate. Can be hemorrhagic (blood), purulent (pus), or serous (serum) | |
| Fissure | • Linear crack in the skin often from excessive dryness | |
| Excoriation | • Traumatic injury to the skin | |
| Erosion | • Partial loss of the epidermis | |
| Ulcer | • Full-thickness loss of the epidermis. Can extend even deeper | 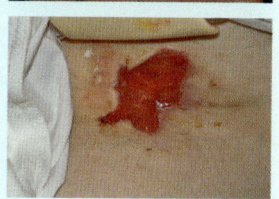 |

| TABLE 1-3 | Patterns of Dermatologic Lesions |
|---|---|
| Linear | 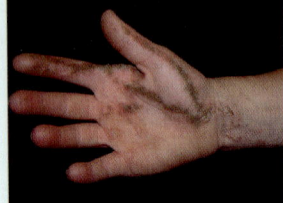 |
| Annular | 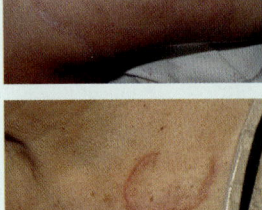 |
| Arcuate | 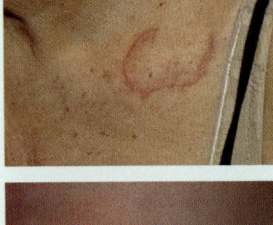 |
| Serpiginous | 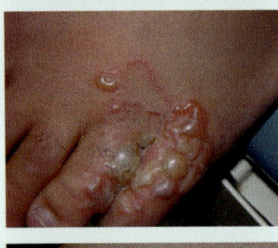 |
| Livedoid | 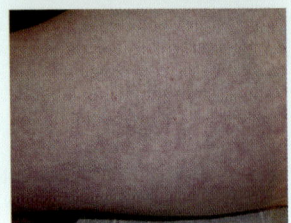 |

# REFERENCES

1. Skin cancer: screening. 2023. https://www.uspreventiveservicestaskforce.org/uspstf/recommendation/skin-cancer-screening
2. Cronin T. 2023. https://www.aad.org/news/aad-statement-uspstf-cancer-screeening
3. US Preventive Services Task Force. Behavioral counseling to prevent skin cancer: US Preventive Services Task Force recommendation statement. *JAMA*. 2018;319(11):1134-1142.

# Basic Science of the Skin

Jennifer Pugh, MD and Joel Adu-Brimpong, MHI

The skin is the largest organ of the human body. It not only serves as a physical barrier but also helps regulate temperature, sensory information, fluid balance, and UV damage.[1] On average, adult skin is 2.1 mm thick and divided into three main layers: the epidermis, dermis, and subcutis. Intermixed between these layers are adnexal structures such as hair follicles, nails, glands, and specialized sensory structures. Additionally, the skin is home to commensal microbiota, including millions of bacteria, fungi, and viruses. These organisms play a significant role in preventing invasion of foreign pathogens, informing innate immunity, and can be implicated in tumorigenesis.[2] Throughout this chapter, the authors discuss the intricate dynamic between the structure and function of healthy skin and how aberrancy contributes to the development and manifestation of clinical disease.

## 1. Basic Anatomy

- **Epidermis**, the outermost layer of the skin, averages 50 μm in thickness, consists principally of keratinocytes and completely turns over approximately every 50 days. The structure of the epidermis allows it to regulate fluid loss and protect against environmental insults. Histologically, the epidermis contains five strata, each representing a different stage of keratinocyte migration and maturation.[3] Also contained within the epidermis are melanocytes, Langerhans cells, and Merkel cells. Each strata are detailed below, starting from the inner- to outer-most layer.
  - **Stratum basale** (innermost): Typically a one- to three-cell layer, the stratum basale contains the basal keratinocytes, the stem cell reserve pool for skin regeneration. The basal keratinocytes attach to the extracellular matrix of the basement membrane via **hemidesmosomes**. The stratum basale also contains pigment-producing **melanocytes**, antigen-presenting **Langerhans cells**, and touch receptor–mediating **Merkel cells**.
  - **Stratum spinosum:** This layer of viable, outward migrating keratinocytes histologically appears "spiny" due to contracted microfilaments in **desmosomes**, structures composed of desmogleins and other molecules critical to epidermal integrity.
  - **Stratum granulosum:** This layer contains maturing keratinocytes filled with lamellar and keratohyalin granules, structures that mediate keratin and lamellar membrane formation, respectively, in the stratum corneum.
  - **Stratum lucidum:** This thin "clear layer" of dead keratinocytes just below the corneum serves as an additional reinforcing layer, found almost exclusively in the thickest skin (eg, palms, soles).
  - **Stratum corneum** (outermost): Composed of approximately 20 flattened anucleated corneocytes strengthened by corneodesmosomes within a network of hydrophobic lipid, including ceramides, cholesterol, and free fatty acids (eg, the "lamellar membrane"). This layer serves as a physical and immunologic barrier, modulates drug penetrance, and provides the microenvironment for commensal microbiota.

*The authors would like to acknowledge the first edition authors Karl Staser and Shadmehr Demehri.*

- **Clinical correlations:** Pathologic processes occurring in the epidermis typically demonstrate scaling, blistering, and/or crusting. **Examples**:
  - **Psoriasis**, which, among other mechanisms, results from increased keratinocyte proliferation and maturation, classically presents with distinctive silver-scaled pink papules and plaques. Histologically, there is parakeratosis containing neutrophils and uniform psoriasiform hyperplasia.
  - **Atopic dermatitis**, which is characterized by epidermal barrier dysfunction and immune dysregulation, has been associated with abnormalities in the filaggrin gene, which encodes for the filaggrin protein, a major structural protein in the stratum corneum. Clinically, patients present with dry, scaly, pruritic patches and plaques and have increased susceptibility to staph infections involving affected skin. Histologically, during the acute and subacute phase, there are varying degrees of spongiosis within the epidermis as well as a mixed superficial perivascular infiltrate.
  - **HSV infection**, which results in keratinocyte necrosis, presents with blistering and crusting. Histologically, viral cytopathic change can be seen involving keratinocytes.
  - **Seborrheic keratosis**, a common benign epidermal neoplasm, presents as a "stuck on," well-demarcated lesion, commonly with a waxy, scaled character due to uniform thickening of the epidermis. Unlike psoriasis, there is not parakeratosis containing neutrophils.
- **Dermis**, the layer located just below the epidermis (Fig. 2-1), provides structural support and facilitates nutrition and immune cell trafficking through its blood

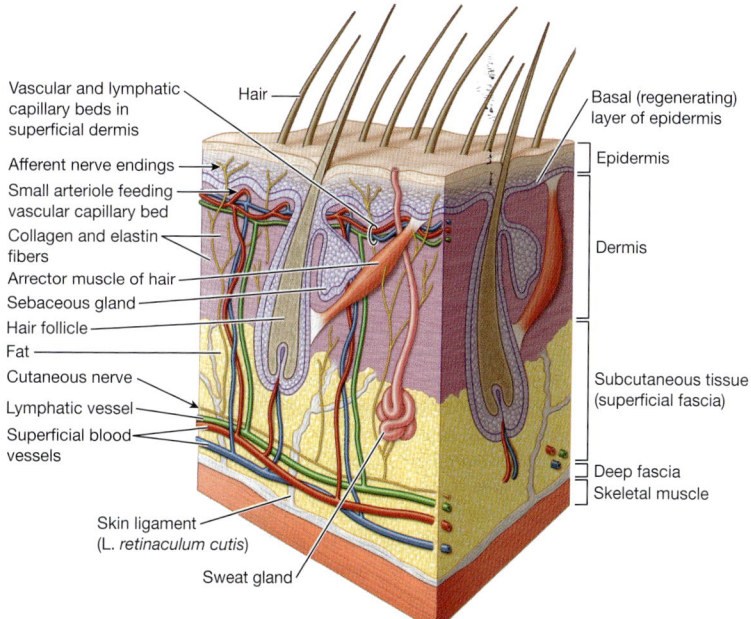

**Figure 2-1.** Anatomy of the skin. (Reprinted with permission from Moore KL, Agur AMR, Dalley AF. *Clinically Oriented Anatomy*. 9th ed. Wolters Kluwer; 2023:13. Figure 1.6.)

supply. Structural components include elastin, collagen, and the extrafibrillar matrix (ie, "ground substance," composed of water, glycosaminoglycans such as hyaluronan, proteoglycans, and glycoproteins). Histologically, the dermis contains three distinct anatomical zones:
- **Papillary dermis:** This uppermost, cellular layer of the dermis intercalates with the rete ridges of the epidermis, increasing the contact surface area between the epidermis and the vascular dermis, thus facilitating fine innervation and the exchange of nutrients, oxygen, and waste. The papillary dermis contains loosely arranged collagen types I, II, III, and VII.
- **Reticular dermis:** Predominantly composed of densely packed collagen type I, this lower layer of the dermis reinforces the skin's structural integrity; contains hair follicles, sweat glands, and nerve fibers; and serves as a critical conduit for the blood and lymphatic supply. Horizontal vessels in the reticular dermis join the subpapillary plexus that give rise to papillary capillaries and lymphatics supplying the epidermis.
- **Subcutaneous tissue:** Histologically, adipocytes and the presence of arteries and veins distinguish this dermal layer. This fatty tissue cushions the skin and provides a conduit for the large vessels that give rise to the horizontal vessels of the reticular dermis. This layer directly connects to the underlying deep fascia via fibrous bands.
- **Clinical correlations:** Pathologic processes confined to the dermis typically present as deeper papules or nodules lacking prominent changes on the skin surface. **Examples:**
  - **Neurofibromas**, a dermal neoplasm, present as prominent papules or nodules but lack discernible scaling, crusting, or blistering.
  - **Panniculitis**, such as **erythema nodosum**, which is considered a septal panniculitis due to inflammation primarily within the septa, may present as very indurated, tender, red-brown nodules or plaques with no overlying epidermal changes.
- **Hair** functions in thermoregulation, hygiene, and social-sexual communication. Individual hairs cycle between anagen (active growth ~85% of hairs), telogen (resting ~15%), and catagen (cessation of growth ~1%). Histologically, the **hair follicle** is composed of the **hair bulb** (deep portion), **isthmus** (middle portion), and the **infundibulum** (superficial portion).
  - The **hair bulb**, the site from which the entire follicle originates in the deep dermis, centers on the hair **papilla**, a nonregenerating structure comprised connective tissue and capillaries. The papilla reinforces and feeds the **hair matrix**, a collection of epithelial cells and melanocytes giving rise to the **hair shaft**.
  - The **hair shaft** contains a medulla, cortex, and cuticle, which, combined with the cuticle and root sheaths, contain at least 54 different keratin proteins. Compared to epidermal keratins, hair keratins contain increased sulfur in head and tail domains, allowing cross-links, which strengthen hair fibers.
  - The **hair bulge** rests at the insertion site of the arrector pili muscle. Multipotent stem cells localized within the hair bulb mediate epidermal regeneration, wound healing, and, possibly, neural regeneration.
  - The **arrector pili** muscles cause hair erection (ie, "goose bumps") and can serve as a source of neoplastic leiomyosarcoma.
  - **Hair follicles** escape immune detection (ie, "immunologically privileged"), similar to the anterior chamber of the eye, testis, brain, and placenta.
  - **Clinical correlations:** The presence and style of hair remain fundamental attributes to self-identity and social communication. As such, disorders related to hair growth can psychosocially devastate patients. **Examples:**
    - **Androgenic alopecia**, or "male pattern baldness," results from dihydrotestosterone stimulation, which promotes facial hair growth but inhibits scalp hair growth.

- **Scarring alopecia** processes include **lichen planopilaris**, **discoid lupus**, and **central centrifugal cicatricial alopecia.** With lichen planopilaris, there is CD8$^+$ predominant inflammatory infiltrate present at the level of the infundibulum and isthmus in contrast to a CD4$^+$ predominant infiltrate in central centrifugal cicatricial alopecia. Discoid lupus is characterized by follicular plugging and a lymphohistiocytic infiltrate at the level of the sebaceous gland and the hair bulge. All result in fibrosis and permanent hair loss.
- **Nonscarring alopecia** processes such as **alopecia areata (AA)**, which results from pathologic T-cell attack on hair matrix cells, do not destroy the stem cell pool, permitting complete regrowth. Inflammation is found at the level of the hair bulb in AA.
- **Neoplasms** such as **trichodiscoma** or **fibrofolliculoma** may arise from cells of the hair follicle.
- **Fungus** (tinea capitis), **lice**, and **crabs** (pediculosis pubis) commonly infest hair-bearing areas. Depending on severity, fungal infections can cause either scarring or nonscarring alopecia.
- The **pilosebaceous unit** describes the anatomical structure comprised the hair follicle, sebaceous glands, and apocrine or eccrine sweat glands.
  - **Eccrine sweat glands**, which are found on every cutaneous surface except the vermilion lip, clitoris, labia minora, and the external auditory canal, originate in perifollicular secretory coils located at the junction of the dermis and subcutaneous tissue. These coils attach to the eccrine duct, which extends upward through the dermis to extrude sweat via the acrosyringium (ie, "sweat pore"). Sweat is a sterile, hypotonic solution consisting of NaCl, $K^+$, $HCO_3^-$, and antimicrobial peptides (AMPs) such as dermcidin. Eccrine sweat glands receive innervation from muscarinic, α1, β2, β3, and purinergic receptors. Histologically, the eccrine sweat gland consists of three cell types: **large clear cells** secrete electrolytes and water, interspersed **dark cells** contain basophilic granules likely composed of sialomucin, and surrounding **myoepithelial cells** promote the outward movement of fluid.
  - **Apocrine sweat glands** are found on the external auditory canal (ceruminous glands), eyelid margins (glands of Moll), portions of the nostril, vermilion border of the lip, axilla, areola, nipple, and anogenital region. Like the eccrine sweat gland, apocrine sweat glands originate at the junction of the dermis and the subcutaneous tissue. In contrast to the eccrine sweat gland, the apocrine duct extends through the mid dermis to directly connect to the hair follicle, where it extrudes its contents. Apocrine sweat contains sterile, odorless, and acidic fluid rich in lipids including cholesterol, cholesterol esters, triglycerides, fatty acids, and squalene. This lipid, when processed by the skin's microbiota, produces bromhidrosis, that is, "body odor." Apocrine sweat glands receive innervation from β2, β3, purinergic, and, to a lesser degree, muscarinic receptors.
  - **Sebaceous glands** produce sebum, an oily substance composed of triglycerides, wax esters, squalene, and free fatty acids. Sebum lubricates the skin and reinforces its barrier function. Sebaceous glands also extrude diverse proteins important to endocrinologic and immunologic function. In most body sites, sebaceous glands associate with and directly connect to the hair follicle. Exceptions include sebaceous glands in the labia (Tyson glands), eyelids (Meibomian glands), areolae (Montgomery tubercles), and vermilion lips/oral mucosa (Fordyce granules).
  - **Clinical correlations:**
    - **Hyperthermia** can result from impaired sweating and cooling.
    - **Hyperhidrosis**, or excessive sweating, can significantly impair quality of life. Commonly affected areas included the axilla, palms, soles, back, buttocks, and groin.

- **Acne vulgaris** correlates with androgen-mediated sebaceous gland activity. Increased sebum production creates the milieu for pustule formation.
- **Sebaceous hyperplasia**, which presents as a pink/yellow crateriform papule typically on the face, can be mistaken for basal and squamous cell carcinoma (SCC).
- **Neoplasms**, including **sebaceous carcinoma**, **eccrine hidradenoma**, and **apocrine gland carcinoma**, arise from adnexal structures.
- **Muir-Torre syndrome**, a heritable variant of hereditary nonpolyposis colorectal carcinoma syndrome that results from mutations in DNA mismatch repair genes, may present as multiple sebaceous gland tumors in the context of a family history of gastrointestinal malignancy.

- **Cutaneous innervation** depends on specialized microanatomical structures with high sensitivity for specific types of sensation. Cutaneous sensation facilitates critical human activities, including feeding, sexuality/mating, and avoiding harm (ie, pain).[4]
  - **Merkel cells**, oval receptor cells located in the epidermal stratum basale, synapse with somatosensory afferents and mediate light touch discrimination. Merkel cells are found in the highest concentration in the fingertips, lips, and external genitalia.
  - **Free nerve endings**, branching, nonencapsulated nerve fibers terminating in the stratum granulosum, detect pain, temperature, and mechanical stimuli including stretch, pressure, and touch.
  - **Tactile (Meissner) corpuscle**, an unmyelinated nerve encapsulated by connective tissue and lamellated Schwann cells, localizes to the papillary dermis and mediates low-frequency (30- to 50-Hz) vibratory sensation. Tactile corpuscles are found in highest concentrations in the fingers, palms, and soles (ie, glabrous or non–hair-bearing skin).
  - **Lamellar (Pacinian) corpuscle**, a single afferent nerve encapsulated in lamellated Schwann cells and fibroblasts, has a distinctive "onionlike" appearance, localizes to the deep dermis, and mediates high-frequency (250- to 350-Hz) vibration of the skin. Lamellar corpuscles are found in the highest concentrations in the hand, where they compose 10% to 15% of cutaneous receptors.
  - **Bulbous (Ruffini) corpuscle**, a spindle-shaped encapsulated receptor with enlarged dendritic endings, localizes to the deep dermis and likely mediates cutaneous stretch sensations. Bulbous corpuscles are found in the highest concentrations in the fingertips, lips, and external genitalia. They compose approximately 25% of cutaneous receptors in the hand.
  - **Clinical correlations:**
    - **Erythromelalgia**, a disorder characterized by burning and erythema of the extremities, results from gain-of-function mutations in *SCN9A*, a gene that encodes a voltage-gated sodium channel subunit.
    - **Autosomal recessive insensitivity to pain** results from loss-of-function mutations of *SCN9A*. This disorder leads to unintentional self-mutilation and, potentially, accidental death.[5]
    - **Schwannomas, neuromas, neurofibromas**, and related tumors arise from Schwann cells (and their precursor cells) encapsulating axons in the cutaneous tissue.
    - **Merkel cell carcinoma**, a highly anaplastic neuroendocrine tumor, classically presents as a rapidly growing red-purple papule or nodule on the head or neck of an older male. However, some pathologists prefer to call these tumors **primary neuroendocrine carcinoma of the skin**, as they do not appear to arise directly from a clonogenic Merkel cell population.

- **Specialized skin sites** include the scalp, nails, palms and soles, and mucous membranes.
  - **Scalp** skin contains a high concentration of hair follicles, sebaceous glands, and blood vessels, explaining hair oiliness and the brisk bleeding of head lacerations.
  - **Volar** skin (palms and soles) contains a prominent keratinized stratum corneum and stratum lucidum and an increased concentration of eccrine sweat glands.
  - **The mucous membranes** lack a stratum corneum and thus are nonkeratinized.
  - **Finger and toenail** skin contains a **nail plate** composed of a thick layer of clear keratin (corresponding to the stratum corneum) overlying the **nail bed**, a thin layer of viable epidermal cells. Other distinctive structures include the **eponychium** (corresponding to the cuticle) and the **hyponychium**, thickened epidermis at the distal aspect of the nail bed reinforcing the nail against exterior insult.

## 2. Cellular and Molecular Biology

- **Epidermal cells** include keratinocytes, melanocytes, Merkel cells, and Langerhans cells.
  - **Keratinocytes** form the substance of the epidermis. These ectoderm-derived cells proliferate and migrate outward from their reserve pool along the stratum basale and, in wound healing, from the bulge of the hair follicle. Keratinocytes produce keratin, the key epidermal structural protein, and rely on specialized adherens junctions for epidermal integrity. There is a growing body of research investigating keratinocyte-derived cytokines, such as tumor necrosis factor (TNF), IL-17C, IL-36, and their implications in inflammatory skin diseases such as psoriasis and hidradenitis suppurativa (HS). These new developments have allowed for more targeted systemic therapies. Finally, keratinocytes, altered molecularly by UV damage or other insults, give rise to **actinic keratosis**, **basal cell**, and **SCC**.
    - **Keratin** intermediate filaments underpin the structural integrity of the epidermis and participate in cellular signaling. Keratins 5 and 14 predominate in the stratum basale, while keratins 1, 2, and 10 predominate in upper epidermal layers. Keratin gene mutations underpin **epidermolysis bullosa** and **epidermolytic ichthyosis** diseases, many of which lead to severe debility or fatality at an early age.[6]
    - **Keratohyalin granules** contain loricrin and profilaggrin, proteins critical to the barrier and water retention functions of the stratum corneum. Filaggrin mutations underlie **ichthyosis vulgaris** and some cases of **atopic dermatitis/eczema**. Hypothetically, in atopic dermatitis, filaggrin dysfunction permits increased antigen penetration, leading to immune hypersensitivity and inflammation.
    - **Hemidesmosomes** connect keratinocytes along the stratum basale to the basement membrane. Autoantibodies directed against hemidesmosome-localized transmembrane collagen XVII (ie, BPAG2) and cytoskeletal linker BP230 (ie, BPAG1) underpin **bullous pemphigoid**, a disease characterized by tense blistering.
    - **Desmosomes**, a specialized adherens junction composed of desmoglein, desmocollin, and plakins, connect keratinocytes to each other within the epidermis. Autoantibodies directed against desmoglein-1 and desmoglein-3 underpin **pemphigus** group (eg, vulgaris, foliaceous), diseases characterized by

flaccid blistering. Desmoglein proteins reinforce hair follicle integrity, just as in the epidermis. Genetic mutations in desmoglein and other desmosome-related proteins underpin some **palmoplantar keratosis, ectodermal dysplasia**, and hair follicle malformation syndromes.

- **E6** and **E7**, viral peptides expressed by the human papillomavirus, inhibit keratinocyte **p53** and **Rb**, promoting malignant transformation in HPV-associated **SCC**. HPV-associated squamous cell hyperplasia also results in verruca vulgaris (warts). **Epidermodysplasia verruciformis** is a rare genetic condition characterized by the inability of the immune system to clear HPV, increasing the risk of mutations accumulating in affected keratinocytes and the development of SCC.

○ **Melanocytes**, neural crest–derived pigmented cells located in the stratum basale, determine skin color through their synthesis of melanin, a product of tyrosine oxidation. Via dendritic processes, melanocytes transfer melanin-containing melanosomes to neighboring keratinocytes in the epidermis. Melanin refracts light and protects against UV damage. Accordingly, dark-skinned individuals, who have the highest concentrations of eumelanin, have the lowest risk of **melanoma**, a common and potentially fatal neoplasm of melanocytes. Fair-skinned red-haired individuals, who have high concentrations of pheomelanin, a relatively poor photoprotective molecule, have the highest risk of melanoma. Of note, melanin production indicates existing UV damage—therefore, one could argue that no tan is a "safe tan." Melanoma is caused by unchecked proliferation of melanocytes with mutations most commonly affecting *CDKN2A*, *PTEN*, *BRAF*, and *N-RAS*. There have been significant advancements in the understanding and management of melanoma with many therapies targeted at preventing tumors from evading the immune system, such as PD1 inhibitors, allowing patients' T cells to identify and attack the cancer cells.

- α-**MSH** (melanocyte-stimulating hormone) activates **MC1-R** (melanocortin-1 receptor), which ultimately transcribes **MITF** (microphthalmia-associated transcription factor). MITF regulates the expression of genes critical to melanin synthesis. Mutations in *MITF* underpin a subtype of **Waardenburg syndrome**, a disease characterized by heterochromia, white forelock, and hearing impairment.
- **Tyrosinase** hydroxylates tyrosine to DOPA, the rate-limiting step in melanin synthesis. Mutations in tyrosinase and associated transporter proteins underlie **oculocutaneous albinism**.
- **C-kit receptor tyrosine kinase** modulates melanocyte migration and survival. Inactivating *KIT* mutations result in **piebaldism** (white forelock, patchy hypopigmentation), while activating mutations correlate with certain forms of **melanoma**.
- **RAS-RAF-MEK-ERK** signaling pathway activating mutations, especially those in *BRAF*, are found in many melanomas.
- **Neurofibromin**, the protein product of the *NF1* gene, negatively regulates RAS-RAF-MEK-ERK signaling. *NF1* mutations underpin **neurofibromatosis type 1**, a disease characterized by multiple neurofibromas and pigmented **café au lait macules**, which contain hyperactive melanocytes. *NF1* mutations also correlate with certain forms of **melanoma**.

○ **Merkel cells** are specialized touch receptors (see **Cutaneous innervation**).
○ **Langerhans cells** are specialized dendritic cells (DCs), antigen-presenting cells of the immune system (see **Adaptive immunity**).

- **Dermal cells** include fibroblasts, endothelial cells, smooth muscle cells, Schwann cells, adipocytes, specialized epithelial cells (eg, eccrine cells, apocrine cells; sebocytes), and inflammatory cells.
  - **Fibroblasts** synthesize and extrude the major components of the extracellular matrix, including collagens, laminins, elastin, fibrillins, and the macromolecules of the extrafibrillary matrix.
    - **Collagen**, a hydroxyproline-enriched α-helix trimer, exits the cell as procollagen before cross-linking with other structural proteins to create collagen fibrils, the backbone of the extracellular matrix. Many of the 28 known collagen types and their isoforms localize to the skin. Of note, collagen types I, III, and V compose much of the dermis, and collagen IV reinforces the basement membrane. **Deficiency in vitamin C**, a cofactor for lysyl and prolyl hydroxylases, results in defective collagen trimer formation and causes **scurvy**, a disease characterized by bleeding mucous membranes, spongy gums, and petechiae, all consequences of impaired wound healing. Genetic mutations in collagen and collagen-related genes result in **Ehlers-Danlos syndrome**, a disease characterized by hyperextensible skin and joints, easy bruising, and vascular anomalies. **Hypertrophic scars** and **keloids** result from increased numbers of fibroblasts and collagen density in the dermis.
    - **Elastin**, a highly cross-linked hydrophobic protein, and **fibrillin**, the main protein constituent of **microfibrils**, form **elastic fibers**, extracellular matrix molecules that allow skin to reform its original shape following stretching. Elastic fibers maintain the structural integrity of many organ systems, a point demonstrated by the systemic consequences of **Marfan syndrome**, a disease resulting from autosomal dominant mutations in **fibrillin** and the resultant increase in TGF-β signaling. Marfan patients present with long slender limbs, arachnodactyly, scoliosis, pes planus, hyperextensible joints, unexplained stretch marks, eye pathology (eg, subluxation or ectopia lentis, glaucoma, cataracts, retinal detachment), mitral valve prolapse, aortic aneurysm or dissection, and spontaneous pneumothorax.
    - **Fibronectin** and **laminin** reinforce cell-to-collagen and cell-to-basement membrane connections, respectively.
    - **Proteoglycans**, negatively charged molecules such as heparan sulfate, chondroitin sulfate, and keratin sulfate, capture nutrients, growth factors, and water by attracting cations such as $Na^+$, $K^+$, and $Ca^{2+}$.
    - **Hyaluronic acid**, a nonproteoglycan polysaccharide, absorbs large amounts of water and resists compressive forces. Hyaluronic acid can be found in most popular dermal fillers used in the United States.
  - **Endothelial cells** form veins, arteries, arterioles, venules, and capillaries. Endothelial cells regulate body temperature, nutrient and oxygen delivery, and waste disposal.
    - **CD31, CD34**, and **PAL-E** mark blood vessels histologically.
    - **FGFR** and **VEGFR** modulate vasculogenesis and angiogenesis. Bevacizumab, a monoclonal antibody against VEGF-A, carries FDA approval in the treatment of several cancers.
    - **Selectins**, **ICAMs**, and **VCAMs** on the endothelial lumen modulate leukocyte chemotaxis.
    - **Vascular neoplasms** include **infantile hemangiomas**, **Kaposi sarcoma**, and **angiosarcoma**.
    - **Vasculitides** result from either immune complex–mediated inflammation or antineutrophil cytoplasmic antibodies, which incite neutrophil-endothelial

adherence and inflammatory effector release. Prominent dermatologic vasculitides include small-vessel (eg, **urticarial, Henoch-Schönlein, drug-** or **infection-induced**), small-to-medium (eg, **cryoglobulinemia, Churg-Strauss, granulomatosis with polyangiitis**), and, less commonly, medium-vessel vasculitis (eg, polyarteritis nodosa). Large-vessel vasculitides (eg, temporal arteritis, Takayasu's) rarely have prominent skin findings, as these vessels localize to deeper tissue.
- **Vasculopathies** result from microvascular occlusion (noninflammatory). The causes are numerous and include platelet plugging (eg, **TTP**), agglutination (noninflammatory **cryoglobulinemia**), infection (eg, **fungal, pseudomonas, strongyloidiasis, leprosy**), embolic (eg, **cholesterol, oxalate**), coagulopathic (eg, **warfarin necrosis**), occlusive (eg, **lymphoma**), and toxic (eg, **brown recluse spider**'s sphingomyelinase D).
○ **Schwann cells**, the principal glial cells of the peripheral nervous system, encase nerve axons to provide growth factors and conductive myelination.
- **S100** antibody detects for Schwann cells as well as melanocytes, adipocytes, Langerhans cells, DCs, myoepithelial cells, and macrophages.
- **Myelin** insulates nerves and is composed of cholesterol, other lipids, water, and proteins, including **myelin basic protein**. Antibodies against myelin basic protein may contribute to **multiple sclerosis**.
- **Neoplasms** arising from Schwann cells and their precursors include **plexiform neurofibromas** and **Schwannoma**.
○ **Adipocytes** contain lipid in the deep dermis. **Panniculitis**, or inflammation of the fat, results from many mechanisms, including autoimmune, infectious, and neoplastic.
○ **Smooth muscle cells** in the skin localize to arterial walls and arrector pili muscle. These structures, as well as the dartos muscle in the scrotum, serve as potential cells of origin for **leiomyoma** and **leiomyosarcoma** arising in the skin.
○ **Specialized epithelial cells** include apocrine cells, eccrine cells, and sebocytes (see **The pilosebaceous unit**).

## 3. Immunology

Cells of the **immune system** defend against pathogens, modulate tumorigenesis, and, in their dysregulation, effect inflammatory disorders such as psoriasis and lupus. Although convention has divided the immune system into the **innate** and **adaptive** systems, we increasingly appreciate the complex and inextricable interaction between all molecules, cells, and tissues of the immune system.[7]
- **Innate immunity** includes immune modalities activating in an antibody-independent fashion: complement, toll-like receptors (TLRs), AMPs, cytokines, and myeloid cells such as macrophages, neutrophils, eosinophils, basophils, mast cells, and innate lymphoid cells (ILCs) (eg, natural killer [NK] cells).
  ○ **Innate antimicrobial molecules** include AMPs, TLRs, and complement.
    - **AMPs**, low molecular weight (~5- to 15-kD) proteins synthesized in the skin by keratinocytes, eccrine/apocrine epithelial cells, and sebocytes, directly defend against bacteria, fungi, and, likely, viruses. Examples include **dermcidin, human β-defensin, lysozyme**, and **psoriasin**. Pathogens and secreted cytokines can induce AMP expression, and AMPs can attract DCs and memory T cells via CCR6.
    - **TLRs** expressed on DCs and keratinocytes recognize pathogen-derived molecules. Once activated, TLRs signal in a similar fashion as the IL-1 receptor, activating NF-κB and subsequent interferon production.

- **Complement** is activated by microbial polysaccharide interactions (alternate pathway), by other microbial carbohydrate interactions (lectin pathway), or by immune complex interactions (classical pathway). All pathways increase C3, and C3 cleaved products attract phagocytes. Moreover, complement C5b assembly with C6 to C9 forms the membrane attack complex, which directly lyses microbial cells.
  - **Macrophages** phagocytize cells labeled with complement as well as cells expressing nonvertebrate carbohydrates. They additionally secrete colony factors (eg, G-CSF), which promote neutrophil production and chemotaxis, present antigen to T and B cells, and critically modulate wound healing and angiogenesis.
  - **Neutrophils**, which activated macrophages can recruit in large numbers from precursor cells in the bone marrow, serve as frontline defenders against microbes. Neutrophils kill via oxygen-dependent (eg, the respiratory burst) and oxygen-independent (eg, myeloperoxidase secretion) mechanisms.
  - **Eosinophils** defend against parasites through IgE receptor (FcεR)-mediated degranulation of cytotoxic molecules and through the secretion of cytokines, leukotrienes, and prostaglandins. Eosinophil-mediated inflammation also underlies asthma and allergy.
  - **Mast cells**, granular myeloid lineage cells, mediate wound healing, host defense, and response to toxic insult. IgE-sensitized mast cells promote inflammation of asthma and allergy, including **urticaria**, through the release of cytokines and vasoactive effectors such as histamine. Cutaneous **mastocytosis** may present as widely distributed red macules and patches.
  - **ILCs**, a recently devised nomenclature with newly discovered cell types, include NK cells and other lymphoid-derived cells that activate in an antibody-independent fashion. Our current understanding of ILCs is rapidly evolving.[8]
    - **Group 1 ILCs** (which includes NK cells) produce TNF and IFN-γ and kill virus-infected and tumor cells.
    - **Group 2 ILCs** produce IL-4, IL-5, IL-9, and IL-13, mediate Th2 responses (see below), and help fight against parasite infection.
    - **Group 3 ILCs** produce IL-17 and IL-22 and likely modulate inflammatory disorders and tumorigenesis.
- **Adaptive immunity**, which regulates both cytotoxic and long-term antibody-dependent immunity (eg, response to vaccination), includes DCs (a key antigen-presenting cell), T lymphocytes, B lymphocytes, and plasma cells or antibody-producing lymphocytes. Multiple subsets of T cells exist, including Th1, Th2, regulatory (or immunosuppressive) T cells, and the more recently described Th17 cells, which appear to critically modulate certain inflammatory disorders such as psoriasis.
  - **DCs** process and present antigen to adaptive immune cells, thus acting as intermediaries between the innate and adaptive immune systems. **Langerhans cells**, DCs located in the epidermis, express major histocompatibility complex (MHC) class II and serve as powerful antigen-presenting cells that, following antigen capture, migrate to the lymphatic tissue to activate naive T cells.
  - **T cells**
    - **CD8⁺ T cells** recognize MHC class I–presented intracellular antigens (eg, virus, fungus, mycobacteria, tumor antigens). Cytotoxic CD8⁺ T cells affect killing through perforins, granzymes, granulysin, and FAS ligand interactions with Fas expressed on the target cell.
    - **CD4⁺ T cells** recognize MHC class II–presented antigens to modulate host defense against intracellular and extracellular antigens.

- CD4⁺IL-12R⁺ **Th1** cells produce IFN-γ, TNF-β, and IL-2, which stimulate macrophages and cytotoxic lymphocytes to fight intracellular pathogens and tumor cells.
- CD4⁺IL-4R⁺ **Th2** cells produce IL-5, IL-4, and IL-13, which stimulate macrophages, eosinophils, and B cells, promoting plasma cell differentiation and antibody production.
- CD4⁺IL-23⁺ **Th17** cells, which have more recently been described, produce IL-17 and help fight *Candida* and *Staphylococcus* infections. Th17 cells also promote psoriasis and eczema, and monoclonal antibodies directed against the Th17 pathway may effectively treat these diseases.
- **Tregs** suppress adaptive immune responses through secretion of IL-10, IL-35, and TGF-β, through conversion of adenosine triphosphate to adenosine (a cytotoxin), and through CTLA-4 interactions with MHC class II complex. **Ipilimumab**, a drug that carries FDA approval for the treatment of metastatic **melanoma**, inhibits CTLA-4 to promote antitumor cytotoxicity.
- **B cells** receive activating signals from T cells, which induce them to plasma cells that secrete antigen-specific immunoglobulin antibodies. **Plasma cells** produce IgM (primary responses), IgG (secondary immune responses, ie, long-term immunity), IgA (mucosal surfaces), IgE (allergy and anaphylaxis), or IgD (function largely unknown).

## 4. Immunomodulating Therapies

- Increased depth of knowledge regarding disease pathogenesis and aberrancies in the immune system have given rise to several systemic and local treatment options. Some therapies cause more broad immunosuppression, while others are more targeted monoclonal antibodies. Some of the more commonly used therapies are detailed below:
  - **TNF-alpha inhibitors**, such as **infliximab, adalimumab**, and **etanercept**, are used to treat psoriasis, psoriatic arthritis, and HS.[9,10] Of note, there have been a few reports of TNF alpha inhibitors leading to worse cardiac outcomes in patients with congestive heart failure NYHA class III or IV.[11]
  - **IL-4/13 inhibitors** are used in the treatment of moderate-to-severe atopic dermatitis. IL-4 acts upstream promoting the differentiation of naive CD4⁺ T cells into Th2 cells.[12] Th2 cells lead to pro-inflammatory cytokine production, such as IL-4 and IL-13.[13] **Dupilumab** inhibits IL-4 and IL-13, while **tralokinumab** only inhibits IL-13.[14,15] Neither have recommendations for routine lab monitoring.
  - **IL-17 inhibitors** such as **ixekizumab, secukinumab, bimekizumab**, and **brodalumab** are indicated for plaque psoriasis.[16-18] Secukinumab is also approved for HS.[19] Ixekizumab and secukinumab inhibit IL-17A; bimekizumab inhibits IL-7A and IL-17F; brodalumab inhibits IL-17RA and IL-17RC. Brodalumab has an FDA-mandated black box warning for suicidal ideation and is contraindicated in Crohn disease.[20]
  - **IL-23 inhibitors** include **guselkumab, tildrakizumab**, and **risankizumab**, which target the p19 domain.[21] **Ustekinumab** has activity against IL-23 and IL-12 as it targets the p40 subunit.[22] These therapies are effective for treatment of moderate-to-severe plaque psoriasis.[21,22]
  - **IL-31 inhibitors**, such as **nemolizumab**, block the proinflammatory cascade associated with itch and is, therefore, approved for the treatment of moderate-to-severe atopic dermatitis and prurigo nodularis.[23]
  - **Tyrosine kinase 2 (TYK2), deucravacitinib**, is an oral TYK2 inhibitor approved for the treatment of moderate-to-severe psoriasis.[24]

- **Anti-IgE antibody, omalizumab,** is used for the treatment of chronic idiopathic or spontaneous urticaria by binding free IgE and downregulating FcεRI.[25]
- **Janus kinase inhibitors (JAKi),** oral and topical, are used to treat dermatologic conditions through varying degrees of inhibition. **Baricitinib**, an oral treatment which inhibits Jak 1/2, is the first systemic JAKi to be approved for atopic dermatitis and the first systemic medication approved for AA.[26] **Ritlecitinib** works by dual JAK3/TEC family kinase inhibition and is indicated for AA.[27] **Upadacitinib** and **abrocitinib** are JAK1 inhibitors for treatment of atopic dermatitis.[28] **Upadacitinib** is indicated for psoriatic arthritis.[29] **Ruxolitinib**, which inhibits JAK1/2, is available as a topical and used to treat mild-to-moderate atopic dermatitis and vitiligo.[30,31] **Oral ruxolitinib** can be used in the treatment of graft versus host disease.[32] Black box warnings for JAKi include thromboembolic events, malignancy, and adverse cardiac events.[33]
- **Programmed cell death 1/programmed cell death ligand 1 (PD1/PDL1)** inhibitors are immune check point inhibitors that allow native cytotoxic T cells to identify and kill cancer cells.[34] PDL1 is located on the surface of the tumor cells, while PD1 is located on the T cells. These therapies are used in the treatment of metastatic melanoma. **Pembrolizumab** and **nivolumab** are PD1 inhibitors. **Cemiplimab** is also a PD1 inhibitor used to treat locally advanced or metastatic squamous cell and basal cell carcinoma.[35,36] **Ipilimumab** is the first approved check point inhibitor used to treat melanoma through CTLA-4 inhibition and is often used in combination with nivolumab for improved 10-year survival.[37] **Nivolumab** and **relatlimab-rmbw** target PD1 and LAG-3, respectively, in patients with untreated advance melanoma.[38] **Avelumab** is approved to treat advanced Merkel cell carcinoma.[39] Immune checkpoint inhibitors can cause immune-related adverse events such as lichenoid dermatoses, vitiligo, pneumonitis, and colitis. Vitiligo has been associated with antitumor efficacy in patient with metastatic melanoma.[40]
- **BRAF/MEK inhibitors** approved to treat melanoma include **dabrafenib/trametinib**, **vemurafenib/cobimetinib**, and **encorafenib/binimetinib**.[41,42] BRAF inhibitors have been associated with resistance and cutaneous SCC due to activation of MAPK pathway, both which are decreased with combination therapy.[41,42]
- **Talimogene laherparepvec (TVEC)** is an oncolytic viral immunotherapy derived from type 1 herpes simplex virus (HSV1). TVEC is currently approved for unresectable metastatic stage IIIB/C–IVM1a melanoma and being used off label for cutaneous SCC.[43] Local injection of TVEC stimulates local and systemic immunologic responses leading to tumor cell lysis, subsequent release of tumor-derived antigens, and activation of tumor-specific effector T cells.[43]
- **Tumor-infiltrating lymphocytes** therapy is an emerging treatment for unresectable stage IIIC or IV melanoma. Tumor-infiltrating lymphocytes therapy involves the ex vivo outgrowth and expansion of tumor-resident T cells and subsequent intravenous adoptive transfer of the cells after preparative lymphodepleting chemotherapy.[44]

# REFERENCES

1. Bolognia JL, Schaffer JV, Cerroni L, eds. *Dermatology*. 5th ed. Elsevier; 2025.
2. Belkaid Y, Segre JA. Dialogue between skin microbiota and immunity. *Science*. 2014;346(6212):954-959.
3. Elston DM, Ferringer T. Dermatopathology. In: *Requisites in Dermatology*. 2nd ed. Elsevier Saunders; 2008. http://hdl.library.upenn.edu/1017.12/1338118
4. Purves D, Williams SM. *Neuroscience*. 2nd ed. Sinauer Associates; 2001.

5. Hoeijmakers JG, Faber CG, Merkies IS, Waxman SG. Painful peripheral neuropathy and sodium channel mutations. *Neurosci Lett.* 2015;596:51-59.
6. Toivola DM, Boor P, Alam C, Strnad P. Keratins in health and disease. *Curr Opin Cell Biol.* 2015;32C:73-81.
7. Parham P, Janeway C, Louis A. Duhring fund. In: *The Immune System.* 3rd ed. Garland Science; 2009.
8. Diefenbach A, Colonna M, Koyasu S. Development, differentiation, and diversity of innate lymphoid cells. *Immunity.* 2014;41(3):354-365.
9. Mease PJ, Ory P, Sharp JT, et al. Adalimumab for long-term treatment of psoriatic arthritis: 2-year data from the Adalimumab Effectiveness in Psoriatic Arthritis Trial (ADEPT). *Ann Rheum Dis.* 2009;68(5):702-709. doi:10.1136/ard.2008.092767. PMID: 18684743; PMCID: PMC2663711.
10. Chung ES, Packer M, Lo KH, Fasanmade AA, Willerson JT; Anti-TNF Therapy Against Congestive Heart Failure Investigators. Randomized, double-blind, placebo-controlled, pilot trial of infliximab, a chimeric monoclonal antibody to tumor necrosis factor-alpha, in patients with moderate-to-severe heart failure: results of the anti-TNF Therapy Against Congestive Heart Failure (ATTACH) trial. *Circulation.* 2003;107(25):3133-3140. doi:10.1161/01.CIR.0000077913.60364.D2. PMID: 12796126.
11. Kimball AB, Okun MM, Williams DA, et al. Two phase 3 trials of adalimumab for hidradenitis suppurativa. *N Engl J Med.* 2016;375(5):422-434. doi:10.1056/NEJMoa1504370. PMID: 27518661.
12. Pappa G, Sgouros D, Theodoropoulos K, et al. The IL-4/-13 axis and its blocking in the treatment of atopic dermatitis. *J Clin Med.* 2022;11(19):5633. doi:10.3390/jcm11195633. PMID: 36233501; PMCID: PMC9570949.
13. Kokubo K, Onodera A, Kiuchi M, Tsuji K, Hirahara K, Nakayama T. Conventional and pathogenic Th2 cells in inflammation, tissue repair, and fibrosis. *Front Immunol.* 2022;13:945063. doi:10.3389/fimmu.2022.945063. PMID: 36016937; PMCID: PMC9395650.
14. Le Floc'h A, Allinne J, Nagashima K, et al. Dual blockade of IL-4 and IL-13 with dupilumab, an IL-4Rα antibody, is required to broadly inhibit type 2 inflammation. *Allergy.* 2020;75(5):1188-1204. doi:10.1111/all.14151. PMID: 31838750; PMCID: PMC7317958.
15. Wollenberg A, Blauvelt A, Guttman-Yassky E, et al. Tralokinumab for moderate-to-severe atopic dermatitis: results from two 52-week, randomized, double-blind, multicentre, placebo-controlled phase III trials (ECZTRA 1 and ECZTRA 2). *Br J Dermatol.* 2021;184(3):437-449. doi:10.1111/bjd.19574. PMID: 33000465; PMCID: PMC7986411.
16. Reich K, Warren RB, Lebwohl M, et al. Bimekizumab versus secukinumab in plaque psoriasis. *N Engl J Med.* 2021;385(2):142-152. doi:10.1056/NEJMoa2102383. PMID: 33891380.
17. Gordon KB, Blauvelt A, Papp KA, et al. Phase 3 trials of ixekizumab in moderate-to-severe plaque psoriasis. *N Engl J Med.* 2016;375(4):345-356. doi:10.1056/NEJMoa1512711. PMID: 27299809.
18. Lebwohl M, Strober B, Menter A, et al. Phase 3 studies comparing brodalumab with ustekinumab in psoriasis. *N Engl J Med.* 2015;373(14):1318-1328. doi:10.1056/NEJMoa1503824. PMID: 26422722.
19. Kimball AB, Jemec GBE, Alavi A, et al. Secukinumab in moderate-to-severe hidradenitis suppurativa (SUNSHINE and SUNRISE): week 16 and week 52 results of two identical, multicentre, randomised, placebo-controlled, double-blind phase 3 trials. *Lancet.* 2023;401(10378):747-761. doi:10.1016/S0140-6736(23)00022-3. Erratum in: *Lancet.* 2024;403(10427):618. doi:10.1016/S0140-6736(24)00266-6. PMID: 36746171.
20. Lebwohl MG, Koo JY, Armstrong AW, et al. Brodalumab: six-year US pharmacovigilance report. *Dermatol Ther (Heidelb).* 2025;15(1):213-222. doi:10.1007/s13555-024-01304-y. PMID: 39589679; PMCID: PMC11785849.
21. Blauvelt A, Chiricozzi A, Ehst BD, Lebwohl MG. Safety of IL-23 p19 inhibitors for the treatment of patients with moderate-to-severe plaque psoriasis: a narrative review. *Adv Ther.* 2023;40(8):3410-3433. doi:10.1007/s12325-023-02568-0. PMID: 37330926; PMCID: PMC10329957.
22. Papp KA, Blauvelt A, Bukhalo M, et al. Risankizumab versus ustekinumab for moderate-to-severe plaque psoriasis. *N Engl J Med.* 2017;376(16):1551-1560. doi:10.1056/NEJMoa1607017. PMID: 28423301.
23. Kabashima K, Matsumura T, Komazaki H, Kawashima M; Nemolizumab-JP01 Study Group. Trial of nemolizumab and topical agents for atopic dermatitis with pruritus. *N Engl J Med.* 2020;383(2):141-150. doi:10.1056/NEJMoa1917006. PMID: 32640132.
24. Strober B, Thaçi D, Sofen H, et al. Deucravacitinib versus placebo and apremilast in moderate to severe plaque psoriasis: efficacy and safety results from the 52-week, randomized, double-blinded, phase 3 Program fOr Evaluation of TYK2 inhibitor psoriasis second trial. *J Am Acad Dermatol.* 2023;88(1):40-51. doi:10.1016/j.jaad.2022.08.061. PMID: 36115523.
25. Maurer M, Rosén K, Hsieh HJ, et al. Omalizumab for the treatment of chronic idiopathic or spontaneous urticaria. *N Engl J Med.* 2013;368(10):924-935. doi:10.1056/NEJMoa1215372. Erratum in: *N Engl J Med.* 2013;368(24):2340-2341. PMID: 23432142.
26. King B, Maari C, Lain E, et al. Extended safety analysis of baricitinib 2 mg in adult patients with atopic dermatitis: an integrated analysis from eight randomized clinical trials. *Am J Clin Dermatol.* 2021;22(3):395-405. doi:10.1007/s40257-021-00602-x. Epub 2021 Apr 7. PMID: 33826132; PMCID: PMC8068648.

27. King B, Zhang X, Harcha WG, et al. Efficacy and safety of ritlecitinib in adults and adolescents with alopecia areata: a randomised, double-blind, multicentre, phase 2b-3 trial. *Lancet.* 2023;401(10387):1518-1529. doi:10.1016/S0140-6736(23)00222-2. Erratum in: *Lancet.* 2023;401(10392):1928. doi:10.1016/S0140-6736(23)01078-4. PMID: 37062298.
28. Wan H, Jia H, Xia T, et al. Comparative efficacy and safety of abrocitinib, baricitinib, and upadacitinib for moderate-to-severe atopic dermatitis: a network meta-analysis. *Dermatol Ther.* 2022;35(9):e15636. doi:10.1111/dth.15636. PMID: 35703351; PMCID: PMC9541568.
29. McInnes IB, Anderson JK, Magrey M, et al. Trial of upadacitinib and adalimumab for psoriatic arthritis. *N Engl J Med.* 2021;384(13):1227-1239. doi:10.1056/NEJMoa2022516. PMID: 33789011.
30. Papp K, Szepietowski JC, Kircik L, et al. Efficacy and safety of ruxolitinib cream for the treatment of atopic dermatitis: results from 2 phase 3, randomized, double-blind studies. *J Am Acad Dermatol.* 2021;85(4):863-872. doi:10.1016/j.jaad.2021.04.085. PMID:33957195.
31. Rosmarin D, Passeron T, Pandya AG, et al.; TRuE-V Study Group. Two phase 3, randomized, controlled trials of ruxolitinib cream for vitiligo. *N Engl J Med.* 2022;387(16):1445-1455. doi:10.1056/NEJMoa2118828. PMID: 36260792.
32. Zeiser R, von Bubnoff N, Butler J, et al. Ruxolitinib for glucocorticoid-refractory acute graft-versus-host disease. *N Engl J Med.* 2020;382(19):1800-1810. doi:10.1056/NEJMoa1917635. PMID:32320566.
33. Ytterberg SR, Bhatt DL, Mikuls TR, et al. ORAL Surveillance Investigators. Cardiovascular and cancer risk with tofacitinib in rheumatoid arthritis. *N Engl J Med.* 2022;386(4):316-326. doi:10.1056/NEJMoa2109927. PMID: 35081280.
34. Wang Y, Zhou S, Yang F, et al. Treatment-related adverse events of PD-1 and PD-L1 inhibitors in clinical trials: a systematic review and meta-analysis. *JAMA Oncol.* 2019;5(7):1008-1019. doi:10.1001/jamaoncol.2019.0393
35. Stratigos AJ, Sekulic A, Peris K, et al. Cemiplimab in locally advanced basal cell carcinoma after hedgehog inhibitor therapy: an open-label, multi-centre, single-arm, phase 2 trial. *Lancet Oncol.* 2021;22(6):848-857. doi:10.1016/S1470-2045(21)00126-1. PMID:34000246.
36. Migden MR, Rischin D, Schmults CD, et al. PD-1 blockade with cemiplimab in advanced cutaneous squamous-cell carcinoma. *N Engl J Med.* 2018;379(4):341-351. doi:10.1056/NEJMoa1805131. PMID: 29863979.
37. Wolchok JD, Chiarion-Sileni V, Rutkowski P, et al. Final, 10-year outcomes with nivolumab plus ipilimumab in advanced melanoma. *N Engl J Med.* 2025;392(1):11-22. doi:10.1056/NEJMoa2407417. PMID:39282897.
38. Tawbi HA, Schadendorf D, Lipson EJ, et al. Relatlimab and nivolumab versus nivolumab in untreated advanced melanoma. *N Engl J Med.* 2022;386(1):24-34. doi:10.1056/NEJMoa2109970. PMID: 34986285; PMCID: PMC9844513.
39. Kaufman HL, Russell J, Hamid O, et al. Avelumab in patients with chemotherapy-refractory metastatic Merkel cell carcinoma: a multicentre, single-group, open-label, phase 2 trial. *Lancet Oncol.* 2016;17(10):1374-1385. doi:10.1016/S1470-2045(16)30364-3. PMID: 27592805; PMCID: PMC5587154.
40. Hua C, Boussemart L, Mateus C, et al. Association of vitiligo with tumor response in patients with metastatic melanoma treated with pembrolizumab. *JAMA Dermatol.* 2016;152(1):45-51. doi:10.1001/jamadermatol.2015.2707. PMID: 26501224.
41. Long GV, Stroyakovskiy D, Gogas H, et al. Combined BRAF and MEK inhibition versus BRAF inhibition alone in melanoma. *N Engl J Med.* 2014;371(20):1877-1888. doi:10.1056/NEJMoa1406037. PMID:25265492.
42. Larkin J, Ascierto PA, Dréno B, et al. Combined vemurafenib and cobimetinib in BRAF-mutated melanoma. *N Engl J Med.* 2014;371(20):1867-1876. doi:10.1056/NEJMoa1408868. PMID:25265494.
43. Ferrucci PF, Pala L, Conforti F, Cocorocchio E. Talimogene laherparepvec (T-VEC): an intralesional cancer immunotherapy for advanced melanoma. *Cancers (Basel).* 2021;13(6):1383. doi:10.3390/cancers13061383. PMID: 33803762; PMCID: PMC8003308.
44. Rohaan MW, Borch TH, van den Berg JH, et al. Tumor-infiltrating lymphocyte therapy or ipilimumab in advanced melanoma. *N Engl J Med.* 2022;387(23):2113-2125. doi:10.1056/NEJMoa2210233. PMID: 36477031.

# 3 Inflammatory Disorders
Amy Musiek, MD

Inflammatory disorders of the skin encompass several common dermatologic complaints. Some conditions, such as allergic contact dermatitis, may be clinically limited while others, such as acne and psoriasis, are chronic conditions that may span the course of years.

## 1. Acne

### 1.1. BACKGROUND

- Acne affects 85% of young adults ages 12 to 24 and may persist into adulthood.[1]
- This multifactorial disorder is driven by genetics, hormonal influences, sebum production, comedone formation, and the bacterium, *Propionibacterium acnes*.
  - Genetics largely determines number and activity of sebaceous glands.
  - Adrenarche heralds the onset of adrenal production of dehydroepiandrosterone sulfate, which leads to increased sebum production.
  - Increased cohesiveness of follicular-based keratinocytes leads to follicular plugging, accumulation of keratin, and proliferation of *P acnes* at the base of the hair follicle.
  - *P acnes*, a gram-positive rod, triggers a robust inflammatory response.
  - Increasing pressure secondary to keratin accumulation can lead to comedone rupture, triggering a vigorous inflammatory reaction.

### 1.2. CLINICAL PRESENTATION

One or more subtypes may be observed in any given patient (Fig. 3-1).
- Comedonal acne
  - Characterized by open and closed comedones.
    - Closed comedones, commonly called whiteheads, are small, round, skin-colored papules.
    - Open comedones, commonly called blackheads, are small, round, skin-colored papules with a central black open core reflective of lipid oxidation of keratin.
  - Lesions are most commonly seen on the forehead, nose, cheeks, and chin. Eyelids are generally spared.
- Inflammatory acne
  - Characterized by erythematous papules, pustules, nodules, and cysts.
  - Inflammatory lesions frequently result in the development of postinflammatory hyperpigmentation and scarring.
  - The violaceous macules of postinflammatory hyperpigmentation may resolve over the course of months.
  - Resultant scarring is permanent and difficult to treat.

---

*The authors would like to acknowledge the first edition authors* Emily Beck and Sena Lee.

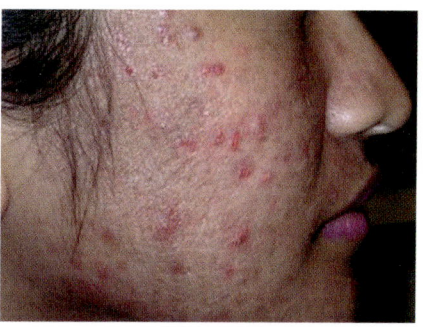

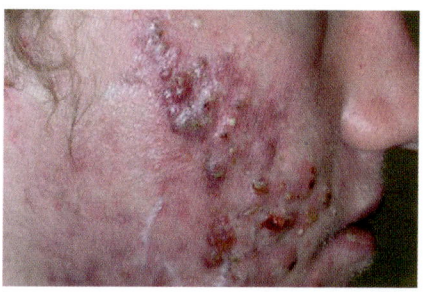

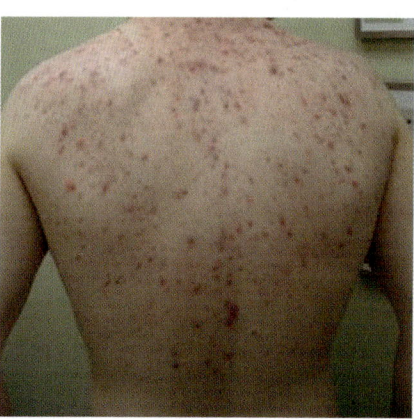

**Figure 3-1.** Forms of acne vulgaris. **A.** Inflammatory acne. **B.** Nodulocystic acne. **C.** Truncal acne. (Courtesy of David Sheinbein, MD.)

- Acne subtypes
  - Acne fulminans
    - Adolescent males are most commonly affected.
    - Symptoms include rapid development of fever, arthralgias, inflammatory papules, cysts, and hemorrhagic crusts.
    - Laboratory abnormalities include elevated erythrocyte sedimentation rate, leukocytosis, proteinuria, and osteolytic lesions.
    - SAPHO syndrome is a subset characterized by synovitis, acne, pustulosis, hyperostosis, and osteitis.
  - Acne conglobata
    - Adolescent males are most commonly affected.
    - Symptoms include severe nodulocystic, scarring inflammatory acne with possible sinus tract formation.
    - Acne conglobata, hidradenitis suppurativa, dissecting cellulitis of the scalp, and pilonidal cysts form the follicular occlusion tetrad.
    - PAPA syndrome is an autosomal dominant variant composed of pyogenic arthritis, pyoderma gangrenosum, and acne conglobata.
  - Postadolescent acne
    - Women with features of hyperandrogenism are most commonly affected.
    - Typical lesions are deep-set, erythematous papules on the lower cheeks and jawline.
    - Lesions tend to flare the week prior to menses.
  - Drug-induced acne
    - Typical lesions are monomorphic papules and pustules distributed on the chest and back.
    - The monomorphic morphology of drug-induced acne allows differentiation from the more heterogeneous appearance of acne vulgaris.
    - The most common drugs associated with acneiform eruptions include oral steroids, topical steroids, corticotropin, lithium, bromide, iodide, isoniazid, phenytoin, and epidermal growth factor receptor inhibitors.

## 1.3. EVALUATION

- Acne is primarily a clinical diagnosis. Presence of comedones, red papules, pustules, and nodules on typically involved areas, such as face, chest, shoulders, and upper back, helps to make the diagnosis. If the pustular component is prominent and patient is unresponsive to typical acne treatment, bacterial culture and KOH prep should be done to rule out gram-negative folliculitis and pityrosporum folliculitis, respectively.
- Careful review of contributing factors is recommended to optimize treatment.
- Check dehydroepiandrosterone sulfate and testosterone in the setting of obesity, hirsutism, irregular menses, and insulin resistance given concern for polycystic ovarian syndrome.
- Review the medication list for contributing drugs.

## 1.4. TREATMENT

Therapy is directed at normalizing keratinization, decreasing inflammation, and decreasing bacterial proliferation. Topical medications are first-line therapy for the management of mild comedonal and inflammatory acne. Oral antibiotics may be added for the control of moderate to severe inflammatory acne. In the event

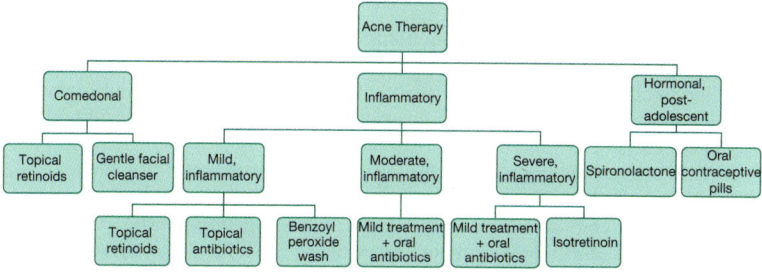

**Figure 3-2.** Overview of acne management based on clinical morphology and severity.

of severe, recalcitrant, nodulocystic, or scarring acne, isotretinoin may be used to prevent further scarring. In female patients with a predominantly hormone-induced cystic acne, oral contraceptive pills (OCPs) or spironolactone may be tried. See Figure 3-2 for an overview of acne management.

- Comedonal acne
  - Topical retinoids
    - Retinoids are vitamin A derivatives that promote normalization of keratinization and exhibit anti-inflammatory effects, which inhibit comedone formation making retinoids particularly effective at treating comedonal acne. Examples include adapalene, tretinoin, and tazarotene.
    - Retinoids are applied once daily at night given concern for inactivation by UV exposure. It may be applied 2 to 3 nights per week, and frequency may be increased, depending on tolerability.
    - Treatment is prophylactic and requires consistent application of affected areas, rather than spot treating active lesions. Initial flare is commonly observed in the first 4 weeks. Improvement is often observed in 8 to 12 weeks.
    - The most common side effects include xerosis, erythema, and photosensitivity. Drying or exfoliating agents should not be used in conjunction with topical retinoids. Daily use of moisturizer and broad-spectrum sunscreen is needed for increasing tolerability and successful treatment.
    - All topical retinoids (except for tazarotene, which is in category X) are in pregnancy category C. Topical retinoids are generally discontinued during pregnancy.
- Inflammatory acne
  - Combination of topical antibiotic and topical retinoid is generally effective in treating inflammatory acne. Oral antibiotic may be added for 3 to 6 months, if needed, to control cystic components. Isotretinoin is reserved for severe nodulocystic, scarring acne, or acne refractory to other therapies.
    - Clindamycin (gel, lotion, foam)
      - Binds bacterial ribosomal 50S subunit and inhibits protein synthesis.
      - An important side effect to be aware of is the development of gram-negative folliculitis.
    - Sodium sulfacetamide (lotion, wash, solution)
      - Inhibits dihydropteroate synthetase, which impairs folic acid synthesis.
      - The most common side effects are pruritus and xerosis.
    - Benzoyl peroxide (gel, wash)
      - Creates reactive oxygen species which directly damage bacterial proteins.
      - The most common side effect is skin irritation. Patients must take caution when using benzoyl peroxide as it is a bleaching agent.

- Oral antibiotics
  - Tetracyclines are the most commonly used class of oral antibiotics for acne treatment. Typically, this is given twice per day for 3 months at a time.
  - Tetracyclines inhibit the bacterial 50S ribosomal subunit, which inhibits protein synthesis. Oral antibiotics exhibit both anti-inflammatory and antibacterial properties.
  - Medication should be taken with a full glass of water to prevent the development of esophagitis.
  - The most common class side effects include gastrointestinal (GI) upset, esophagitis, and photosensitivity. Pseudotumor cerebri is a rare side effect.
    - Minocycline can cause blue-gray or muddy brown discoloration, autoimmune hepatitis, drug-induced lupus, or a drug hypersensitivity reaction.
    - Minocycline produces less photosensitivity than doxycycline, which may be advantageous in the summer.
- Isotretinoin
  - Isotretinoin is generally reserved for severe nodulocystic scarring acne due to its side effect profile. It is the only medication that offers a potential cure, meaning that other prescription acne medications would not be needed after treatment. It is given 0.5 to 1 mg/kg/d in divided doses twice daily. Cumulative dose of 150 mg/kg is generally needed to reduce the risk of relapse.
  - Isotretinoin is a vitamin A derivative that normalizes epithelial keratinization, differentiation, and proliferation, decreases sebum production, and induces apoptosis of sebocytes.
  - Side effects include xerosis, xerophthalmia, exacerbation of eczema, muscle and joint aches, mood changes, depression, anxiety, liver toxicity, and pseudotumor cerebri.
  - Complete blood count (CBC), fasting lipid profile, and hepatic function panel should be checked before initiating therapy and monthly during therapy with dose changes. Lab abnormalities, such as elevated cholesterol, triglycerides, and transaminases, can be seen. Diet modification, omega-3 fatty acid supplementation, or dose modification may be help in hyperlipidemia, which generally self-resolves after completing therapy. Dose reduction or cessation of therapy may be required in cases of elevated transaminases.
  - Isotretinoin is a potent teratogen and requires enrollment in the iPledge pregnancy prevention program to ensure appropriate administration.
    - Females of child-bearing potential are required to have two documented negative pregnancy tests 1 month apart prior to starting therapy. Two contraceptive measures must start 1 month prior to initial dose, and monthly negative pregnancy tests (serum beta-human chorionic gonadotropin) thereafter are required to continue therapy.
- Postadolescent acne
  - Oral contraceptive pills (OCPs)
    - Most OCPs are composed of both an estrogen and a progestin component. Older progestins have androgenic activity, but newer progestins have low or antiandrogenic activity.
    - Several OCP formulations are food and drug administration approved for acne treatment: Ortho Tri-Cyclen, Estrostep, Yaz, Loryna, and Beyaz.
    - Side effects include nausea, vomiting, breast tenderness, and weight gain. More serious side effects include hypertension and thromboembolism. Cardiovascular risk must be assessed to weigh risk versus benefit in each patient before starting OCP.

- Spironolactone
  - Spironolactone blocks androgen receptors and inhibits the conversion of testosterone to dihydrotestosterone.
  - Dose of 50 to 200 mg a day divided in q12h doses for 3 to 6 months is generally needed to achieve improvement. Therapy may be continued for a few years, if needed.
  - Side effects include irregular menses, breast tenderness, hyperkalemia, headache, fatigue, and drug hypersensitivity reaction.
  - Given its antiandrogenic effects, spironolactone is a teratogen that may cause feminization of a male fetus. Contraceptive measures should be advised.

# 2. Rosacea

## 2.1. BACKGROUND

- Rosacea is more common in women than men and in those with Fitzpatrick skin types I and II. The estimated prevalence in Caucasians is 14% in women and 5% in men.[2]
- Rosacea is a multifactorial disorder modulated by UV exposure, innate immune system dysfunction, epidermal barrier dysfunction, and Demodex mite infestation.
- Exacerbating factors include sunlight, strong wind, hot or spicy foods, alcohol, emotional distress, and topical skin irritants.

## 2.2. CLINICAL PRESENTATION

- Erythrotelangiectatic rosacea (Fig. 3-3A)
  - Symptoms include persistent centrofacial erythema, flushing, telangiectasias, and increased skin sensitivity to irritants.
- Papulopustular rosacea
  - Symptoms include erythematous, dome-shaped papules, and pustules in the centrofacial region.
  - Papules last several weeks and fade to residual background erythema.
  - Lack of comedones helps distinguish papulopustular rosacea from acne.
- Phymatous rosacea
  - Men are more commonly affected than women.
  - Phymatous rosacea is characterized by nodular, soft tissue hypertrophy classically of the nose (rhinophyma, Fig. 3-3B).
  - Patients may also develop phymatous changes of the chin (gnathophyma), ears (otophyma), glabella (glabellophyma), or forehead (metophyma).
- Ocular rosacea
  - Ocular manifestations of rosacea are common. Studies have shown a prevalence of ocular rosacea in 20.8% of patients with other features of rosacea.[3]
  - Manifestations of ocular rosacea include xerosis, pruritus, stinging, burning, conjunctivitis, blepharitis, hordeola, chalazia, and rarely keratitis.

## 2.3. EVALUATION

- Rosacea is a clinical diagnosis that generally does not require laboratory evaluation. Patients exhibit erythema and telangiectases on the glabella, nose, cheeks, and chin in addition to erythematous papules in the papulopustular variant of rosacea.

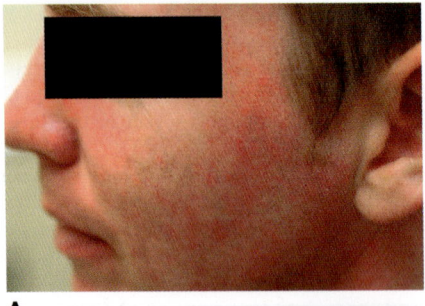

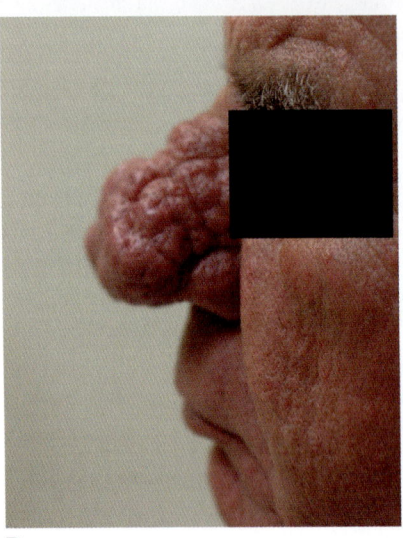

**Figure 3-3.** Rosacea. **A.** Erythrotelangiectatic rosacea. **B.** Rhinophymatous rosacea. (**A:** Courtesy of M. Laurin Council, MD; **B:** courtesy of Eva Hurst, MD.)

- Differential diagnosis includes conditions that exhibit centrofacial erythema, such as seborrheic dermatitis or lupus erythematosus.
- If patients complain of photophobia, they should be evaluated by ophthalmology.

## 2.4. TREATMENT

Treatment focuses primarily on prevention. Patients should be advised to avoid common rosacea triggers and wear sunscreen daily. Centrofacial erythema and telangiectasia may be treated with topical antibiotics or vasoconstrictive agents or lasers. Papules and pustules may be prevented with the use of topical or oral antibiotics, or low-dose isotretinoin, if refractory to antibiotics. Phymatous rosacea treatment centers largely on surgical procedures for revision. Ocular rosacea treatment begins with warm compresses and gentle soap. If persistent, topical or oral antibiotics may be prescribed.

- Erythrotelangiectatic rosacea: This is the most difficult type to control. In addition to sun protection and trigger avoidance, topical antibiotics and vasoconstrictors are tried to varying degrees of success. Vascular lasers are often helpful.
  - Sunscreen with sun protection factor 30+ daily
  - Trigger avoidance
  - Vasoconstrictors
  - Topical antibiotic/inflammatory (metronidazole, sulfacetamide-sulfur, azelaic acid)
  - Topical brimonidine tartrate (0.33% gel) daily
    - Alpha-2 adrenergic agonist.
    - Decreases centrofacial erythema for 12 or more hours when applied once daily. No rebound or worsening of disease was noted.[4]
  - Topical oxymetazoline (0.05% solution) daily
    - Imidazoline vasoconstrictor.
    - Case report demonstrates decreased centrofacial erythema in two patients when applied once daily. No rebound or sporadic flares were noted.[5]
  - Laser therapy
    - Pulsed dye laser, potassium titanyl phosphate laser, and intense pulsed light can be used to treat telangiectasias and persistent centrofacial erythema.
    - Multiple treatments are often required to produce good cosmetic outcomes.
    - Patients reported a statistically significant increased quality of life via the Dermatology Life Quality Index score after three pulsed dye laser treatments.[6]
- Papulopustular rosacea
  Topical medications, one or a combination, should be tried first. Improvement is generally seen in 1 to 2 months. Oral antibiotic may be added for 2 to 3 months, if needed. A low-dose, submicrobial dose of doxycycline is also an option.
  - Topical treatments
    - Metronidazole gel or cream once or twice daily
    - Azelaic acid gel or cream twice daily
    - Sodium sulfacetamide—sulfur lotion, solution, or wash, once or twice daily
    - Clindamycin 1% gel, solution, or lotion once or twice daily
  - Systemic treatments
    - Oral antibiotics have been shown to decrease the appearance of papules and pustules. A short course of 4 to 12 weeks rapidly decreases inflammation.
    - Tetracycline antibiotics
      - Doxycycline 50 to 100 mg once or twice daily
      - Minocycline 50 to 100 mg once or twice daily
      - Tetracycline 250 to 500 mg once or twice daily
    - Macrolide antibiotics
      - Erythromycin 250 to 500 mg once or twice daily
      - Azithromycin 250 to 500 mg three times per week
    - Other antibiotics
      - Metronidazole 200 mg once or twice daily
    - Isotretinoin
      - Lower doses of isotretinoin achieve acceptable therapeutic results (10-40 mg once daily), as compared to isotretinoin dose in acne.
      - Requires strict counseling on avoidance of pregnancy, avoidance of blood donation, and possible side effects.
- Phymatous rosacea
  - Surgical revision debulks and recontours the nose. Revision options include partial-thickness excision, electrosurgery, and ablative laser.[7,8]

- Ocular rosacea
  - Artificial tears, warm compresses, and gentle lid washing
  - Metronidazole 0.75% gel
  - Cyclosporine 0.5% ophthalmic emulsion
  - Oral antibiotics as above if severe
  - Ophthalmologist evaluation if photophobia is present

# 3. Atopic Dermatitis

## 3.1. BACKGROUND

- Atopic dermatitis (AD) affects 19.3% of children 0 to 3 years old and gradually declines to 14.5% in children 10 to 13 years old.[9]
- Prior helminth infection has been associated with a decreased risk of AD.[10] Exposure to animals, endotoxin, and early daycare correlated with lower rates of AD.[11]
- Though the prevalence of AD declines with age, a substantial percentage continue to have symptoms into adulthood.[12]
- AD has a significant impact on quality of life in children secondary to chronic pruritus and sleep disturbance.[13]
- Children with AD are more prone to develop food allergies, asthma, and rhinitis.
- AD is a multifactorial disease based on genetics, epidermal barrier dysfunction, and environmental exposures as mentioned above.
  - Twins of affected individuals have a sevenfold increased risk of developing AD as compared to the general population.[14]
  - Epidermal skin barrier dysfunction promotes transepidermal water loss, which contributes to lesion development.[15]
  - Loss of filaggrin, a protein involved in skin barrier formation, has been described in the development of AD.[16]

## 3.2. CLINICAL PRESENTATION

- Skin lesions (Fig. 3-4)
  - Acute
    - More common in infants and young children

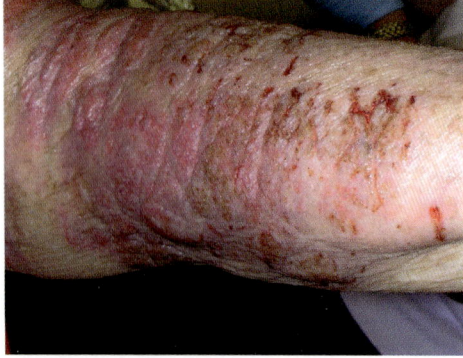

**Figure 3-4.** Severe atopic dermatitis. (Courtesy of David Sheinbein, MD.)

- Scaly, red papules and plaques with variable presence of vesicles, bullae, serosanguineous drainage, and excoriations
  - Subacute
    - May be seen in any age group
    - Scaly, red papules and plaques with variable crusting and excoriations
  - Chronic
    - More commonly seen in adolescents and adults.
    - Thickened, scaly, hyperpigmented plaques with accentuation of skin lines.
    - Patients may also form prurigo nodules in response to chronic rubbing and scratching.
- Lesions by age
  - Infantile AD
    - Characterized by acute and subacute lesions.
    - Distributed on the cheeks, scalp, neck, trunk, and extensor surfaces of the extremities. The diaper area is usually spared given the retention of moisture.
  - Childhood AD
    - Characterized primarily by acute and subacute lesions with some development of chronic lesions.
    - Lesions assume a more classic AD pattern, affecting the flexural surfaces, neck, hands, feet, ankles, and wrists.
  - Adolescent and adult AD
    - Characterized primarily by subacute and chronic lesions.
    - Lesions are distributed in a classic AD pattern, with the hands and feet frequently being affected.
- Symptoms
  - Lesions are extremely pruritic and cause a significant disruption in quality of life.[17]
  - Given the child's distress and frustration of treating a chronic disease, parents of children with AD have a similarly decreased quality of life.[18]

## 3.3. EVALUATION

- AD is a clinical diagnosis, though patch testing, prick testing, and serology may be considered to identify contributing factors.

## 3.4. TREATMENT

Given the chronicity of AD, treatment requires dedication and patient compliance. Patients should be advised to avoid triggers and perform good dry skin care habits.[19]
- Avoidance of triggering factors
  - Decrease shower length and temperature
  - Decrease soap usage
  - Avoid products with fragrance
  - Avoid smoking
  - Avoid wool fabrics
- Emollients
  - Skin barrier dysfunction and increased transepidermal water loss require compensation in the form of ointment-based emollients.
  - Petroleum jelly should be applied, ideally to wet skin, multiple times daily.

- Topical steroids
  - Steroids are the mainstay of acute flare treatment. Steroids interact with nuclear receptors to decrease transcription of inflammatory mediators.
  - The potency should be based on the severity of the lesion. The steroid chosen should be able to quickly clear the lesion. Rapid clearance with an appropriately potent steroid helps prevent side effects of prolonged steroid application including atrophy, striae, skin fragility, and telangiectasias.
  - Steroids should be tapered as lesions resolve, though complete cessation may lead to rebound flares. Studies have shown that prophylactic maintenance application of steroids twice weekly in addition to emollients may prevent recurrence.[20]
  - Steroids should be avoided on the face given concern for side effects.
  - In infants and young children, low-potency, class V, VI, and VII steroids should be attempted before escalating therapy.
  - See Table 3-1 for a listing of corticosteroids by potency.

### TABLE 3-1  Topical Corticosteroid Potency

**Class I (superpotent)**

Clobetasol propionate ointment, cream, gel, and foam 0.05%
Betamethasone dipropionate gel and ointment 0.05%
Fluocinonide cream 0.1%
Flurandrenolide tape 4 µg/cm$^2$

**Class II (high potency)**

Clobetasol solution 0.05%
Betamethasone dipropionate cream 0.05%
Desoximetasone ointment and cream 0.25% and gel 0.05%
Fluocinonide gel, ointment, cream, and solution 0.05%
Mometasone furoate ointment 0.1%
Triamcinolone acetonide ointment 0.5%

**Class III (high potency)**

Triamcinolone acetonide ointment 0.1% and cream 0.5%
Betamethasone valerate ointment 0.1%
Fluticasone propionate ointment 0.005%

**Class IV (medium potency)**

Fluocinolone acetonide ointment 0.025%
Desoximetasone cream 0.05%
Fluocinolone acetonide ointment 0.025%
Hydrocortisone valerate ointment 0.2%
Mometasone furoate cream and lotion 0.1%

**Class V (medium potency)**

Fluocinolone acetonide cream 0.025% or oil and shampoo 0.01%
Fluticasone cream and lotion 0.05%
Hydrocortisone butyrate ointment, cream, and lotion 0.1%
Hydrocortisone valerate cream 0.2%

| TABLE 3-1 | Topical Corticosteroid Potency (*continued*) |
|---|---|

**Class VI (low potency)**
Alclometasone dipropionate ointment and cream 0.05%
Betamethasone valerate lotion 0.1%
Desonide gel, ointment, cream, lotion, and foam 0.05%
Fluocinolone cream and solution 0.01%

**Class VII (low potency)**
Hydrocortisone ointment 2.5%
Hydrocortisone ointment 1%

- Topical calcineurin inhibitors
  - Tacrolimus and pimecrolimus are unique anti-inflammatory agents most commonly used on the face. Topical calcineurin inhibitors allow control of inflammation while avoiding the side effects of steroids on the face including acneiform eruptions, perioral dermatitis, and skin thinning.
  - The most common side effects are transient stinging and burning. The sensation should fade with repeated application.
  - Topical Janus kinase (JAK) inhibitors.
    - Ruxolitinib cream is FDA approved in patients ages 12 years and older. It inhibits JAK1 and JAK2.[21]
- Light therapy
  - Narrowband UVB (NB UVB) therapy may be used to treat severe or recalcitrant AD in older children; however, little is known of the long-term safety of light therapy in children. NB UVB therapy requires multiple visits to achieve a durable response.
  - A study of 25 AD patients demonstrated a 68% clearance rate after a mean of 24 NB UVB treatments. Side effects were generally mild and included erythema, herpes simplex virus reactivation, and anxiety.[22]
  - Children receiving NB UVB therapy should have yearly skin screenings given the concern for increased risk of skin cancer.
- Biologic therapy
  - Dupilumab is FDA approved for 6 months and older. It is a human monoclonal IgG4 antibody that inhibits the IL4R alpha subunit of IL-4 and IL13.[23,24] Tralokinumab is approved for children ages 12 years and older. It is an IgG4 monoclonal antibody that binds to IL-13.[25]
  - Lebrikizumab is approved in children 12 years and older. It functions as a IgG4 monoclonal antibody that inhibits IL-13.[26]
- Systemic JAK inhibitors
  - Upadacitinib and abrocitinib are JAK1 inhibitors approved for patients 12 years and older.[27,28]
  - Baricitinib is a JAK1 and JAK inhibitor approved for adults with AD.[29]
- Cyclosporine
  - Cyclosporine rapidly clears severe, diffuse skin disease and may be considered an option to achieve short-term rapid control.
  - Long-term low-dose cyclosporine may also be used to control recalcitrant AD. Long-term courses have proven beneficial but are limited by side effects: hypertension, GI upset, hypertrichosis, and renal dysfunction.[30]

- Other immunomodulatory agents
  - Azathioprine and methotrexate may be considered as alternate systemic treatment options second to cyclosporine, producing similar results with a reported reduction in disease severity of 40%.[31]
  - Omalizumab, an anti-IgE antibody, has shown potential for the treatment of AD.[32]
  - Rituximab, an anti-CD20 antibody, has also shown potential for treatment-resistant AD.[33]

## 4. Contact Dermatitis

### 4.1. BACKGROUND

- Contact dermatitis is characterized by a pruritic, eczematous eruption in a body distribution correlated with the area of exposure. The acute phase manifests as vesicles on a well-defined erythematous patch or plaque with variable serosanguineous drainage and crusting. Chronic lesions present as well-demarcated, hyperpigmented, lichenified plaques with accentuation of skin lines.
- Lesions are most commonly found on the hands, feet, face, and arms and in a generalized eruptive pattern.[34]
- Contact dermatitis is divided into two broad categories: allergic contact dermatitis and irritant contact dermatitis.
  - Allergic contact dermatitis results from repeated exposure to a sensitizing agent. A rash is produced via a delayed type IV hypersensitivity reaction mediated primarily by T cells.
  - Irritant contact dermatitis does not require repeated exposures and is the result of local inflammation secondary to irritants such as soap, solvents, alkali, and acid.
- There is no age, gender, nor racial predilection for contact dermatitis, though different exposures predominate in different populations. For example, women have higher incidence of nickel allergy than men likely secondary to jewelry exposure.[35]
- The most common allergic contact allergens are nickel and poison ivy. Balsam of Peru is another important contact allergen.
  - Nickel allergic contact dermatitis
    - Nickel allergy was found in 34.4% of women and 8.9% of men in a European study by patch testing.[35] It is commonly found in costume jewelry, watches, denim snaps, and belt buckles. Lesions are commonly found on sites of nickel exposure such as the earlobes, around the umbilicus, wrists, and back of the neck.
    - Cell phones are a newer source of nickel exposure that may lead to development of lesions on the cheek and ear.
    - It is postulated that ear piercing in particular contributes to nickel allergy formation given the chronic exposure of nickel to a damaged cutaneous surface.[36]
    - Patients should be advised to wear nickel-free jewelry, snaps, and buckles. If unavoidable, they may try painting nickel-containing objects with clear nail polish to decrease the level of exposure. Sweating in the area of contact with nickel will aggravate the allergic dermatitis.
  - Poison ivy, poison oak, and poison sumac
    - These three plants are members of the family Anacardiaceae, genus *Toxicodendron*, and cause more allergic contact dermatitis than all other plants combined. In the United States, there are two varieties of poison ivy, two of poison oak, and one of poison sumac.

- These plants contain urushiol and laccase, which oxidizes the urushiol to produce a black resin commonly observed as black spots on plants and areas of dermatitis.
- Identification
  - Poison ivy and poison oak produce leaves with three green leaflets. "Leaves of three; let them be" is a common pneumonic used to remember avoidance.
  - Poison sumac has leaves with five or seven leaflets that angle upward.
  - All three members of the *Toxicodendron* genus produce small green fruit that ripen to off-white to light tan fruit when mature.
- Geographic distribution
  - Poison ivy is found across the United States. In the West, it is found as a low-growing shrub, whereas in the East, it is found as a climbing vine.
  - Poison oak is found primarily in the Western United States.
  - Poison sumac is largely found in the Southeastern United States.
- Lesions are characterized by weeping vesicles arranged in a linear fashion on an erythematous base. Shiny black dots may be present, reflecting the oxidation of urushiol. Lesions are very pruritic.
- Balsam of Peru
  - Balsam of Peru is complex resin comprised over 400 chemicals derived from the tree *Myroxylon pereirae*. It is one of the most common allergens identified by the North American Contact Dermatitis Group.
  - Allergenic components of Balsam of Peru are found in fragrances, cosmetics, medicinal products, and food. Food sources may include vanilla, cinnamon, cloves, carbonated beverages, vermouth, and tomatoes.[37,38]
- Other common allergens include topical antibiotic (eg, neomycin), fragrance, adhesives, rubber, latex, hair dye, nail polish, and metals (eg, gold). See Table 3-2 for commonly patch tested substances.
- Some are photocontact allergens and cause allergic dermatitis only when exposed to sunlight. Common ones include sunscreens (oxybenzone, octyl

| TABLE 3-2 | Components of the NACDG and True Test Patch Test Series |
|---|---|
| Compound | Sources |
| **NACDG and True Test** | |
| 2-Mercaptobenzothiazole | Rubber, shoes |
| Colophony | Adhesives, chewing gum, violin bows |
| 4-Phenylenediamine base | Hair dye, rubber |
| Neomycin sulfate | Topical antibiotics |
| Thiuram mix | Latex, rubber, adhesives |
| Formaldehyde | Preservatives, wrinkle-free clothing, cosmetics, shampoo, household cleaners |
| Epoxy resin | Uncured epoxy glue, adhesives, dental bonding agents, appliance finishes, varnish |
| Quarternium-15 | Cosmetics, creams, lotions, shampoo, sunscreen |
| 4-Tert-butylphenol formaldehyde resin | Adhesives, shoes |

*(continued)*

## TABLE 3-2  Components of the NACDG and True Test Patch Test Series (*continued*)

| Compound | Sources |
|---|---|
| Mercapto mix | Rubber, gloves, boots, shoes, safety goggles |
| Potassium dichromate | Wet cement, welding fumes, chrome tanned leather, antirust paint |
| Balsam of Peru | Fragrances, pharmaceutical products, flavorings, sunscreen, shampoo |
| Nickel sulfate hexahydrate | Jewelry, snaps, zippers, buttons |
| Methylchloroisothiazolinone/methylisothiazolinone | Cosmetics, shampoo, skin care products |
| Paraben mix | Cosmetics, skin care products |
| Fragrance mix I | Perfume, cologne, skin care products |
| Cobalt chloride | Nickel-plated objects, jewelry, cosmetics |
| Tixocortol-21-pivalate | Nasal spray |
| Budesonide | Asthma inhalers |
| Carba mix | Rubber, adhesives, gloves, safety goggles |
| Ethylenediamine dihydrochloride | Medicated skin creams |
| Imidazolidinyl urea | Cosmetics, shampoo, nail polish, deodorant |
| Diazolidinyl urea | Cosmetics, skin creams, pharmaceuticals |
| **NACDG Only** | |
| Benzocaine | Topical anesthetics |
| *N*-Isopropyl-*N*-phenyl-4-phenylenediamine | Black rubber |
| Sesquiterpene lactone mix | Cosmetics, creams, lotions, Asteraceae family plants (artichokes, chamomile, chrysanthemums, sunflowers, marigolds, and dandelions) |
| Methyldibromoglutaronitrile | Latex paint, adhesives, moist toilet wipes, cosmetics |
| Fragrance mix II | Perfume, cologne, skin care products |
| Cinnamic aldehyde | Perfume, cologne, flavoring agents |
| Amerchol L-101 | Medicated ointments, furniture polish, cosmetics, textiles |
| DMDM hydantoin | Cosmetics, shampoos |
| Bacitracin | Topical antibiotics |
| Mixed dialkyl thioureas | Rubber, neoprene, shoes, wet suits |
| Glutaraldehyde | Disinfectants, leather and clothing tanners, dyes |
| 2-Bromo-2-nitropropane-1,3-diol | Cosmetics, conditioner, shampoo, moisturizers, cleansing lotions |
| Propylene glycol | Cosmetics, personal lubricants, deodorant, hand sanitizers, food coloring |
| 2-Hydroxy-4-methoxybenzophenone | Textiles, rubber, plastic, cosmetics, sunscreen |

### TABLE 3-2 Components of the NACDG and True Test Patch Test Series (*continued*)

| Compound | Sources |
|---|---|
| 4-Chloro-3,5-xylenol | Creams, deodorants, disinfectants, conditioner |
| Ethyleneurea/melamine-formaldehyde mix | Textiles, draperies |
| Ethyl acrylate | Perfume, rubber, adhesives |
| Glyceryl monothioglycolate | Hair acid permanent wave solution |
| Tosylamide/formaldehyde resin | Nail polish |
| Methyl methacrylate | Dentures, fillings, fragrances |
| Disperse 106/124 mix | Blue linens, clothes |
| Iodopropynyl butyl carbamate | Cosmetics, water-based paint, wood preservatives |
| Compositae mix II | Cosmetics, shampoo, conditioner, oils, lotions |
| Hydrocortisone-17-butyrate | Topical steroids |
| Dimethylol dihydroxyethyleneurea | Draperies, permanent press clothing |
| Cocamidopropyl betaine | Shampoos, detergents, cleansing lotions |
| Triamcinolone acetonide | Topical steroids |
| **True Test Only** | |
| Caine mix | Topical anesthetics, cough syrup |
| Black rubber mix | Black rubber, boots, tires, scuba equipment, shoes, gloves |
| Thimerosal | Eye drops, ear drops, vaccines, cosmetics |
| Quinoline mix | Topical antibiotics |

dimethyl para-aminobenzoic acid, and cinnamate), fragrance, and plants (lime, celery, parsnip).
- Airborne contact dermatitis is most commonly seen with plant allergens with diffuse involvement of exposed skin. It is most frequently seen with outdoor exposure to allergens carried by wind, but indoor exposure in the setting of a fireplace may also be seen.

### 4.2. CLINICAL PRESENTATION

- Allergic contact dermatitis
  - Given the mechanism of delayed type IV hypersensitivity reaction, lesions develop days to weeks after exposure.
  - Characteristic features vary by chronicity.
    - Acute lesions are characterized by pruritic, erythematous, well-demarcated patches and plaques with variable vesicle formation and serosanguineous drainage (Fig. 3-5).

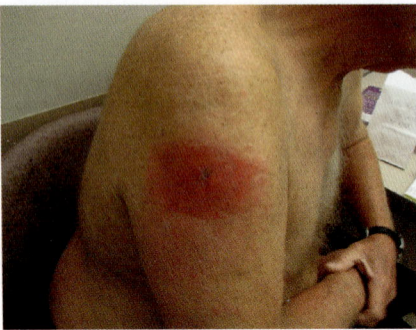

**Figure 3-5.** Allergic contact dermatitis, to adhesive in bandage. (Courtesy of David Sheinbein, MD.)

- Chronic lesions are characterized by pruritic, hyperpigmented, thickened plaques with accentuation of skin lines.
  ○ Geometric or linear morphologic patterns are strongly suggestive of contact dermatitis; however, certain diffuse exposures such as shampoo may produce a widespread distribution pattern. In cases of severe localized contact dermatitis, id reaction, a diffuse nonspecific reactive dermatitis involving nonexposed areas, may be seen.
- Irritant contact dermatitis
  ○ Clinical presentation of irritant contact dermatitis may be subdivided into acute contact dermatitis, acute delayed irritant contact dermatitis, and cumulative irritant contact dermatitis.
    - Acute contact dermatitis
      □ Characterized by rapid development of pain, burning, erythema, edema and variable vesiculation, bullae formation, and necrosis.
      □ Potent acute irritants include acids, alkali solutions, and solvents.
    - Acute delayed irritant contact dermatitis
      □ Characterized by the development of pain, burning, pruritus, xerosis, scaling, and fissuring on an erythematous background.
      □ Results from exposure to moderate irritants such as benzalkonium chloride, which is a commonly used disinfectant.
      □ Lesions may develop 8 to 24 hours after exposure.
    - Cumulative irritant contact dermatitis
      □ Characterized by the gradual development of burning, pruritus, erythema, xerosis, fissuring, hyperkeratosis, and accentuation of skin lines. Lesions tend to be less well defined than those of acute irritant dermatitis.
      □ Results from repetitive exposure to mild irritants with insufficient time between exposures for restoration of skin barrier function.
      □ Lesions develop days to weeks after chronic exposure.
      □ Examples of mild irritants producing cumulative irritant contact dermatitis include soap and water.

## 4.3. EVALUATION

- A careful history is critical in diagnosing either allergic or irritant contact dermatitis. Questions should be asked about all possible topical exposures. A history of exposure to known allergens versus irritants helps differentiate the two.

- The differential diagnosis includes AD, stasis dermatitis, seborrheic dermatitis, psoriasis, tinea, and rosacea. History and clinical examination are crucial in differentiating these diagnoses.
  - AD is more frequently widespread, symmetric, and found in a classic distribution pattern on flexor surfaces.
  - Stasis dermatitis found on lower legs frequently has associated edema, varicosities, and hyperpigmentation. It is important to note that along with stasis dermatitis, one could also develop contact dermatitis, since chronicity and frequency of exposure to topical antibiotic, steroids, and emollients are increased.
  - Seborrheic dermatitis is more frequently symmetric and produces less well-defined erythematous patches with greasy, yellow scale.
  - Psoriasis is differentiated by the presence of erythematous plaques with adherent silvery scale.
  - A potassium hydroxide preparation may be performed to rule out tinea on the hands and feet.
  - Rosacea produces centrofacial erythema that may be confused with contact dermatitis, but the associated findings of telangiectasia, phymatous changes, and history of flushing help reach the correct diagnosis.
- Patch testing is the gold standard for identifying contact allergens (Fig. 3-6). The North American Contact Dermatitis Group's standard screening tray and True Test are most frequently used to screen for common allergens. See Table 3-2 for a list of included allergens.

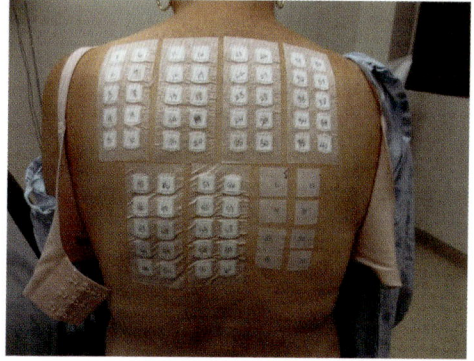

A

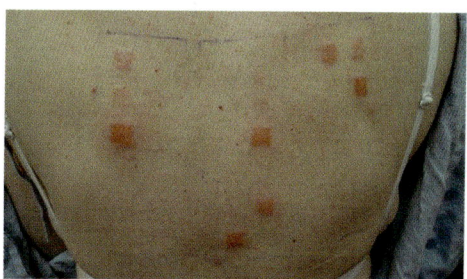

B

**Figure 3-6. A.** Patch test in place. **B.** Positive patch test results. (Courtesy of David Sheinbein, MD.)

| TABLE 3-3 | International Grading System for Patch Tests |
| --- | --- |
| Grade | Reaction |
| − | None |
| +/− | Unlikely reaction. Faint erythema |
| + | Weak reaction. Erythema, possible papules |
| ++ | Strong reaction. Erythema, infiltration, papules |
| +++ | Very strong reaction. Erythema, bullae, ulcers, spreading |
| IR | Irritant reaction |

- Patch test trays are placed on the upper back, and the patient is instructed to return in 48 hours for removal. Patients should not get the patches wet or perform activities resulting in excessive sweating.
- Patches are removed at 48 hours, allergens are marked, and any positive reactions are noted and scored. The patient is then asked to come back for a final read 72 hours to 1 week after initial patch placement.
- Reactions are graded according to the international grading system for patch tests. See Table 3-3.

## 4.4. TREATMENT

The primary goal of treatment is to identify causative allergens and irritants and avoid exposure. Cessation of exposure will prevent further flares, though current episodes of dermatitis may take weeks to resolve. To hasten resolution of active lesions, clinicians may use topical steroids. If the reaction is particularly severe or diffuse, patients may take a short course of oral steroids to expedite clearance.

- Topical steroids
  - Topical steroids are first-line therapy for mild-to-moderate, localized contact dermatitis. Generally, mid- to superpotent topical steroids are needed to resolve allergic contact dermatitis; for irritant contact dermatitis, high potency is rarely needed.
  - High-potency to superpotent topical steroids may be applied twice daily until lesions clear. Ointments are more effective than creams. One week of midpotency steroid is generally used on the face, if needed. Use of high potency on the face should be avoided.
  - Side effects include atrophy, striae formation, telangiectasias, perioral dermatitis, purpura, acneiform, and rosacealike lesions; however, given the transient nature of the disease, side effects are less common than when treating chronic conditions such as AD.
  - Examples in order of increasing potency:
    - Triamcinolone 0.1% ointment BID
    - Desoximetasone 0.05% ointment BID
    - Clobetasol 0.05% ointment BID
- Oral steroids
  - A short course of oral steroids is effective in achieving rapid improvement of severe contact dermatitis. There is no difference in time to improvement, percentage with complete clearance, or recurrence between 5- and 15-day courses of prednisone observed in treatment of severe poison ivy.[39]

- Side effects of oral steroids include hypertension, hyperglycemia, hyperlipidemia, cataracts, myopathy, striae formation, adrenal axis suppression, mood changes, insomnia, osteoporosis, and osteonecrosis; however, given the very short duration of therapy, side effects are limited.
- Example
  - Prednisone 40 mg PO daily × 5 days

# 5. Pityriasis Rosea

## 5.1. BACKGROUND

- Pityriasis rosea (PR) is an acute, self-limited entity that commonly presents in young adults as a red, scaly rash. PR is slightly more common in females.
- The pathogenesis has not been definitively identified, but a viral etiology has been suggested based on the transient nature, case clustering, possible prodrome, and lack of recurrence suggesting immunity.
- Human herpesvirus 6 and 7 have been extensively studied as the causative agents of PR; however, evidence is inconsistent.[40,41]

## 5.2. CLINICAL PRESENTATION (FIG. 3-7)

- Onset typically begins with a solitary pink or salmon-colored, round to oval, patch or plaque with fine, trailing scale on the trunk. This is called the "herald patch."
- The herald patch slowly expands over the course of several days, after which, similar smaller lesions appear on the trunk and extremities. Lesions often follow Langer lines of cleavage and produce a "Christmas tree" pattern on the back.
- Patients may have a mild prodrome, but otherwise, lesions are typically asymptomatic and last 6 to 8 weeks. Lesions resolve completely without scarring.

## 5.3. EVALUATION

- Diagnosis is largely clinical, though laboratory testing and biopsy may be helpful. Rapid plasma reagin or the Venereal Disease Research Laboratory test is generally

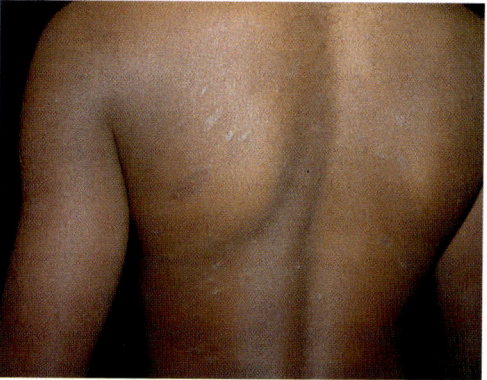

**Figure 3-7.** Pityriasis rosea. (Courtesy of Susan Bayliss, MD.)

recommended for those who are sexually active to rule out secondary syphilis, which resembles PR. Follow-up with confirmatory testing, if positive. If the eruption does not resolve within 3 months, a skin punch biopsy should be done to rule out other diagnoses on the differential.
- KOH preparation may be done to rule out tinea.
- Drug reactions can produce a similar rash, so a careful review of the medication list is important.

## 5.4. TREATMENT

Since PR is a self-limited, generally asymptomatic disease, most cases require only education and reassurance. Patients suffering from pruritus may benefit from topical steroids, NB UVB, or oral antibiotics.
- Medium or high potency topical steroids applied twice daily may decrease pruritus. See Table 3-1 for a listing of corticosteroids by potency.
- NB UVB decreases extent of lesions and pruritus.[42]
- Erythromycin has been shown to speed resolution in some studies.[43]

# 6. Psoriasis

## 6.1. BACKGROUND

- Psoriasis is an immune-mediated disorder characterized by the development of thick, red plaques with adherent silvery scale commonly found on the scalp, extensor surfaces, hands, feet, and gluteal cleft.
- Worldwide prevalence in the adult population ranges from 0.91% to 8.5%.[44]
- Psoriasis can develop at any age; however, there are three peak ages of onset around puberty and fourth and sixth decades of life.[45]
- Systemic manifestations of psoriasis include psoriatic arthritis, increased risk of cardiovascular disease, and increased prevalence of metabolic syndrome.
  - Psoriatic arthritis can lead to crippling, erosive joint disease most commonly in the proximal interphalangeal (PIP) joints and distal interphalangeal (DIP) joints of the fingers and toes.
  - Patients with psoriasis have a two times increased risk of myocardial infarction and cardiovascular disease.[46]
  - Meta-analysis of over 1.4 million patients revealed an odds ratio of 2.1 in psoriatic patients for the development of metabolic syndrome, defined as a combination of three of five criteria including elevated fasting glucose, elevated triglycerides, hypertension, decreased high-density lipoprotein, and elevated waist circumference.[47]
- Patients also suffer from psychosocial manifestations of their disease.
  - Patients with psoriasis report physical discomfort, impaired emotional functioning, negative body and self-image, and limitations in daily activities, social contacts, (skin-exposing) activities, and work.[48]
- Psoriasis results from a complex interplay between genetics, the innate and adaptive immunity, and triggering factors.
  - Twin association studies have demonstrated an increased prevalence of psoriasis in fraternal twins and an even higher prevalence in monozygotic twins, suggesting a strong genetic component.[49] Furthermore, a study of 5,197 families with psoriasis showed that 36% of the probands had one or more parents with psoriasis.[50]

- HLA-Cw6 is the most commonly associated histocompatibility antigen. Its presence heralds an increased relative risk of development of psoriasis and earlier age of onset. Approximately 10% of HLA-Cw6–positive individuals will develop psoriasis.[51]
- T lymphocytes drive inflammation in psoriasis. Supporting evidence includes association with specific HLA alleles, presence of oligoclonal lesional T cells, and response to T-cell–suppressive agents.[52-54]
- Natural killer (NK) cells, part of the innate immune system, are increased in psoriatic lesions.[55] NK cells interact with CD1d receptors on keratinocytes. Activation of these receptors stimulates NK cells to produce IFN-gamma, which stimulates antigen presenting cells.[56]
- Innate and adaptive-derived cytokines and chemokines stimulate inflammation and keratinocyte proliferation.
  - Cytokines including IFN-gamma, IL-2, IL-12, IL-23, and IL-15 are increased in psoriatic skin. Anti-inflammatory cytokines such as IL-10 are decreased.
  - IL-12 and IL-23 are postulated to play a central role in lesion development, supported by the profound response to IL-12 and IL-23 inhibitors such as ustekinumab.
  - Proinflammatory innate cytokines including IL-1, IL-6, and tumor necrosis factor (TNF)-alpha are also increased in lesional skin.
- Triggering factors include infection, stress, drugs, trauma, and hypocalcemia.
  - Bacterial infections such as streptococcal pharyngitis are commonly implicated in the onset of guttate psoriasis.
  - High stress has been correlated with increased severity of skin lesions and joint symptoms.[57]
  - Medications such as angiotensin-converting enzyme inhibitors, lithium, β-blockers, antimalarials, and nonsteroidal anti-inflammatory drugs have been shown to worsen psoriasis.
  - Psoriasis is well known to exhibit the Koebner phenomenon, meaning that cutaneous injury may trigger development of psoriatic lesions.
  - Hypocalcemia is associated primarily with the development of pustular psoriasis.[58]

## 6.2. CLINICAL PRESENTATION (FIG. 3-8)

There are several clinical variants of psoriasis. The main subtypes are chronic plaque psoriasis, guttate psoriasis, pustular psoriasis, and inverse psoriasis. Each of these variants may be associated with the development of psoriatic arthritis.
- Chronic plaque psoriasis
  - Characterized by erythematous, scaly, well-demarcated plaques.
  - Lesions are frequently found on the scalp, elbows, knees, hands, feet, and gluteal cleft.
  - Disease may be localized or widespread.
- Guttate psoriasis
  - Characterized by scattered small round to oval-shaped, erythematous, scaly, well-demarcated papules and plaques covering a widespread distribution.
  - Onset is frequently preceded by streptococcal pharyngitis, and lesions may spontaneously resolve. Neither penicillin nor erythromycin directed at streptococcal infection hastens resolution of lesions.[59]
  - This pattern is more frequently seen in children and young adults.
- Pustular psoriasis
  - Characterized by sterile, neutrophil-derived pustules in a generalized or localized pattern.

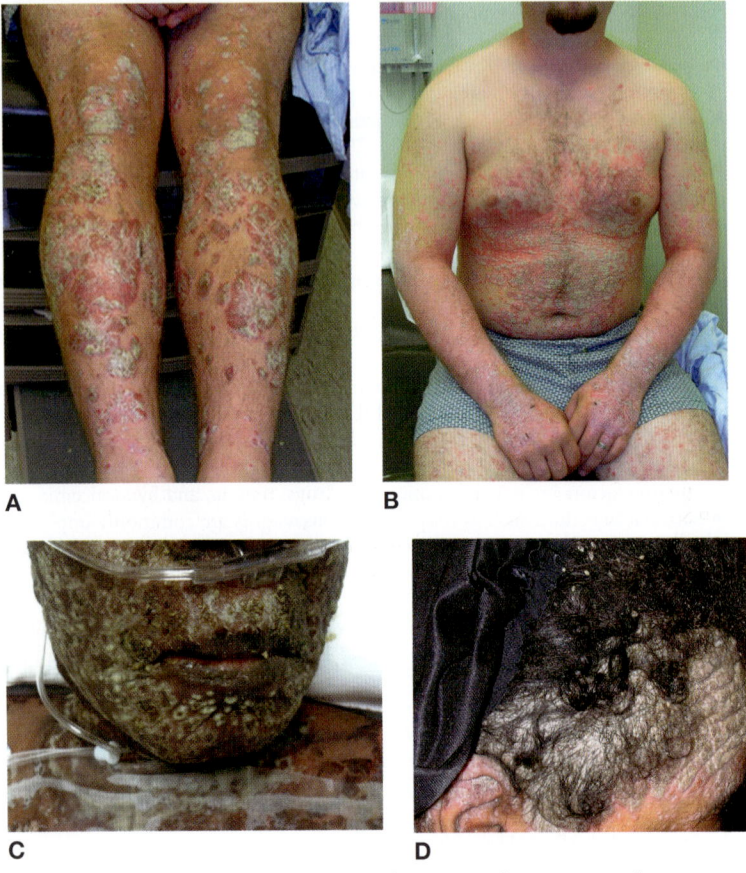

**Figure 3-8.** Variants of psoriasis. **A.** Psoriasis vulgaris. **B.** Moderate-to-severe plaque psoriasis. **C.** Pustular psoriasis. **D.** Scalp psoriasis. (Courtesy of David Sheinbein, MD.)

- Several variants exist, including palmoplantar pustulosis, acute generalized von Zumbusch, annular pattern, exanthematic type, and localized pattern.
  - Palmoplantar psoriasis is defined by the presence of sterile, pustules on the palms and soles on a background of erythematous, scaly plaques.
  - Von Zumbusch pattern is characterized by acute, generalized eruption of pustules on an erythematous background with pain and fever.
  - Annular pattern demonstrates pustules arranged in an annular fashion at the advancing edge of erythematous plaques.
  - Exanthematic type shows acute, widespread eruption of small pustules without background erythema, fever, or systemic symptoms.
  - Localized pattern is characterized by the development of pustules in pre-existing lesions of chronic plaque psoriasis.
- Inverse psoriasis
  - Lesions are typically located in the axillae, inguinal crease, inframammary folds, and gluteal cleft.

- Characterized by well-demarcated thin red plaques with minimal scale.
- Lesions may demonstrate fissures.
- Psoriatic arthritis
  - Characterized by progressive, erosive joint disease.
  - Estimates of the prevalence of psoriatic arthritis widely vary but is felt to be about 30%.[60]
  - Arthritis is more common in patients with more severe skin disease. However, it can also be seen in patients with none to minimal skin disease.
  - Several patterns exist including asymmetric mono- and oligoarthritis of the DIP and PIP joints, rheumatoidlike arthritis, arthritis mutilans, and spondylitis with sacroiliitis.
    - Asymmetric mono-/oligoarthritis of the DIP and PIP joints is the most common form of psoriatic arthritis. "Sausage digits" may result from vigorous inflammation of the distal digits.
    - Rheumatoidlike psoriatic arthritis produces symmetric polyarthritis of the hands, wrists, ankles, and elbows as in rheumatoid arthritis. Patients may have a positive or negative rheumatoid factor.
    - Arthritis mutilans is the most severe form of psoriatic arthritis characterized by progressive, destructive joint disease resulting in permanent deformity.
    - Spondylitis and sacroiliitis are more common in patients with HLA-B27 alleles. Prominent symptoms include axial joint pain with morning stiffness.

## 6.3. EVALUATION

- Psoriasis is largely a clinical diagnosis, though careful review of contributing factors and screening for psoriatic arthritis is important. Psoriasis must be differentiated from other papulosquamous disorders including seborrheic dermatitis, cutaneous T-cell lymphoma (CTCL), and chronic eczema.
  - Sharp demarcation and thick, scaly, red plaques characteristic of psoriasis help to differentiate psoriatic lesions from those of seborrheic dermatitis, which are less well demarcated.
  - Epidermal atrophy and wrinkling followed by subsequent infiltration suggests CTCL. Biopsy would be warranted to rule out CTCL.
  - Chronic eczema may produce scaly plaques, but they are frequently less well demarcated and less erythematous, allowing differentiation from psoriasis.
- Review the medication list for contributing factors.
- Check antistreptolysin O titer in guttate psoriasis given possibility of streptococcal infection as an inciting factor.
- Check radiographs for erosion if psoriatic arthritis is suspected.
- Check rheumatoid factor and cyclic citrullinated peptide antibodies to help distinguish psoriatic arthritis from rheumatoid arthritis.
- Consider rheumatology referral if joint pain is not well controlled with standard therapies.

## 6.4. TREATMENT

Therapy is directed at effectively managing acute flares and maintaining a limited or disease-free maintenance phase.[61] Both topical and systemic medications are enlisted. Topical medications comprise first-line therapy for limited disease. Steroids and calcineurin inhibitors reduce inflammation, while vitamin D analogues and retinoids help normalize epidermal differentiation. Topical therapies are often combined for treatment of mild to moderate psoriasis. Phototherapy is beneficial adjuvant therapy for treatment of plaques resistant to topical therapy or for more diffuse skin involvement. Systemic therapy should be utilized in those with recalcitrant, extensive disease and is mandated in patients with significant psoriatic arthritis.

- Topical therapy
  - Corticosteroids
    - Inhibit inflammation by interacting with nuclear receptors to decrease production of inflammatory cytokines.
    - Ointments have the highest efficacy, but creams may be better tolerated. Solutions and oils may be used on the scalp for increased ease of application.[62]
    - Patients may wrap steroid ointment under plastic wrap to increase penetration and enhance efficacy.
    - Steroids should be applied twice daily until lesions resolve. Intermittent application thereafter several times per week helps maintain remission.[62]
    - Examples in order of increasing potency:
      - Fluocinolone 0.1% solution
      - Desonide 0.05% cream
      - Triamcinolone 0.1% cream
      - Triamcinolone 0.1% ointment
      - Fluocinonide 0.05% solution
      - Clobetasol 0.05% solution
      - Clobetasol 0.05% ointment
    - Side effects of topical steroid application include atrophy, striae formation, telangiectasia, perioral dermatitis, purpura, acneiform, and rosacealike lesions. Application should be performed twice daily to areas of active inflammation. Maintenance therapy should be decreased to twice-weekly application to limit risks of cutaneous side effects.
  - Vitamin D analogues: calcipotriene
    - Inhibits epidermal proliferation, normalizes differentiation, and inhibits neutrophils.
    - Calcipotriene ointment applied twice daily resulted in a 70% reduction in lesion severity score after 8 weeks of treatment. Side effects were minimal, and there was no significant difference in serum calcium levels between active and vehicle-only treatment groups.[63]
    - Vitamin D analogues are frequently used in combination with topical steroids.
    - Example
      - Calcipotriene 0.005% ointment or cream BID
  - Topical retinoids: tazarotene
    - Inhibits epidermal proliferation and normalizes differentiation by binding to retinoic acid receptor (RAR)-beta and RAR-gamma.
    - Tazarotene gel application reduces erythema, plaque elevation, and pruritus as compared to vehicle.[64]
    - Tazarotene is less effective than topical steroids, though may be used in combination as a second-line therapy.
    - Side effects include burning, pruritus, and irritation.
    - Example
      - Tazarotene 0.1% or 0.05% gel once daily
  - Calcineurin inhibitors
    - Inhibits production of proinflammatory cytokine IL-2.

- Calcineurin inhibitors are particularly beneficial in the treatment of facial, genital, and intertriginous psoriasis given the absence of steroid-associated side effects in these sensitive areas.
- Tacrolimus and pimecrolimus are both beneficial, though tacrolimus is somewhat more effective.[65]
- Side effects including burning and irritation.
- Examples
  - Tacrolimus 0.1% and 0.3% ointment BID
  - Pimecrolimus 1% cream BID

• Phototherapy

NB UVB has become the phototherapy treatment of choice for diffuse cutaneous psoriasis, as its efficacy is nearly comparable to that of psoralen-UVA (PUVA) while demonstrating a superior safety profile. Phototherapy is administered two to three times per week, and the dose is gradually titrated to produce minimally perceptive erythema. Generally, 20 to 40 treatments over the course of a few months are required to achieve remission or significant improvement. Afterward, phototherapy can be tapered off or maintained at a less frequent schedule. For all wavelengths, eyes and genitalia are shielded in the light box, in addition to any unaffected areas.

- Narrowband UVB (NB UVB)
  - 311- to 313-nm light.
  - Absorbed by chromophores including nuclear DNA resulting in the formation of pyrimidine dimers and expression of p53. Both result in arrest of proliferation, and p53 can lead to apoptosis. NB UVB also reduces production of inflammatory cytokines.
  - NB UVB may be combined with calcipotriene or acitretin to increase efficacy.[66,67]
  - Side effects include erythema, xerosis, blistering, and reactivation of herpes simplex virus.
  - Long-term side effects include photoaging and potential increased risk of skin cancer; however, a study of 3,867 patients did not show any increased risk of basal cell carcinoma, squamous cell carcinoma, or melanoma in association with NB UVB treatment.[68]
- Psoralen with UVA (PUVA)
  - 320- to 400-nm light in combination with topical or oral psoralens.
  - Psoralens are photosensitizing agents that intercalate with DNA. UVA absorption stimulates DNA helix cross-linking, which inhibits DNA replication and leads to cell cycle arrest. Cells may then proceed through apoptosis.
  - Studies have shown that PUVA with oral psoralens is more effective than NB UVB as monotherapy. NB UVB was more effective than PUVA with topical psoralens.[69]
  - PUVA may be combined with other medications to increase efficacy and reduce side effects.
    - Methotrexate combined with PUVA resulted in faster clearing and decreased number of PUVA treatments compared to either monotherapy alone.[70]
    - Oral retinoids combined with PUVA resulted in a 30% improvement in clearance rate as compared to PUVA alone.[71]
  - Cutaneous side effects include delayed erythema peaking at 72 to 96 hours posttreatment, persistent erythema, blistering, edema, pruritus, and stinging. Oral psoralen side effects include nausea and vomiting. PUVA induces cataract formation, so eye shielding during treatment as well as up to 24 hours posttreatment with UVA- and UVB-protective sunglasses is mandatory.

- Long-term side effects include photoaging, actinic keratosis formation, lentigo formation, and increased risk of nonmelanoma skin cancers.
- Systemic therapy
  - Methotrexate
    - Inhibits dihydrofolate reductase, which impairs purine nucleotide synthesis, halting DNA and RNA synthesis.
    - Generally, 15 to 20 mg weekly is needed to provide good control. Start at 7.5 mg weekly and titrate up by 2.5 mg every 2 weeks to achieve the required dose while checking complete blood count (CBC) and liver function tests (LFTs) weekly. Administer the weekly dose in three divided doses every 12 hours (eg, 15 mg/week dosing would give 5 mg every 12 hours for 3 doses per week).
    - Folic acid 1 mg PO daily may be administered on off days to mitigate side effects.
    - Side effects include hepatotoxicity, pancytopenia, nausea, mucositis, and photosensitivity. Potential for hepatotoxicity and pancytopenia requires laboratory monitoring with CBC and LFTs. Risk of hepatotoxicity is related to cumulative dose.
  - Cyclosporine
    - Binds cyclophilin and inhibits production of IL-2.
    - Results in rapid improvement of severe disease. Given its ability to produce rapid clearance, it is often used for short durations to achieve quick control of extensive, severe disease.
    - Long-term, low-dose cyclosporine may be used for control of persistent psoriasis not cleared by other medicines but is limited by side effects: nephrotoxicity, hypertension, increased risk of skin cancers, GI disturbance, hypertrichosis, gingival hyperplasia, headache, and tremor.[72]
    - Laboratory abnormalities include hyperkalemia, hyperuricemia, hypomagnesemia, and elevated lipid profile.
  - Systemic retinoids: acitretin
    - Normalizes proliferation and differentiation via activation of RARs.
    - Acitretin is indicated for use as first-line therapy for pustular or erythrodermic psoriasis or as second-line therapy for chronic plaque psoriasis.
    - May be combined with NB UVB as above to increase efficacy of both treatments.
    - Acitretin may be re-esterified to a related systemic retinoid called etretinate, particularly in the presence of alcohol. The half-life of etretinate is 120 days.
    - Side effects include xerosis, xerophthalmia, exacerbation of eczema, headaches, muscle and joint aches, mood changes, depression, and anxiety.
    - Laboratory abnormalities include increased cholesterol, triglycerides, and aminotransferases. Labs should be checked prior to, during, and after therapy.
    - Oral retinoids are potent teratogens. Pregnancy should be avoided for 3 years after stopping acitretin given re-esterification to etretinate as mentioned. For this reason, acitretin is generally avoided in women of child-bearing age.
  - Biologics
    - TNF inhibitors
      - Bind to TNF-alpha and impede its binding to TNF-alpha receptors.
      - Excellent efficacy for treatment of skin lesions and psoriatic arthritis. Cost and side effects limit its use to those with moderate-to-severe psoriasis.
      - Prior to treatment, patients should obtain a purified protein derivative, CBC, comprehensive metabolic panel, human immunodeficiency virus, and hepatitis B virus and hepatitis C virus serologic testing. While on treatment, patients should obtain a purified protein derivative annually and CBC and comprehensive metabolic panel every 3 to 12 months.

- Side effects include increased risk of infection, reactivation of latent tuberculosis, autoimmune antibodies, congestive heart failure, palmoplantar pustulosis, and hypersensitivity reactions.
- Examples
  - Etanercept 25 to 50 mg subcutaneously twice weekly
  - Infliximab 5 mg/kg IV infusion at 0, 2, and 6 weeks, and then every 8 weeks thereafter
  - Adalimumab 80 mg subcutaneously for the first dose, and then 40 mg subcutaneously at day 8 and every other week thereafter
- IL-12/IL-23 inhibitors: ustekinumab
  - Binds to the p40 subunit of IL-12 and IL-23.
  - Ustekinumab produces excellent clearance of skin lesions but is not effective for psoriatic arthritis. 67.1% of patients receiving ustekinumab 45 mg achieved 75% improvement in their lesion severity by 12 weeks.[73]
  - Side effects include increased risk of infections, reactivation of latent tuberculosis, and hypersensitivity reactions. Further studies are needed to evaluate the risks of cardiovascular disease and malignancy.
  - Examples:
    - Ustekinumab 40 to 90 mg subcutaneously at 0 weeks, 4 weeks, and then every 12 weeks thereafter
- IL-17 inhibitors[74]:
  - Highly effective for psoriasis and psoriatic arthritis.
  - May worsen inflammatory bowel disease.
  - Examples include secukinumab, ixekizumab, and brodalumab.
- IL-23 inhibitors:
  - Highly effective for psoriasis. Inferior to IL-17 inhibitors for psoriatic arthritis.
  - Examples include guselkumab, risankizumab, and tildrakizumab.
- JAK inhibitors:
  - Deucravacitinib works by inhibiting TYK2 and therefore, inhibiting signaling through the JAK/STAT pathway.[75]
  - Baricitinib is a JAK1/JAK2 inhibitor. Side effects of JAK inhibitors include blood clots and infection.[76]

# 7. Seborrheic Dermatitis

## 7.1. BACKGROUND

- Seborrheic dermatitis is a mild eczematous process characterized by greasy, flaky, yellow scales on an erythematous background. Pruritus is a common symptom. It predominates on areas of high sebum production, including the face, scalp, and upper trunk.
- There are two peak age distributions in infancy and later between the ages of 40 to 60 years old. Seborrheic dermatitis is more common in men than women.
- Seborrheic dermatitis in babies is often called "cradle cap." Cradle cap is very common, and studies have shown a prevalence of 71.7% in children less than 3 months old with that number declining to 44.5% of children at 1 year of age.[77] The peak in infancy correlates with a transient period of sebaceous gland activity.
- The pathogenesis of seborrheic dermatitis is multifactorial and involves increased sebum production, *Malassezia globosa*, and an altered host immune response.[78-80]

## 7.2. CLINICAL PRESENTATION

- Seborrheic dermatitis is characterized by greasy, flaky, yellow scales on poorly demarcated erythematous patches or thin plaques. Vesicles, crusting, and secondary infection are less frequently seen manifestations (Fig. 3-9).
- Lesions are most commonly found on areas of high sebum production including the face, scalp, and upper trunk. The eyebrows, nasal sidewalls, nasolabial folds, and glabella are classic areas of facial involvement.
- The rash is typically localized and follows a mild course; however, rarely, it may become generalized and produce erythroderma.
- Dandruff is a milder version with less inflammation. Pruritus is common.

## 7.3. EVALUATION

- Seborrheic dermatitis is primarily a clinical diagnosis with key features that distinguish it from other eczematous processes seen in a similar distribution.
- The differential diagnosis varies by age group.
  - The differential diagnosis of infantile and childhood seborrheic dermatitis includes AD, psoriasis, and tinea capitis.

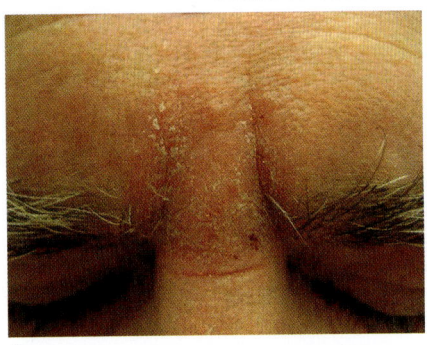

**A**

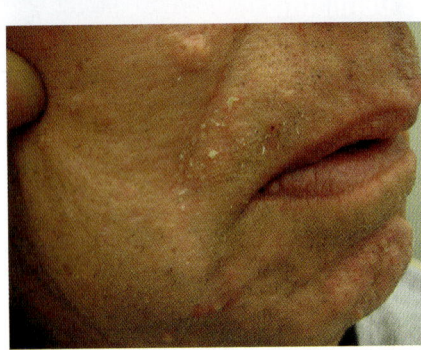

**B**

**Figure 3-9. A, B.** Seborrheic dermatitis. (Courtesy of David Sheinbein, MD.)

- AD is associated with more intense inflammation, higher degree of pruritus, later age of onset, and more widespread distribution on the face, scalp, and extensor surfaces. AD also produces higher morbidity with greater disturbance in patient quality of life.
- Psoriasis tends to have more well-demarcated, thick plaques with silvery, adherent scale as opposed to the greasy, flaky scale of seborrheic dermatitis.
- Tinea capitis may produce a more robust inflammatory reaction and lead to hair loss. Fungal culture should be performed to rule out tinea capitis in high-risk populations.
- The adult seborrheic dermatitis differential includes psoriasis, AD, contact dermatitis, rosacea, and acute lupus erythematosus.
  - Psoriasis is distinguishable as mentioned above by more well-demarcated thick, red plaques with adherent silvery scale. Distribution is often more widespread and includes the extensor surfaces. Nail findings and symptoms of inflammatory joint disease further distinguish psoriasis from seborrheic dermatitis (SD).
  - AD in the adult population is differentiated by its common distribution pattern on the flexor surfaces and hands.
  - Contact dermatitis typically follows a less symmetric pattern. Geometric or linear patterns in particular suggest contact dermatitis over SD. A history of exposure to potential allergens and irritants is key in differentiating contact dermatitis from seborrheic dermatitis.
  - Rosacea produces centrofacial erythema similar to SD, but the lack of scale differentiates rosacea from SD.
  - Similarly, acute lupus erythematosus produces centrofacial erythema as in SD, but it classically spares the nasolabial folds, allowing simple differentiation from SD.

## 7.4. TREATMENT

Seborrheic dermatitis is a chronic condition requiring routine application of therapeutic shampoos, solutions, and creams for continued control. Treatment is directed at minimizing erythema, scale, and pruritus. Topical products including antifungals and steroids are the mainstays of treatment. Topicals may be applied once or twice daily during acute flares and once or twice weekly thereafter for maintenance.
- Antifungal agents decrease the load of *Malassezia* yeast on affected skin.
  - Ketoconazole (KC) 2% shampoo or cream once or twice daily
  - Zinc pyrithione 1% shampoo once or twice daily
    - KC and zinc pyrithione have similar efficacy in SD management with a reported 73% and 67% reduction in total dandruff scores, respectively.[81]
  - Ciclopirox olamine (CPO) 1.5% shampoo once or twice daily
    - Comparison of CPO shampoo with KC shampoo demonstrated similar reductions in affected areas of 41.4 and 48.2 cm$^2$, respectively. Patients reported higher levels of satisfaction in signs and symptoms with CPO shampoo.[82]
- Topical steroids decrease inflammation. Mild- and moderate-potency topical steroids were found to have a similar degree of efficacy.[83] Given their similar efficacy and decreased side effect profile, low-potency steroids should be tried first.
  - Steroids may be applied once or twice daily during the acute phase.
  - Maintenance should be attempted with antifungal agents. If unable to achieve disease-free maintenance state with antifungal agents alone, a topical steroid may be added with once- or twice-weekly application.

- Examples
  - Hydrocortisone 2.5% cream once or twice daily
  - Desonide 0.05% cream once or twice daily
  - Fluocinolone 0.01% solution once or twice daily

# REFERENCES

1. Collier CN, Harper JC, Cafardi JA, et al. The prevalence of acne in adults 20 years and older. *J Am Acad Dermatol.* 2008;58:56-59.
2. Berg M, Liden S. An epidemiological study of rosacea. *Acta Derm Venereol.* 1989;69:419-423.
3. Spoendlin J, Voegel JJ, Jick SS, Meier CR. A study on the epidemiology of rosacea in the UK. *Br J Dermatol.* 2012;167:598-605.
4. Fowler J Jr, Jackson M, Moore A, et al. Efficacy and safety of once-daily topical brimonidine tartrate gel 0.5% for the treatment of moderate to severe facial erythema of rosacea: results of two randomized, double-blind, and vehicle-controlled pivotal studies. *J Drus Dermatol.* 2013;12:650-656.
5. Shanler SD, Ondo AL. Successful treatment of the Erythema and flushing of Rosacea using a topically applied selective α1-adrenergic receptor agonist, oxymetazoline. *Arch Dermatol.* 2007;143:1369-1371.
6. Shim TN, Abdullah A. The effect of pulsed dye laser on the dermatology life quality index in erythematotelangiectatic rosacea patients: an assessment. *J Clin Aesthet Dermatol.* 2013;6:30-32.
7. Bassi A, Campolmi P, Dindelli M, et al. Laser surgery in rhinophyma. *G Ital Dermatol Venereol.* 2016;151(1):9-16.
8. Prado R, Funke A, Bingham J, Brown M, Mellette JR. Treatment of severe rhinophyma using scalpel excision and wire loop tip electrosurgery. *Dermatol Surg.* 2013;39:807-810.
9. Hong S, Son DK, Lim WR, et al. The prevalence of atopic dermatitis, asthma, and allergic rhinitis and the comorbidity of allergic diseases in children. *Environ Health Toxicol.* 2012;27:e2012006.
10. Flohr C, Yeo L. Atopic dermatitis and the hygiene hypothesis revisited. *Curr Probl Dermatol.* 2011;41:1-34.
11. Flohr C, Pascoe D, Williams HC. Atopic dermatitis and the 'hygiene hypothesis': too clean to be true? *Br J Dermatol.* 2005;152:202-216.
12. Margolis JS, Abuabara K, Bilker W, Hoffstad O, Margolis DJ. Persistence of mild to moderate atopic dermatitis. *JAMA Dermatol.* 2014;150:593-600.
13. Chang YS, Chou YT, Lee JH, et al. Atopic dermatitis, melatonin, and sleep disturbance. *Pediatrics.* 2014;134:e397-e405.
14. Thomsen SF, Ulrik CS, Kyvik KO, et al. Importance of genetic factors in the etiology of atopic dermatitis: a twin study. *Allergy Asthma Proc.* 2007;28:535-539.
15. Elias PM, Schmuth M. Abnormal skin barrier in the etiopathogenesis of atopic dermatitis. *Curr Asthma Allergy Rep.* 2009;9:265-272.
16. Palmer CN, Irvine AD, Terron-Kwiatkowski A, et al. Common loss-of-function variants of the epidermal barrier protein filaggrin are a major predisposing factor for atopic dermatitis. *Nat Genet.* 2006;38:441-446.
17. Lewis-Jones S. Quality of life and childhood atopic dermatitis: the misery of living with childhood eczema. *Int J Clin Pract.* 2006;60:984-992.
18. Gelmetti C, Boralevi F, Seité S, et al. Quality of life of parents living with a child suffering from atopic dermatitis before and after a 3-month treatment with an emollient. *Pediatr Dermatol.* 2012;29:714-718.
19. Davis DMR, Drucker AM, Alikhan A, et al. Executive summary: guidelines of care for the management of atopic dermatitis in adults with phototherapy and systemic therapies. *J Am Acad Dermatol.* 2024;90(2):342-345.
20. Peserico A, Städtler G, Sebastian M, Fernandez RS, Vick K, Bieber T. Reduction of relapses of atopic dermatitis with methylprednisolone aceponate cream twice weekly in addition to maintenance treatment with emollient: a multicentre, randomized, double-blind, controlled study. *Br J Dermatol.* 2008;158:801-807.
21. Papp K, Szepietowski JC, Kircik L, et al. Efficacy and safety of ruxolitinib cream for the treatment of atopic dermatitis: results from 2 phase 3, randomized, double-blind studies. *J Am Acad Dermatol.* 2021;85(4):863-872. doi:10.1016/j.jaad.2021.04.085
22. Jury CS, McHenry P, Burden AD, Lever R, Bilsland D. Narrowband ultraviolet B (UVB) phototherapy in children. *Clin Exp Dermatol.* 2006;31:196-199.
23. Simpson EL, Bieber T, Guttman-Yassky E, et al. Two phase 3 trials of dupilumab versus placebo in atopic dermatitis. *N Engl J Med.* 2016;375(24):2335-2348. doi:10.1056/NEJMoa1610020
24. Blauvelt A, de Bruin-Weller M, Gooderham M, et al. Long-term management of moderate-to-severe atopic dermatitis with dupilumab and concomitant topical corticosteroids (LIBERTY AD

CHRONOS): a 1-year, randomised, double-blinded, placebo-controlled, phase 3 trial. *Lancet.* 2017;389(10086):2287-2303. doi:10.1016/S0140-6736(17)31191-1
25. Wollenberg A, Blauvelt A, Guttman-Yassky E, et al. Tralokinumab for moderate-to-severe atopic dermatitis: results from two 52-week, randomized, double-blind, multicentre, placebo-controlled phase III trials (ECZTRA 1 and ECZTRA 2). *Br J Dermatol.* 2021;184(3):437-449. doi:10.1111/bjd.19574
26. Silverberg JI, Guttman-Yassky E, Thaçi D, et al. Two phase 3 trials of lebrikizumab for moderate-to-severe atopic dermatitis. *N Engl J Med.* 2023;388(12):1080-1091. doi:10.1056/NEJMoa2206714
27. Guttman-Yassky E, Thyssen JP, Silverberg JI, et al. Safety of upadacitinib in moderate-to-severe atopic dermatitis: an integrated analysis of phase 3 studies. *J Allergy Clin Immunol.* 2023;151(1):172-181. doi:10.1016/j.jaci.2022.09.023
28. Simpson EL, Sinclair R, Forman S, et al. Efficacy and safety of abrocitinib in adults and adolescents with moderate-to-severe atopic dermatitis (JADE MONO-1): a multicentre, double-blind, randomised, placebo-controlled, phase 3 trial. *Lancet (London, England).* 2020;396(10246):255-266. doi:10.1016/S0140-6736(20)30732-7
29. Simpson EL, Lacour JP, Spelman L, et al. Baricitinib in patients with moderate-to-severe atopic dermatitis and inadequate response to topical corticosteroids: results from two randomized monotherapy phase III trials. *Br J Dermatol.* 2020;183(2):242-255. doi:10.1111/bjd.18898
30. Haw S, Shin MK, Haw CR. The efficacy and safety of long-term oral cyclosporine treatment for patients with atopic dermatitis. *Ann Dermatol.* 2010;22:9-15.
31. Thomsen SF, Karlsmark T, Clemmensen KK, et al. Outcome of treatment with azathioprine in severe atopic dermatitis: a five-year retrospective study of adult outpatients. *Br J Dermatol.* 2015;172(4):1122-1124.
32. Sheinkopf LE, Rafi AW, Do LT, Katz RM, Klaustermeyer WB. Efficacy of omalizumab in the treatment of atopic dermatitis: a pilot study. *Allergy Asthma Proc.* 2008;29:530-537.
33. Simon D, Hösli S, Kostylina G, Yawalkar N, Simon H-U. Anti-CD20 (rituximab) treatment improves atopic eczema. *J Allergy Clin Immunol.* 2008;121:122-128.
34. Nethercott JR, Holness DL, Adams RM, et al. Patch testing with a routine screening tray in North America, 1985 through 1989: I. Frequency of response. *Dermatitis.* 1991;2:122-129.
35. Teixeira V, Coutinho I, Gonçalo M. Allergic contact dermatitis to metals over a 20-year period in the Centre of Portugal: evaluation of the effects of the European directives. *Acta Med Port.* 2014;27:295-303.
36. Larsson-Stymne B, Widström L. Ear piercing—a cause of nickel allergy in schoolgirls? *Contact Dermatitis.* 1985;13:289-293.
37. Srivastava D, Cohen DE. Identification of the constituents of Balsam of Peru in tomatoes. *Dermatitis.* 2009;20:99-105.
38. Cheman A, Rakowski EM, Chou V, Chhatriwala A, Ross J, Jacob SE. Balsam of Peru: past and future. *Dermatitis.* 2013;24:153-160.
39. Curtis G, Lewis AC. Treatment of severe poison ivy: a randomized, controlled trial of long versus short course oral prednisone. *J Clin Med Res.* 2014;6:429-434.
40. Yildirim M, Aridogan BC, Baysal V, Inaloz HS. The role of human herpes virus 6 and 7 in the pathogenesis of pityriasis rosea. *Int J Clin Pract.* 2004;58:119-121.
41. Chuh AA, Peiris JS. Lack of evidence of active human herpesvirus 7 (HHV-7) infection in three cases of pityriasis rosea in children. *Pediatr Dermatol.* 2008;18:381-383.
42. Arndt KA, Paul BS, Stern RS, Parrish JA. Treatment of pityriasis rosea with UV radiation. *Arch Dermatol.* 1983;119:381-382.
43. Bigby M. A remarkable result of a double-masked, placebo-controlled trial of erythromycin in the treatment of Pityriasis rosea. *Arch Dermatol.* 2000;136:775-776.
44. Parisi R, Symmons DP, Griffiths CE, Ashcroft DM; Identification and Management of Psoriasis and Associated ComorbidiTy (IMPACT) project team. Global epidemiology of psoriasis: a systematic review of incidence and prevalence. *J Investig Dermatol.* 2013;133:377-385.
45. Swanbeck G, Inerot A, Martinsson T, et al. Age at onset and different types of psoriasis. *Br J Dermatol.* 1995;133:768-773.
46. Lin HW, Wang KH, Lin HC, Lin H-C. Increased risk of acute myocardial infarction in patients with psoriasis: a 5-year population-based study in Taiwan. *J Am Acad Dermatol.* 2011;64:495-501.
47. Armstrong AW, Harskamp CT, Armstrong EJ. Psoriasis and metabolic syndrome: a systematic review and meta-analysis of observational studies. *J Am Acad Dermatol.* 2013;68:654-662.
48. de Korte J, Sprangers MA, Mombers FM, Bos JD. Quality of life in patients with psoriasis: a systematic literature review. *J Invest Dermatol.* 2004;9:140-147.
49. Grjibovski AM, Olsen AO, Magnus P, Harris JR. Psoriasis in Norwegian twins: contribution of genetic and environmental effects. *J Eur Acad Dermatol Venereol.* 2007;21:1337-1343.
50. Swanbeck G, Inerot A, Martinsson T, et al. A population genetic study of psoriasis. *Br J Dermatol.* 1994;13:32-39.
51. Elder JT, Henseler T, Christophers E, Voorhees JJ, Nair RP. Of genes and antigens: the inheritance of psoriasis. *J Investig Dermatol.* 1994;103:150S-153S.

52. Conrad C, Boyman O, Tonel G, et al. Alpha1beta1 integrin is crucial for accumulation of epidermal T cells and the development of psoriasis. *Nat Med.* 2007;13:836-842.
53. Lin WJ, Norris DA, Achziger M, Kotzin BL, Tomkinson B. Oligoclonal expansion of intraepidermal T cells in psoriasis skin lesions. *J Investig Dermatol.* 2001;117:1546-1553.
54. Kryczek I, Bruce AT, Gudjonsson JE, et al. Induction of IL-17+ T cell trafficking and development by IFN-gamma: mechanism and pathological relevance in psoriasis. *J Immunol.* 2008;18:4733-4741.
55. Cameron AL, Kirby B, Fei W, Griffiths CEM. Natural killer and natural killer-T cells in psoriasis. *Arch Dermatol Res.* 2002;294:363-369.
56. Bonish B, Jullien D, Dutronc Y, et al. Overexpression of CD1d by keratinocytes in psoriasis and CD1d-dependent IFN-gamma production by NK-T cells. *J Immunol.* 2000;165:4076-4085.
57. Harvima RJ, Viinamäki H, Harvima IT, et al. Association of psychic stress with clinical severity and symptoms of psoriatic patients. *Acta Derm Venereol.* 1996;76:467-471.
58. Kawamura A, Kinoshita MT, Suzuki H. Generalized pustular psoriasis with hypoparathyroidism. *Eur J Dermatol.* 1999;9:574-576.
59. Dogan B, Karabudak O, Harmanyeri Y. Antistreptococcal treatment of guttate psoriasis: a controlled study. *Int J Dermatol.* 2008;47:950-952.
60. Mease PJ, Gladman DD, Papp KA, et al. Prevalence of rheumatologist-diagnosed psoriatic arthritis in patients with psoriasis in European/North American dermatology clinics. *J Am Acad Dermatol.* 2013;69:729-735.
61. van de Kerkhof PCM. From empirical to pathogenesis-based treatments for psoriasis. *J Invest Dermatol.* 2022;142(7):1778-1785.
62. Katz HI, Hien NT, Prawer SE, Scott JC, Grivna EM. Betamethasone dipropionate in optimized vehicle. Intermittent pulse dosing for extended maintenance treatment of psoriasis. *Arch Dermatol.* 1987;123:1308-1311.
63. Highton A, Quell J. Calcipotriene ointment 0.005% for psoriasis: a safety and efficacy study. *J Am Acad Dermatol.* 1995;32:67-72.
64. Weinstein GD, Krueger GG, Lowe NJ, et al. Tazarotene gel, a new retinoid, for topical therapy of psoriasis: vehicle-controlled study of safety, efficacy, and duration of therapeutic effect. *J Am Acad Dermatol.* 1997;37:85-92.
65. Wang C, Lin A. Efficacy of topical calcineurin inhibitors in psoriasis. *J Cutan Med Surg.* 2014;18:8-14.
66. Takahashi H, Tsuji H, Ishida-Yamamoto A, Iizuka H. Comparison of clinical effects of psoriasis treatment regimens among calcipotriol alone, narrowband ultraviolet B phototherapy alone, combination of calcipotriol and narrowband ultraviolet B phototherapy once a week, and combination of calcipotriol and narrowband ultraviolet B phototherapy more than twice a week. *J Dermatol.* 2013;40:424-427.
67. Spuls PI, Rozenblit M, Lebwohl M. Retrospective study of the efficacy of narrowband UVB and acitretin. *J Dermatol Treat.* 2003;14:17-20.
68. Hearn RM, Kerr AC, Rahim KF, Ferguson J, Dawe RS. Incidence of skin cancers in 3867 patients treated with narrow-band ultraviolet B phototherapy. *Br J Dermatol.* 2008;159:931-935.
69. Almutawa F, Alnomair N, Wang Y, Hamzavi I, Lim HW. Systematic review of UV-based therapy for psoriasis. *Am J Clin Dermatol.* 2013;14:87-109.
70. Shehzad T, Dar NR, Zakria M. Efficacy of concomitant use of PUVA and methotrexate in disease clearance time in plaque type psoriasis. *J Pak Med Assoc.* 2004;54:453-455.
71. Heidbreder G, Christophers E. Therapy of psoriasis with retinoid plus PUVA: clinical and histologic data. *Arch Dermatol Res.* 1979;264:331-337.
72. Lowe NJ, Wieder JM, Rosenbach A, et al. Long-term low-dose cyclosporine therapy for severe psoriasis: effects on renal function and structure. *J Am Acad Dermatol.* 1996;35:710-719.
73. Leonardi CL, Kimball AB, Papp KA, et al. Efficacy and safety of ustekinumab, a human interleukin-12/23 monoclonal antibody, in patients with psoriasis: 76-week results from a randomised, double-blind, placebo-controlled trial (PHOENIX 1). *Lancet.* 2008;371:1665-1674.
74. Wride AM, Chen GF, Spaulding SL, Tkachenko E, Cohen JM. Biologics for psoriasis. *Dermatol Clin.* 2024;42(3):339-355. doi:10.1016/j.det.2024.02.001
75. Strober B, Thaçi D, Sofen H, et al. Deucravacitinib versus placebo and apremilast in moderate to severe plaque psoriasis: efficacy and safety results from the 52-week, randomized, double-blinded, phase 3 program for evaluation of TYK2 inhibitor psoriasis second trial. *J Am Acad Dermatol.* 2023;88(1):40-51. doi:10.1016/j.jaad.2022.08.061
76. Papp KA, Menter MA, Raman M, et al. A randomized phase 2b trial of baricitinib, an oral janus kinase (JAK) 1/Jak2 inhibitor, in patients with moderate-to-severe psoriasis. *Br J Dermatol.* 2016;174(6):1266-1276. doi:10.1111/bjd.14403
77. Foley P, Zuo Y, Plunkett A, Merlin K, Marks R. The frequency of common skin conditions in preschool-aged children in Australia: seborrheic dermatitis and pityriasis capitis (cradle cap). *Arch Dermatol.* 2003;139:318-322.
78. Ostlere LS, Taylor CR, Harris DW, Rustin MH, Wright S, Johnson M. Skin surface lipids in HIV-positive patients with and without seborrheic dermatitis. *Int J Dermatol.* 1996;35:276-279.

79. McGinley KJ, Leyden JJ, Marples RR, Kligman AM. Quantitative microbiology of the scalp in non-dandruff, dandruff, and seborrheic dermatitis. *J Investig Dermatol.* 1975;64:401.
80. Sud N, Shanker V, Sharma A, Sharma NL, Gupta M. Mucocutaneous manifestations in 150 HIV-infected Indian patients and their relationship with CD4 lymphocyte counts. *Int J STD AIDS.* 2009;20:771-774.
81. Piérard-Franchimont C, Goffin V, Decroix J, Piérard GE. A multicenter randomized trial of ketoconazole 2% and zinc pyrithione 1% shampoos in severe dandruff and seborrheic dermatitis. *Skin Pharmacol Appl Skin Physiol.* 2002;15:434-441.
82. Ratnavel RC, Squire RA, Boorman GC. Clinical efficacies of shampoos containing ciclopirox olamine (1.5%) and ketoconazole (2.0%) in the treatment of seborrhoeic dermatitis. *J Dermatolog Treat.* 2007;18:88-96.
83. Kastarinen H, Oksanen T, Okokon EO, et al. Topical anti-inflammatory agents for seborrhoeic dermatitis of the face or scalp. *Cochrane Database Syst Rev.* 2014;(5):CD009446.

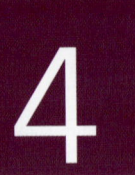

# Infections and Infestations

Rabia Mayer, MD, PhD

Infections and infestations are common dermatologic concerns. Some viral, bacterial, and fungal infections are limited to the skin, whereas others are systemic illnesses with more serious consequences. This chapter covers those conditions that affect patients of any age; additional information about childhood infections can be found in Chapters 5 and 14, Reactive Disorders and Pediatric Dermatology, respectively.

## 1. Verrucae

### 1.1. BACKGROUND

- Papillomaviruses are nonenveloped, double-stranded DNA viruses that infect the skin and induce common warts, palmar and plantar warts, and flat warts.[1]

### 1.2. CLINICAL FEATURES

- Common warts
  - Common warts are hyperkeratotic, exophytic, dome-shaped papules or plaques (Fig. 4-1).
  - Most frequently located on the fingers and dorsal surfaces of the hands but may occur anywhere on the skin.
  - Punctate black dots that represent thrombosed capillaries are characteristic. Shaving the surface results in bleeding.
  - Human papillomavirus (HPV) associations—HPV-1, HPV-2, HPV-4, HPV-27, and HPV-57.
- Palmar and plantar warts
  - Palmar and plantar warts appear as thick, endophytic papules with a central depression.
  - Plantar warts are often painful when walking due to deep inward growth.
  - HPV types 1, 2, 27, and 57 cause the majority of palmoplantar warts.[2]
- Flat warts
  - Flat warts are skin-colored to pinkish, smooth-surfaced, slightly elevated, flat-topped papules most commonly located on dorsal hands, arms, or face.
  - HPV associations—HPV types 3 and 10 and less commonly 28 and 29.
- Condyloma acuminata
  - Condylomata are discrete, sessile, smooth-surfaced exophytic papillomas, which may be skin colored, brown, or whitish.
  - Lesions are located on the external genitalia and perineum and may measure one to several millimeters in diameter.
  - HPV associations—HPV types 6 and 11.

---

*The authors would like to acknowledge the first edition authors* Heather Jones, Jason Burnham, and Kara Blackwell.

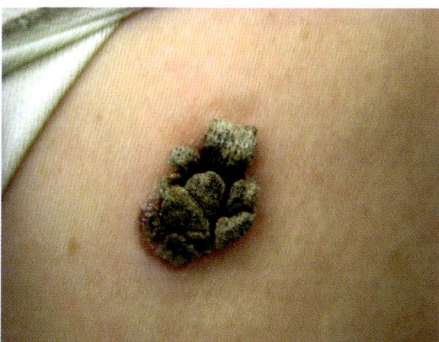

**Figure 4-1.** Common wart. (Courtesy of David Sheinbein, MD.)

### 1.3. EVALUATION

- Warts are diagnosed based on morphology and anatomic location.
- Differential diagnosis
  - Seborrheic keratoses, squamous cell carcinomas, hypertrophic lichen planus, and corns.
  - Condyloma acuminata can be rarely confused with condyloma lata of secondary syphilis.

### 1.4. TREATMENT

- There is no specific antiviral therapy to cure HPV. Current treatment modalities focus on destruction of visible lesions or induction of cytotoxicity against infected cells.
- Destruction is performed with cryotherapy or cantharidin.
  - Considerations include discomfort with cryotherapy and potential for formation of "doughnut" wart formation with cantharidin.
  - If lesions are many or recalcitrant to therapy, clinicians can combine therapy with salicylic acid preparations, intralesional candida or bleomycin, or topical imiquimod, or 5-fluorouracil.
- Genital HPV infection is typically widespread throughout the anogenital tract, and recurrence rates are high.
  - Clinician-applied therapy includes cryotherapy, excision, and curettage.
  - Imiquimod, a topical immunomodulator approved for the treatment of genital HPV lesions, can be applied by patients.
  - HPV infection may cause cervical, vulvar, vaginal, penile, and anal malignancies. Patients with external HPV infection should be screened with Pap smears and physical examinations for signs of dysplasia or malignancy.
  - Gardasil is a vaccine that protects against HPV types 6, 11, 16, and 18.

## 2. Molluscum Contagiosum

### 2.1. BACKGROUND

- Family Poxviridae, double-stranded DNA virus.

- After the eradication of smallpox, molluscum contagiosum (MC) became the only remaining poxvirus to afflict humans.
- MC is a common, self-limited disease in children; however, in adults, it is usually considered a sexually transmitted disease.

## 2.2. CLINICAL PRESENTATION

- MC lesions are firm, umbilicated, flesh-colored papules (see Fig. 14-20).
- Can occur anywhere on the skin. Widespread or large lesions may be seen in the setting of human immunodeficiency virus (HIV) or immunosuppression.

## 2.3. EVALUATION

- MC is diagnosed clinically.
- Differential diagnosis: verrucae, condyloma acuminata, basal cell carcinoma, melanocytic nevi, and pyogenic granuloma. In immunocompromised patients, *Cryptococcus* or *Histoplasma* infections can mimic MC.

## 2.4. TREATMENT

- MC resolves spontaneously in immunocompetent children; however, the time interval between onset and clearance of infection can range from months to years.
- Therapeutic options include curettage, cryotherapy, or cantharidin (a blistering agent). Recently, the FDA has approved Ycanth (0.7% cantharidin) for in-office use and berdazimer gel for at-home treatment of MC.
- Treatment of associated dermatitis with a topical corticosteroid can reduce itching and avoid autoinoculation.

# 3. Superficial Dermatophytes

## 3.1. BACKGROUND

- Dermatophytoses are fungal infections caused by three genera of fungi—*Microsporum*, *Trichophyton*, and *Epidermophyton*[3]—that invade and multiply within keratinized tissue.

## 3.2. CLINICAL FEATURES (FIG. 4-2)

- Tinea corporis
  - Dermatophyte infection of the skin of the trunk and extremities, excluding hair, nails, palms, soles, and groin.
  - Infection is generally restricted to the stratum corneum.
  - *Trichophyton rubrum* is the most common pathogen worldwide followed by *Trichophyton mentagrophytes*.
  - The typical incubation period is 1 to 3 weeks.
  - Characteristic lesions are sharply demarcated with a raised, erythematous, scaly, advancing border and central clearing. Scale may be diminished or absent if topical corticosteroids have been used (tinea "incognito").

- Differential diagnosis: eczematous dermatitis, seborrheic dermatitis, pityriasis rosea, psoriasis, and contact dermatitis.
- Tinea cruris
  - Dermatophyte infection of the inguinal region.
  - The three most common causative agents are *Epidermophyton floccosum*, *T rubrum*, and *T mentagrophytes*.
  - Predisposing factors: obesity, excessive perspiration, and male sex.
  - Often coexistent with tinea pedis.
  - The first signs of infection are often erythema and pruritus in the perineal area.
  - Characteristic lesions are sharply demarcated erythematous plaques with peripheral scale. The scrotum is generally spared.
  - Differential diagnosis: cutaneous candidiasis, intertrigo, psoriasis, contact dermatitis, and mycosis fungoides.

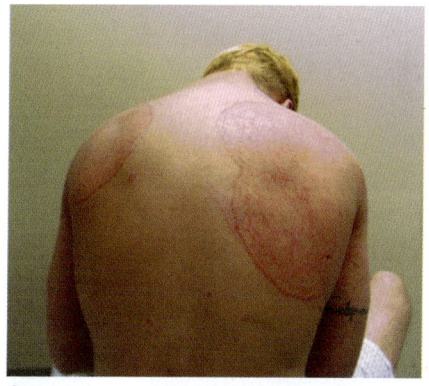

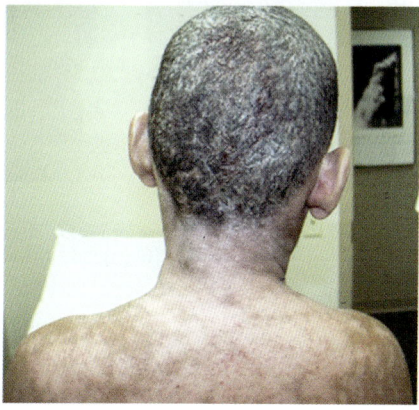

**Figure 4-2.** Tinea. **A.** Tinea corporis. **B.** Tinea capitis.

*(continued)*

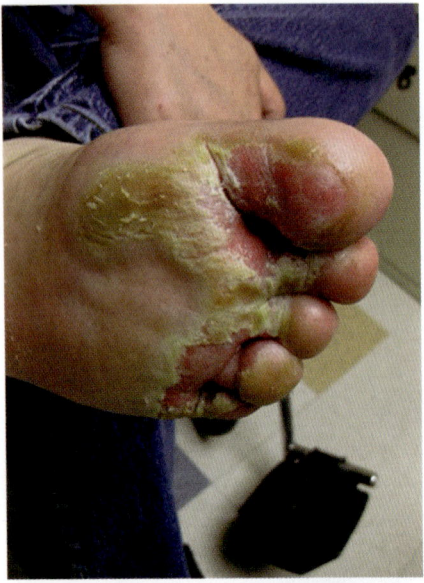

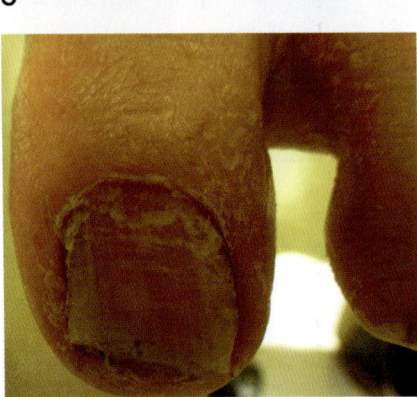

**Figure 4-2.** (*Continued*) **C.** Tinea pedis. **D.** Tinea unguium (onychomycosis). (Courtesy of David Sheinbein, MD.)

- Tinea manuum
  - Dermatophyte infections of the palm and interdigital web spaces.
  - The typical causative organisms are the same as those for tinea pedis and cruris.
  - Infection is usually noninflammatory with hyperkeratosis on the palms, recalcitrant to treatment with emollients.

- It is often unilateral and found in association with tinea pedis ("one-hand, two-foot disease").
- Differential diagnosis: psoriasis, irritant or allergic contact dermatitis, and eczematous dermatitis.
- Tinea capitis
  - Dermatophyte infection of the scalp in children and adults.
  - The typical causative organisms are in two genera, *Trichophyton* and *Microsporum*, with *Trichophyton tonsurans* accounting for more than 90% of cases of tinea capitis in the United States.[4]
  - Presentations of tinea capitis can range from noninflammatory scaling to a severe pustular eruption, with alopecia being the most common presentation.
  - Advanced disease associated with an exaggerated host response to the organism can result in formation of boggy, purulent plaques with abscess formation and alopecia, known as a kerion.
  - Occasionally, patients may become systemically ill with posterior cervical or postauricular lymphadenopathy.
  - Differential diagnosis: seborrheic dermatitis, pustular psoriasis, and alopecia areata.
- Tinea pedis
  - Dermatophyte infection of the soles and interdigital web spaces on the feet.
  - The three most common organisms responsible for tinea pedis are *T rubrum*, *T mentagrophytes*, and *E floccosum*.[5]
  - There are four major clinical types of tinea pedis—moccasin, interdigital, inflammatory, and ulcerative.
    - Moccasin—diffuse hyperkeratosis, erythema, and scaling on one or both plantar surfaces; may be associated with cell-mediated immunodeficiency
    - Interdigital—most common type with erythema, scaling, fissures, and maceration in web spaces
    - Inflammatory—vesicles and bullae on medial foot
    - Ulcerative—exacerbation of interdigital tinea pedis with ulcers and erosions in web spaces, seen in immunocompromised and diabetic patients
  - Differential diagnosis: eczematous dermatitis, tinea pedis caused by nondermatophytes including *Scytalidium dimidiatum*.
- Tinea unguium
  - Dermatophyte infection of the nail unit.
  - The most common causative pathogens are *T rubrum*, *T mentagrophytes*, and *E floccosum*.
  - Toenail infections are more common than fingernail infections. With progression of infection, there is yellowing and thickening of the distal nail plate as well as onycholysis.
  - Differential diagnosis: candidiasis and onychodystrophy.

## 3.3. DIAGNOSIS

- Potassium hydroxide prep (KOH) (Fig. 1-1)
  - Direct microscopy can be performed from a scraping of the scaly advancing border of a lesion.
  - In the case of tinea pedis, KOH preparation has a sensitivity of 77% and a specificity of 62%.[6] A negative test does not rule out the diagnosis, and

a culture should follow the potassium hydroxide examination even if it is positive.

## 3.4. TREATMENTS

- Topical therapies—first line for uncomplicated, localized infections of tinea corporis, cruris, and pedis
  - These agents are generally applied twice daily until clinical signs and symptoms are improved, typically up to 4 weeks.
    - Clotrimazole—1% lotion, solution, or cream. Pregnancy category B. Over the counter (OTC) or by prescription (Rx)
    - Ketoconazole—2% cream, foam, gel, shampoo. Pregnancy category C. Rx
    - Econazole—1% cream. Pregnancy category C. Rx
    - Miconazole—2% cream, lotion, powder. Pregnancy category C. OTC/Rx
    - Terbinafine—1% cream. Pregnancy category B. OTC
- Systemic agents
  - Terbinafine—indicated for onychomycosis and superficial fungal infections unresponsive to topical agents. Mycological cure rates of 70% for toenails after 12 weeks and 80% for fingernails after 6 weeks. Pregnancy category B
  - Ketoconazole—indicated for superficial fungal infections unresponsive to topical therapy. Pregnancy category C
  - Griseofulvin—indicated for tinea capitis or onychomycosis. Drug of choice for treating dermatophyte infections resistant to topical agents in children with mycologic cure rates of 80% to 95%. Pregnancy category C

# 4. Tinea Versicolor

## 4.1. BACKGROUND

- Caused by *Malassezia furfur*, a microbe present in normal skin flora.
- *Malassezia* requires oil to grow, which accounts for its increased incidence in adolescents and preference for sebum-rich areas of the skin.

## 4.2. CLINICAL FEATURES

- Usually presents with multiple oval to round patches or thin plaques with mild, fine scale. The lesions are often confluent centrally within areas of involvement, and seborrheic areas are the favored sites (Fig. 4-3).
- The most common colors are brown and whitish tan.
- Infection is generally asymptomatic.

## 4.3. DIAGNOSIS

- KOH with visualization of both hyphal and yeast forms
- Differential diagnosis: pityriasis alba and postinflammatory hypopigmentation

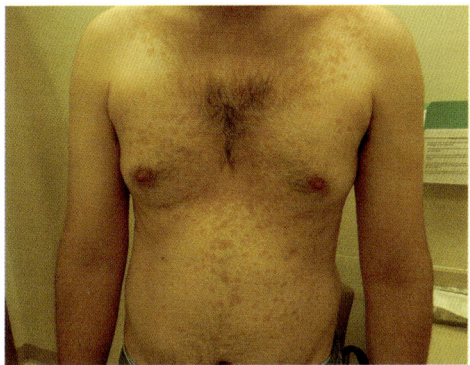

**Figure 4-3.** Tinea versicolor. (Courtesy of David Sheinbein, MD.)

### 4.4. TREATMENT

- Patients usually respond to topical antimycotic treatments including 2% ketoconazole or selenium sulfide shampoo, or topical azole cream.
- Systemic therapy is not generally indicated.

## 5. Candidiasis

### 5.1. BACKGROUND

- *Candida* species are responsible for mucocutaneous infections in immunocompetent hosts and disseminated infections in immunocompromised patients.
- Mucocutaneous candidiasis and disseminated infection are most commonly caused by *Candida albicans*, with *Candida tropicalis* being the second most common cause.
- Predisposing factors for mucocutaneous infection: diabetes mellitus, dry mouth, excessive sweat production, and use of corticosteroids or broad-spectrum antibiotics.
- Primary and secondary immunosuppression are the primary predisposing factors for disseminated candidiasis.
- *Candida glabrata* and *Candida krusei* have intrinsic fluconazole resistance that may be increasing in prevalence with the use of broad-spectrum antifungal agents.

### 5.2. CLINICAL FEATURES

- Mucocutaneous *Candida* infection
  - Oral infection often presents with a white exudate resembling cottage cheese or thrush. Other presentations include adherent white plaques, denture stomatitis, angular cheilitis (perleche), and vulvovaginal infection.

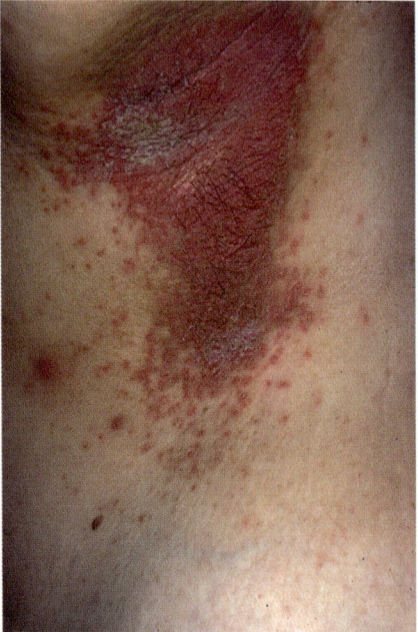

**Figure 4-4.** Candida. (Courtesy of Arthur Eisen, MD.)

- Cutaneous infections present with markedly erythematous, occasionally erosive patches accompanied by satellite papules, most commonly involving the intertriginous areas (Fig. 4-4).
- Infection can also occur in the periungual area and the diaper area in infants.
- Opportunistic *Candida* infection
  - Cutaneous lesions of disseminated candidiasis often present as firm pink papules or nodules on the trunk and extremities.
  - Other presentations include ecthyma gangrenosum–like lesions consisting of hemorrhagic bullae with necrotic eschar, pustules, and abscesses.

## 5.3. DIAGNOSIS

- Mucocutaneous *Candida* infection—diagnosed with KOH examination demonstrating presence of budding yeast and pseudohyphae and by positive fungal culture
- Opportunistic *Candida* infection—diagnosed with positive tissue or blood culture and demonstration of budding yeast and pseudohyphae in dermis

## 5.4. TREATMENT

- Mucocutaneous *Candida* infection—removal of the predisposing factor is of primary importance. Topical nystatin and azole antifungals are generally effective. When oral therapy is required, systemic azoles are used.

- Opportunistic *Candida* infection—consultation with an infectious disease specialist is recommended.

# 6. Herpes Simplex Viruses (HSV-1 and HSV-2)

## 6.1. BACKGROUND

- Herpes simplex virus type 1 (HSV-1) and type 2 (HSV-2) are large, double-stranded DNA viruses of the *Herpesviridae* family[7] with a worldwide distribution.
- HSV-2 is the cause of most genital herpes and is almost always sexually transmitted.[8]
- HSV-1 is usually transmitted during childhood nonsexually.
  - Recent studies have shown an increasing proportion of new genital herpes infections due to HSV-1 in the United States.[9]
- Genital HSV-2 infection increases the risk of HIV infection by at least twofold.[10]
- Host interaction—virus-host interaction includes three stages.
  - First stage: primary and nonprimary infections, which may be symptomatic or asymptomatic
    - Primary infections are first HSV infections in patients without preexisting antibodies to HSV-1 or HSV-2.
    - Nonprimary infections are infections with one HSV type in patients with preexisting antibodies to other HSV types.
  - Second stage: latency stage, in which the virus remains quiescent in the sensory ganglia
  - Third stage: reactivation resulting in recurrent infection with asymptomatic viral shedding or clinical manifestations

## 6.2. CLINICAL FEATURES

- In primary genital infections, symptoms usually appear 4 to 7 days after sexual exposure.[7]
  - A prodrome of tender lymphadenopathy, malaise, anorexia, and fever followed by localized pain, tenderness, or burning often precedes mucocutaneous findings.
  - Painful grouped vesicles appear on an erythematous base and may become umbilicated. Vesicles progress to pustules, erosions, or ulcerations with a characteristic scalloped border before crusting and healing.
- Approximately 70% to 90% of people with symptomatic HSV-2 and 20% to 50% with symptomatic genital HSV-1 will have recurrence in the first year.[7]
  - A similar prodrome can precede recurrent lesions; however, the lesions are often fewer in number, with decreased severity and duration compared to the primary infection.
- HSV lesions can manifest in areas adjacent to the genitalia and should be considered in patients presenting with lesions on the abdomen, thighs, and buttocks (Fig. 4-5).
- The majority of primary orolabial infections are asymptomatic.
  - The most common sites of involvement are the mouth and lips, with recurrent lesions appearing on the vermillion border of the lip.
- Differential diagnosis
  - Orolabial herpes: aphthous ulcers, oral candidiasis, or erythema multiforme major or Stevens-Johnson syndrome
  - Genital herpes: trauma, Lipschütz ulcer, syphilitic chancres, chancroid, and lymphogranuloma venereum

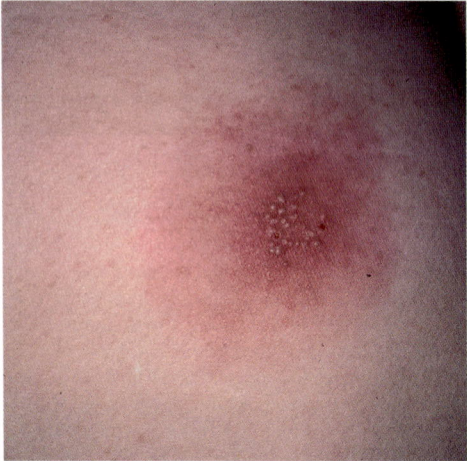

**Figure 4-5.** Primary herpes simplex virus. (Courtesy of Arthur Eisen, MD.)

## 6.3. DIAGNOSIS

Viral culture, direct fluorescent antibody assays, molecular techniques, serology, polymerase chain reaction (PCR)—most sensitive and specific and Tzanck smear can all be utilized for diagnosis.

## 6.4. TREATMENT

- FDA-approved treatment of recurrent orolabial herpes in immunocompetent patients includes oral valacyclovir (2 g twice daily for 1 day), oral famciclovir (single dose of 1.5 g), and topical 1% penciclovir.
  - These treatments result in decreased duration of mucocutaneous lesions and decreased viral shedding, especially if taken at the first symptom or sign of recurrence.
- Intravenous acyclovir is used to treat severe infections in immunocompromised patients.
- Chronic suppressive therapy with oral antiviral agents is usually reserved for those with greater than six outbreaks per year. In addition to reducing outbreaks, chronic suppressive therapy reduces asymptomatic viral shedding and can prevent transmission of infection to susceptible partners.[11]

# 7. Varicella-Zoster Virus

## 7.1. BACKGROUND

- Varicella-zoster virus (VZV) is a herpesvirus with a worldwide distribution that causes two distinct clinical syndromes.
- Since the introduction of the varicella vaccine in 1995, the overall incidence of varicella has decreased approximately 85%.

- Herpes zoster develops in approximately 30% of people over a lifetime,[12] with the risk of disease increasing with age.
- Transmission is usually via airborne droplets; however, direct contact with vesicular fluid represents another mode of spread.
- The incubation period ranges from 11 to 20 days.
- VZV travels to the epidermis via capillary endothelial cells and subsequently travels from mucocutaneous lesions to dorsal root ganglion cells where it remains latent.
- Herpes zoster represents reactivation of VZV, which may occur spontaneously or be triggered by stress, fever, illness, trauma, or immunosuppression.
  - During a zoster outbreak, the virus replicates in the dorsal root ganglion resulting in neuronal inflammation and painful ganglionitis.
  - Severe neuralgia worsens as the virus spreads down the sensory nerve.
  - Fluid from zoster vesicles can transmit VZV to seronegative individuals, leading to primary varicella infection.

## 7.2. CLINICAL FEATURES

- Varicella
  - Begins with a prodrome of fever, malaise, and myalgia followed by an eruption of pruritic, erythematous macules, and papules (Fig. 4-6).
  - Lesions start on the head and spread downward to the trunk and extremities, rapidly evolving over 12 to 14 hours into clear vesicles surrounded by erythema.
  - The presence of lesions in all stages of development is a hallmark of varicella.
  - The disease is usually self-limited, and within 7 to 10 days, lesions crust over and heal.
  - Varicella in adolescents and adults is often more severe than in children, with increased number of skin lesions and more frequent complications.
  - Maternal varicella during the first 20 weeks of pregnancy is associated with a risk of congenital varicella syndrome with defects including low birth weight, cutaneous scarring, ocular abnormalities, psychomotor retardation, and hypoplastic limbs.
  - Severe neonatal varicella can occur when maternal infection develops between 5 days before and 2 days after delivery.
  - Immunocompromised patients can have more extensive and atypical eruptions with higher morbidity and mortality.
- Herpes zoster—reactivation of VZV may occur any time after primary varicella infection (Fig. 4-7).
  - Zoster outbreaks begin with a prodrome of pruritus, tingling, and pain.
  - While most patients develop a painful eruption of grouped vesicles on an erythematous base in a dermatomal distribution, a few patients have the prodrome without subsequent skin findings.
  - Lesions can involve more than one contiguous dermatome and occasionally cross midline.
  - Postherpetic neuralgia is the most common complication, characterized by dysesthetic pain that persists after cutaneous lesions have healed. More than 40% of people older than 50 years of age who have had zoster have postherpetic neuralgia.[13]
  - Additional complications from reactivation of VZV include involvement of the ophthalmic division of the trigeminal nerve with increased risk of ocular involvement.

**70** | The Washington Manual® of Dermatology Diagnostics

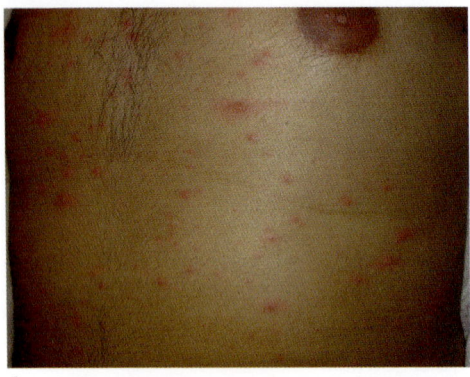

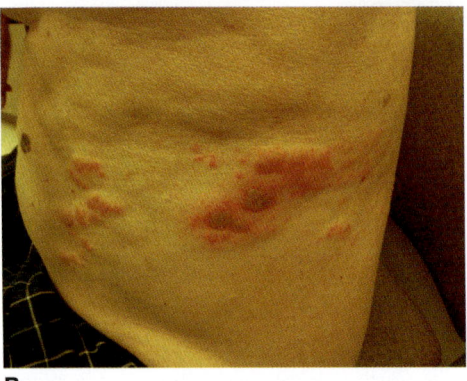

**Figure 4-6.** Varicella-zoster virus. **A.** Varicella. **B.** Zoster. (**A:** courtesy of Susan Bayliss, MD; **B:** courtesy of David Sheinbein, MD.)

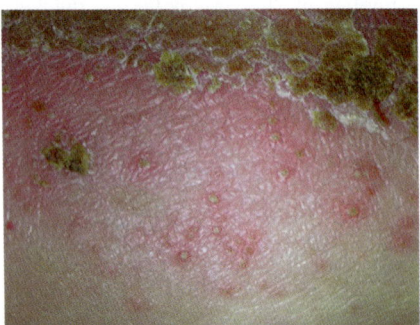

**Figure 4-7.** Impetigo. (Courtesy of David Sheinbein, MD.)

- When skin lesions are in the distribution of the nasociliary nerve, involving the nasal tip, dorsum, and root of the nose, ophthalmologic referral is necessary.
- Involvement of the geniculate ganglion of the facial nerve with lesions affecting the external auditory canal, tympanic membrane, and anterior two-thirds of the tongue may result in partial facial paralysis, hearing loss, or vertigo.
- Differential diagnosis
  - Varicella: viral exanthems, bullous arthropod reactions, and scabies
  - Herpes zoster: cellulitis, bullous impetigo, and localized contact dermatitis

## 7.3. DIAGNOSIS

- Clinical diagnosis can usually be made with a thorough history and physical examination.
- Additional testing includes viral culture, serology, and PCR.

## 7.4. TREATMENT

- Varicella in immunocompetent patients can be treated symptomatically.
- Acyclovir can be used to decrease the duration and symptoms of disease if started within 24 to 72 hours of symptom onset.
  - Oral acyclovir and valacyclovir are FDA approved for treatment of varicella in children (ages 2-17), while acyclovir is approved for adults.
  - In immunocompromised patients, intravenous acyclovir is indicated due to the increased risk of more severe disease and complications.
- Acyclovir, famciclovir, and valacyclovir are FDA approved for treatment of herpes zoster in immunocompetent patients to decrease duration and severity of skin findings and pain.
  - Antiviral therapy is best initiated within 72 hours of symptom onset; however, initiation up to 7 days after onset appears to be beneficial.

# 8. Impetigo

## 8.1. BACKGROUND

- Impetigo is a common, contagious skin infection most commonly caused by *Staphylococcus aureus*. Infection can present in bullous and nonbullous forms.
- Group A beta-hemolytic *Streptococcus* (*Streptococcus pyogenes*) represents an important cause of nonbullous impetigo.

## 8.2. CLINICAL FEATURES

- Nonbullous impetigo—early erythematous macules evolve into vesicles or pustules with late manifestations characterized by superficial erosions with "honey-colored" yellow crust (Fig. 4-5). Accounts for approximately 70% of cases.
  - Local production of exfoliative toxins (ETA, ETB), which binds and cleaves desmosomal protein desmoglein-1. Less common.
  - Most commonly affected sites are the face and extremities.
  - Clinical course is usually self-limited, resolving without scarring.
- Bullous impetigo—early vesicles enlarge into flaccid bullae with little surrounding erythema. After blisters are broken, they develop a collarette of scale without yellow crusting.

- *S aureus* or *S pyogenes* infection at sites of trauma with disruption of skin barrier. Represents 70% of cases.
- The most commonly affected sites are the face, trunk, buttocks, axillae, and extremities.
- Infection typically resolves in 3 to 6 weeks without treatment.
- Differential diagnosis
  - Nonbullous impetigo: insect bites, atopic dermatitis, inflamed dermatophytosis, and herpes simplex
  - Bullous impetigo: bullous insect bite reactions, thermal injury, and autoimmune bullous dermatoses

## 8.3. DIAGNOSIS

- Impetigo is diagnosed clinically and with bacterial Gram stain and culture.

## 8.4. TREATMENT

- In otherwise healthy patients, topical mupirocin 2% ointment can be prescribed.
- Second-line treatment for uncomplicated disease includes oral first-generation cephalosporins, clindamycin, macrolides, or beta-lactamase–resistant penicillins. Topical agents are often equally effective for limited disease.
- For complicated infection, intravenous antibiotics may be required.

# 9. Cellulitis

## 9.1. CELLULITIS BACKGROUND

- Cellulitis is a pyogenic infection of the deep dermis and subcutaneous tissue.
- The most commonly implicated organisms are *S aureus* and group A *Streptococcus*. A mixture of gram-positive cocci and gram-negative anaerobes and aerobes is often found in cellulitis surrounding diabetic or decubitus wounds.
- Bacteria gain entry through breaks in the skin barrier.
- Predisposing factors: chronic lymphedema, diabetes, and peripheral neuropathy.

## 9.2. CLINICAL FEATURES (FIG. 4-8)

- Cellulitis may be preceded by systemic signs or symptoms of infection including fever, chills, and malaise.
- Areas of infection present with inflammation, erythema, warmth, and pain. The borders are often ill defined.
- Severe infection can result in vesicles, pustules, or necrotic eschars.
- Occasionally ascending lymphangitis may be seen.
- Differential diagnosis
  - Lower extremity cellulitis: deep venous thrombosis, lipodermatosclerosis, and stasis dermatitis

## 9.3. DIAGNOSIS

- Cultures of blood or cutaneous aspirates are not routinely recommended but should be considered in patients with malignancy on chemotherapy, neutropenia, severe cell-mediated immunodeficiency, or animal bites.[14]

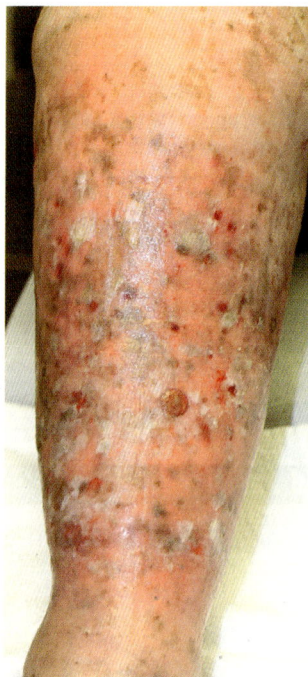

**Figure 4-8.** Cellulitis on severely actinic damaged skin. (Courtesy of M. Laurin Council, MD.)

## 9.4. TREATMENT

- For uncomplicated infection, a 5-day course of antimicrobials covering group A streptococci and *S aureus* is recommended; however, treatment can be extended at clinician discretion.
  - If methicillin-resistant *S aureus* (MRSA) is not suspected, treatment with clindamycin, dicloxacillin, or cephalexin can be initiated.
- For patients with evidence of MRSA infection elsewhere, nasal colonization, history of intravenous drug abuse, or those fitting systemic inflammatory response syndrome criteria, MRSA coverage is recommended.
  - Vancomycin plus either piperacillin-tazobactam or meropenem is recommended for empiric treatment in severe infections.

# 10. Erysipelas

## 10.1. ERYSIPELAS BACKGROUND

- Erysipelas is a superficial variant of cellulitis caused primarily by group A streptococci, affecting the dermis with prominent lymphatic involvement.
- Infection tends to occur in patients at the extremes of age, either very young or very old, and those severely debilitated or with chronic lymphedema or ulcers.

## 10.2. CLINICAL FEATURES

- Infection classically involved the face; however, the most common location affected is the lower extremities.
- An abrupt onset of systemic symptoms occurs including fever, chills, and malaise.
- An erythematous plaque develops that is well-demarcated from uninvolved skin, unlike in cellulitis. The affected area is warm, tense, painful to palpation, and indurated.
- Regional lymphadenopathy may be present, and in severe disease, pustules, vesicles, and areas of hemorrhage and necrosis can develop.
- Differential diagnosis: cellulitis, inflammatory disorders, Sweet syndrome, and drug reactions.

## 10.3. TREATMENT

- Treatment is similar to that of cellulitis (see above).

# 11. Furuncles and Abscesses

Abscesses and furuncles are collections of purulent material separated from the surrounding tissue. By definition, furuncles involve a hair follicle, whereas abscesses can occur anywhere on the body.

## 11.1. BACKGROUND

- Furuncles occur most often in adolescents and young adults.
- *S aureus* is the most common causative organism.
- Predisposing factors: chronic colonization with *S aureus*, diabetes mellitus, obesity, and certain immunodeficiency syndromes including chronic granulomatous disease.

## 11.2. CLINICAL FEATURES (FIG. 4-9)

- Abscesses present as inflamed, erythematous, and fluctuant collections of pus in a cutaneous site.

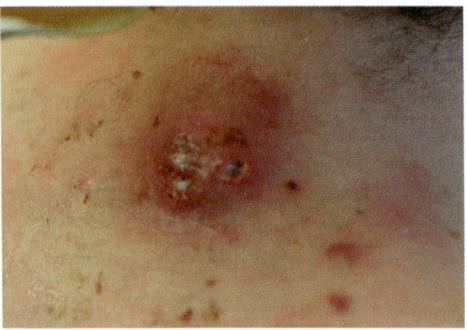

**Figure 4-9.** Abscess. (Courtesy of M. Laurin Council, MD.)

- Furuncles most commonly occur on the face, neck, axillae, buttocks, thighs, and perineum, presenting as firm, painful, erythematous nodules that progressively enlarge.
- Systemic symptoms are typically absent.
- Differential diagnosis
  - Abscesses or furuncles presenting in the axillae and groin may be mistaken for hidradenitis suppurativa.

### 11.3. DIAGNOSIS

- Can often be diagnosed by history and physical examination. Incision and drainage with culture can provide definitive diagnosis and guide antimicrobial therapy.

### 11.4. TREATMENT

- Uncomplicated furuncles may be treated with incision and drainage without additional systemic antimicrobials.
- The decision to administer antimicrobials directed against *S aureus* in addition to incision and drainage should be based on presence of systemic inflammatory response criteria or a history of marked immunosuppression.[14]
- Given the prevalence of MRSA, empiric coverage with doxycycline, trimethoprim-sulfamethoxazole, or clindamycin is appropriate depending on local resistance patterns.
- For recurrent abscesses at sites of previous infection, Gram stain and culture of purulent material may be obtained to guide therapy and consideration given to decolonization with intranasal mupirocin or daily chlorhexidine washes.

## 12. Methicillin-Resistant *Staphylococcus aureus*

### 12.1. BACKGROUND

- MRSA refers to isolates that are resistant to all available beta-lactam antibiotics, including penicillins and cephalosporins.[15]
- First recognized in the early 1960s, MRSA was largely confined to health care facilities; however, since the mid-1990s, it has been increasing in prevalence in the community.[16]
- Skin and soft tissue infections (SSTIs) represent the majority of community-acquired MRSA (CA-MRSA) infections, with furunculosis being the most common manifestation.
- Methicillin resistance is caused by altered penicillin-binding protein (PBP2a) resulting in decreased affinity for beta-lactam antibiotics.

### 12.2. DIAGNOSIS AND TREATMENT

- When an *S aureus* infection is suspected, culture and susceptibility testing should be performed.
- For uncomplicated, nonpurulent cellulitis, empiric treatment for beta-hemolytic streptococci is recommended as the role of CA-MRSA is unknown.
  - Empiric therapy for CA-MRSA is recommended for patients who do not respond to initial treatment or develop systemic toxicity.

- For purulent cellulitis, empiric therapy for CA-MRSA is recommended pending culture results.[17]
- Empiric coverage of CA-MRSA in outpatients with SSTIs includes clindamycin, trimethoprim-sulfamethoxazole, tetracyclines, and linezolid.
- For hospitalized patients with complicated SSTIs, MRSA should be considered pending culture results.
  - Treatment options include intravenous vancomycin, oral or intravenous linezolid, intravenous daptomycin, or intravenous ceftaroline.

## 13. Necrotizing Fasciitis

### 13.1. BACKGROUND

- Necrotizing fasciitis is a severe infection of the subcutaneous tissue that results in rapidly progressive destruction of fat and fascia.
- There are two clinical types, both associated with high mortality, up to 70%.
  - Type I necrotizing fasciitis is a polymicrobial infection with aerobic and anaerobic bacteria.
  - Type II necrotizing fasciitis is due to group A streptococci.

### 13.2. CLINICAL PRESENTATION

- Predisposing factors, type I: diabetes, surgery, trauma, immunosuppression, alcoholism, nonsteroidal anti-inflammatory drugs, peripheral vascular disease, chronic venous insufficiency, decubitus ulcers, Bartholin or vulvovaginal abscesses, and malignancy.[18]
  - Type I infections tend to occur on the lower extremities.
- Predisposing factors, type II: trauma, muscle strain, childbirth, varicella infection, intravenous drug use, and surgery.[18]
- Initially, necrotizing fasciitis may mimic cellulitis, muscle strain, or uncomplicated minor trauma.
- The site of initial bacterial invasion is often minor and is undetectable in 20% of cases.
- Inoculation can occur at the site of minor abrasions, insect bites, splinters, or injection drug sites.
- Pain out of proportion to physical examination findings is characteristic of necrotizing fasciitis. However, physical examination may reveal anesthesia of affected areas due to destruction of superficial nerves.
- Tissue destruction can progress at rates of 1 in per hour.
- Systemic symptoms are common but nonspecific, including fever, chills, malaise, fatigue, myalgias, and anorexia.
- Erythema is the most common cutaneous manifestation, which can progress to a reddish-purple discoloration associated with blisters or bullae.
  - Development of bullae signifies extensive tissue destruction.
  - Lesions can have dusky blue central discoloration, weeping blisters or bullae, and border cellulitis.[19]
  - Subcutaneous tissue may have a wooden feel.
- *Aeromonas hydrophila* infections can occur in patients with trauma and exposure to a water source or rarely in patients who use leeches.
- *Vibrio vulnificus* is a cause of necrotizing fasciitis in patients exposed to warm salt water, typically from the Gulf of Mexico.

- Infection is more likely to occur in immunosuppressed patients. Inoculation can occur via exposure of small abrasions and wounds to contaminated salt water. Puncture wounds from fish, crustaceans, or other sea creatures can also result in infection when they occur in colonized water sources.

### 13.3. EVALUATION

- Necrotizing fasciitis is suggested by history, physical examination, and imaging findings.
- Gas (though not in type II infections) or subcutaneous edema may be seen on computed tomography, magnetic resonance imaging, or ultrasonography.
  - No imaging studies can definitively rule out necrotizing fasciitis. Therefore, when suspicion of the diagnosis is high, surgical exploration should occur. Surgical exploration provides definitive diagnosis.
- Laboratory findings suggestive of necrotizing fasciitis include elevated levels of creatinine, aspartate aminotransferase, creatine phosphokinase, and leukocytosis with a left shift.

### 13.4. TREATMENT

- The mainstay of treatment is surgical débridement.
- Empirically, broad-spectrum antibiotics should be initiated with vancomycin or linezolid plus piperacillin-tazobactam or a carbapenem, or plus ceftriaxone and metronidazole.[14]
  - Antibiotic treatment should be directed toward pathogens cultured intraoperatively.
  - Mixed infections should be treated with broad-spectrum antibiotics, as previously mentioned.
- In confirmed cases of group A streptococcal or *Clostridium* infections, penicillin plus clindamycin is the treatment of choice.[14]
  - For staphylococcal infections, vancomycin should be used in the presence of methicillin resistance, while nafcillin, oxacillin, cefazolin, and clindamycin are all reasonable in its absence.[14]
  - *A hydrophila* infections are best treated with doxycycline plus ciprofloxacin or ceftriaxone.[14]
  - *V vulnificus* infection is best treated with doxycycline plus ceftriaxone or cefotaxime.[14]
- Family members and close contacts of patients with group A streptococcal infections should be considered for prophylactic administration of penicillin (or other agent to which the index organism is susceptible) to prevent a serious infection as their risk is increased 50-fold compared to the general population.[20]
- Supportive care with intravenous fluids is often required due to copious fluid losses from wound sites. In severe or refractory cases of group A streptococcal infection, intravenous immunoglobulin may be of benefit.[21]

## 14. Scabies

### 14.1. BACKGROUND

- Scabies is caused by the mite *Sarcoptes scabiei* var. *hominis* and has a worldwide distribution.

- The entire life cycle of the host-specific mite is completed in the epidermis.
- Transmission occurs via direct contact with an infested person and less frequently by sexual contact or fomites.
- The number of mites living on an affected person is typically less than 15; however, individuals with crusted scabies may have thousands of mites on the skin surface.

## 14.2. CLINICAL FEATURES

- The incubation period between exposure and symptom onset can range from days to months, with the immune system taking 2 to 6 weeks to become sensitized to the mite during a first infestation.
- Pruritus can develop before the onset of skin findings and can be severe.
- Skin findings consist of small erythematous papules symmetrically distributed and typically involve the web spaces of the hands, flexural aspects of the wrists, axillae, waist, ankles, feet, and buttocks.
  - Infants, older adults, and immunocompromised patients may have involvement of the scalp and face.
- The pathognomonic sign is the burrow, representing the tunnel through which the female mite traveled while laying eggs.
- Crusted scabies is found in patients with compromised immune systems, including the older adults, HIV-positive or transplant recipients, and those with decreased sensory functions. Infestation in this population can exceed one thousand mites on the skin surface and presents with marked acral hyperkeratosis.
- Differential diagnosis: atopic dermatitis, arthropod bites, and allergic contact dermatitis.

## 14.3. DIAGNOSIS

- Diagnosis is confirmed by light microscopy examination of skin scrapings from infested areas. Visualization of adult mites, eggs, or fecal pellets confirms diagnosis (Fig. 4-10).

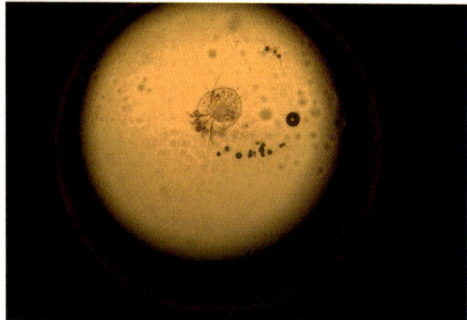

**Figure 4-10.** Scabies mite under light microscopy. (Courtesy of Rabia Mayer, MD, PhD.)

### 14.4. TREATMENT

- Two topical treatments, 1 week apart, with permethrin 5% cream is recommended. The topical agent is applied to entire body surface, excluding the face, and left on overnight.
  - At the time of treatment, all clothing and linens should be washed in hot water or stored in a sealed bag for 10 days.
- Skin lesions and pruritus may persist for 2 to 4 weeks or longer after successful treatment, referred to as "postscabetic" dermatitis.

## 15. Lice (Pediculosis)

### 15.1. BACKGROUND

- Body lice—aka pediculosis corporis
  - Pediculosis corporis is caused by *Pediculus humanus* var. *corporis*.
  - Important human diseases are transmitted via the body louse including *Rickettsia prowazekii*, responsible for endemic typhus; *Borrelia* species, responsible for relapsing fever; and *Bartonella* species, the causative agent for trench fever, bacillary angiomatosis, and endocarditis.
  - Transmission of organisms occurs when lice fecal pellets cross the skin barrier due to excoriations.
- Head lice—aka pediculosis capitis
  - Pediculosis capitis is caused by the head louse, *Pediculus capitis*, an obligate human parasite that lives only on the hairs of the scalp.
  - Head lice have a worldwide distribution. Children aged 3 to 11 years have the highest incidence. Infestation is more frequently seen in girls.
  - Transmission is via direct head-to-head contact or contact with fomites such as brushes and hair accessories.
  - The nits (eggs) are cemented to hair shafts.
  - Females may live up to 30 days, taking blood meals every 4 to 6 hours.

### 15.2. CLINICAL FEATURES

- Body lice
  - Body lice primarily reside on the clothing of their host, rather than the skin.
  - Infestation results in severe pruritus with the most commonly affected areas being the back, neck, shoulders, and waist.
  - Skin lesions present as erythematous macules or papules, crusts, or excoriations.
- Head lice
  - During a first infestation, symptoms may not appear until 2 to 6 weeks after exposure as an immunologic response must develop to lice saliva and excreta.
  - Pruritus then develops and excoriations, erythema, and scaliness are common findings, limited in distribution to the scalp and neck.
  - In repeat infestations, symptoms appear within the first 24 to 48 hours after exposure.

### 15.3. DIAGNOSIS

- Diagnosis is made by direct visualization of the louse or eggs.
  - Inspection of clothing and especially clothing seams is required for diagnosis of body lice.
  - For head lice, diagnosis is made by visual identification of lice or eggs on scalp hair.

## 15.4. TREATMENT

- Body lice
  - First-line treatment is eliminating clothing and bedding of infested persons in tightly sealed bags. If this is not possible, topical treatment with permethrin 5% cream and fumigating or laundering clothes in hot water is recommended.
- Head lice
  - Topical treatments include permethrin 1% rinse or lotion or permethrin 5% cream; however, resistance is common. No resistance in the United States has been found against malathion 0.5% lotion or gel, and this remains a good option. Oral ivermectin and ivermectin lotion are alternative therapeutic options. With all topical preparations, two applications performed 1 week apart are advised.

# 16. Syphilis

## 16.1. BACKGROUND

- Syphilis is a sexually transmitted infection caused by *Treponema pallidum* subspecies *pallidum* and is associated with various dermatologic manifestations depending on the stage of disease.
- Globally, syphilis is a leading cause of ulcerative genital disease, particularly in low-income countries.
- In the United States, syphilis is a male-predominant disease due to its high incidence in men who have sex with men.

## 16.2. CLINICAL PRESENTATION

- Incubation period varies inversely with inoculum size (10-90 days), but on average, primary lesions appear 21 days after exposure.[18]
  - Three to ten weeks after the appearance of the primary painless chancre, hematogenous dissemination of bacteria results in secondary syphilis.
  - Untreated, the lesions of secondary syphilis will spontaneously disappear in 3 to 12 weeks.
  - Approximately 25% of patients will have a recurrence of secondary syphilis in the absence of treatment, 90% of which occur in the first year.[22]
  - Patients then enter the latent stage of syphilis. Over a period of years, patients have either spontaneous cure or progression to tertiary syphilis.
- Syphilis can be transmitted during the primary and secondary stages via direct contact with infective tissue.
- Syphilis facilitates the transmission of HIV.[23-25]
- Primary syphilis (Fig. 4-11A)
  - The initial lesion of primary syphilis can be papular but quickly ulcerates to form the characteristic chancre with a clean base and raised edges.
    - Chancres occur at the site of inoculation, typically sites of intimate contact including the genitals and oropharynx, though they can occur at any site on the skin or mucous membranes.
    - Lesions are typically nontender.
    - Regional lymph nodes may be enlarged.
    - Chancres heal spontaneously over a period of weeks but can leave a scar.
  - Differential diagnosis: other ulcerative genital diseases, including genital herpes, HIV, trauma, aphthous ulcers, malignancy, fixed drug eruption, primary

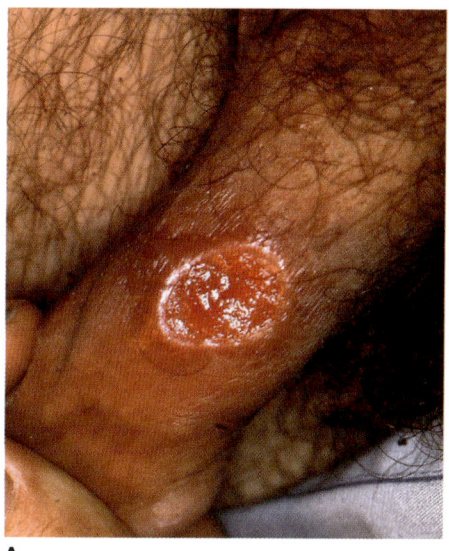

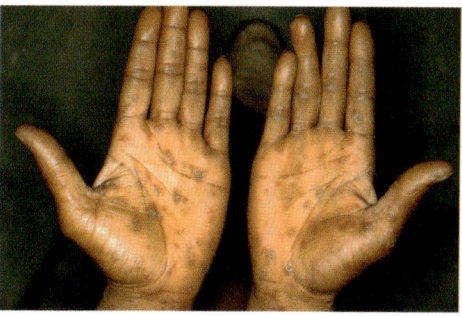

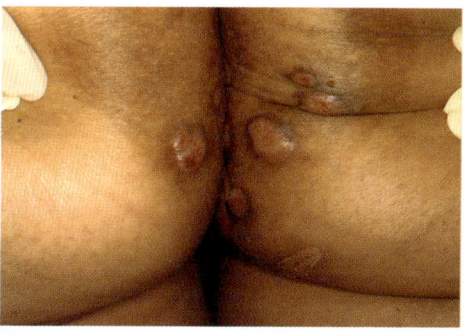

**Figure 4-11.** Syphilis. **A.** Primary chancre. **B.** Secondary syphilis. **C.** Condyloma lata. (Courtesy of Arthur Eisen, MD.)

Epstein-Barr virus, and Behçet disease. In patients with the right exposure and travel history, chancroid, lymphogranuloma venereum, and donovanosis.
- Secondary syphilis (Fig. 4-11B)
  - Secondary syphilis is typically the first symptomatic phase of syphilis infection.
    - Systemic symptoms can include fevers, myalgias and joint pains, malaise, sore throat, and headaches.
    - Rash typically appears about 8 weeks after infection. The rash can be diverse in appearance, usually beginning on the upper trunk, palms and soles, and flexural surfaces of the extremities. Initial lesions are macular but can progress to papules by 3 months.
    - Generalized lymphadenopathy can occur, as opposed to the regional lymphadenopathy of primary syphilis.
  - The most common presentation (~80%) is a nonpruritic papulosquamous eruption. Lesions can range from 1 to 20 mm with color variability from pink to violaceous to red-brown.
    - Differential diagnosis: pityriasis rosea, guttate psoriasis, viral exanthems, lichen planus, pityriasis lichenoides chronica, primary HIV, drug eruption, nummular eczema, and folliculitis[26]
  - Mucosal lesions can vary from aphthous appearance to gray plaques.
    - Differential diagnosis of mucosal lesions: lichen planus; chronic aphthae; hand, foot, and mouth disease; herpangina; and perleche[26]
  - Condyloma lata occur in anogenital regions (Fig. 4-11C).
    - Differential diagnosis: HPV, bowenoid papulosis, condyloma acuminata, and squamous cell carcinoma[26]
  - Some less common manifestations include annular plaques with central hyperpigmentation, granulomatous nodules, necrotic lesions with scale crust, and necrotic, ulcerated, and crusted lesions with constitutional symptoms ("malignant" syphilis).[26] Patchy alopecia results from toxic telogen effluvium.
- Latent syphilis
  - Patients are by definition asymptomatic during the latent stage.
  - Latent syphilis occurs after spontaneous resolution of secondary syphilis.
    - Early latent syphilis is defined as the year following the onset of latency.
    - If time of latency cannot be determined and neurosyphilis is not present, patients are considered to be in the late latent stage.
    - Diagnosis is often incidental by serologic testing.
- Tertiary syphilis
  - In those who progress to tertiary syphilis, about half will develop gummas in various organs (skin, bones, liver, heart, testis, brain, respiratory tract, and others).
    - When present in the skin, gummas are erythematous, nodular, or noduloulcerative plaques, frequently with an arciform pattern.
    - Differential diagnosis: lupus vulgaris, chromoblastomycosis, endemic mycoses, leishmaniasis, systemic lupus erythematosus, mycosis fungoides, sarcoidosis, and benign and malignant tumors.[26]
  - The complications of tertiary syphilis are cardiovascular and neurologic, including aortic aneurysms, tabes dorsalis, general paresis (formerly generalized paresis of the insane), and a form of dementia.
- Congenital syphilis
  - Maternal-fetal transmission can occur via the transplacental route or via infective birth canal.
  - Perhaps, one of the most important reasons to recognize syphilis in adults is to prevent its transmission to a fetus because of the severe consequences.

- When transmitted via transplacental route, there is an approximately 10% risk of spontaneous abortion, 10% risk of stillbirth, and 20% risk of infant death.[26]
  ○ Twenty percent of children develop congenital syphilis, with its own set of severe consequences.
    - Early congenital syphilis has wide-ranging manifestations including marasmic syphilis, a rash similar in appearance to secondary syphilis, bloody or purulent mucinous nasal discharge ("snuffles"), perioral and perianal fissures, lymphadenopathy, hepatosplenomegaly, osteochondritis, anemia, thrombocytopenia, pneumonitis, hepatitis, nephropathy, and neurosyphilis.[26]
    - Rash tends to be more bullous and erosive as compared to adults.
    - Late congenital syphilis is the equivalent of tertiary syphilis in adults.
    - Hutchinson triad is a combination of interstitial keratitis, neural deafness, and Hutchinson teeth.

### 16.3. EVALUATION

- In general, in patients with a high index of suspicion for syphilis, a single negative darkfield microscopy examination does not rule out syphilis. Darkfield microscopy is used for diagnosis of primary or secondary syphilis.
  ○ If microscopy is negative and suspicion is still high, repeat specimen collection and darkfield microscopy should be performed, in addition to serologic testing.
  ○ Positive serologic testing should be confirmed with treponemal tests. Treponemal tests include TPHA, MHA-TP, TPPA, FTA-ABS, SPHA, and FTA-ABS-19S-IgM (for congenital syphilis). Antibody titers correlate with disease activity.
    - Treponemal tests can confirm reactive nontreponemal tests but generally remain positive for life (except in very early treated syphilis) and therefore are not useful in monitoring treatment response.
    - Treponemal tests do not differentiate from other treponemes or spirochetes.
    - Sensitivity of treponemal tests varies based on the stage: 70% to 100% in primary, 100% in secondary and latent, and 95% in late.[27]
      □ In patients with high pretest probability for syphilis, but negative serologic tests, the prozone phenomenon must be kept in mind (falsely negative serologic testing that occurs in the presence of high antibody titers).
  ○ All patients who present with ocular or neurologic symptoms should have a lumbar puncture performed to rule out central nervous system involvement, as this changes treatment.
- Latent syphilis
  ○ Diagnosis is established by positive serologic titers.
  ○ Treatment response is assessed by monitoring titers of RPR or VDRL. Titers should decline fourfold or greater in 12 to 24 months to be considered successful treatment. In the absence of a fourfold decline, treatment is considered a failure and examination of the cerebrospinal fluid should be performed.
- Tertiary syphilis
  ○ Diagnosis is made with positive serologic tests.
  ○ All patients suspected of having tertiary syphilis require a lumbar puncture to guide treatment.
- Congenital syphilis
  ○ Diagnosis is by PCR, serologic titers that are at least fourfold higher than the mother's titers, or FTA-ABS-19S-IgM testing.
- All patients diagnosed with syphilis should be tested for HIV infection.

## 16.4. TREATMENT

- Primary, secondary, and early latent syphilis
  - Adults: Benzathine penicillin G 2.4 million units IM as a single dose.
  - Children ≥1 month of age: Benzathine penicillin G 50,000 units/kg IM, up to the adult dose of 2.4 million units in a single dose.
  - In penicillin-allergic adults, doxycycline 100 mg orally twice daily for 14 days is likely the best alternative.
    - Pregnant patients with penicillin allergies should be desensitized and treated with penicillin.[28]
- Late latent syphilis
  - Adults: Benzathine penicillin G 2.4 million units IM as three doses administered at 1-week intervals.
  - Children ≥1 month of age: Benzathine penicillin G 50,000 units/kg IM, up to the adult dose of 2.4 million units, administered as three doses at 1-week intervals
  - In penicillin-allergic adults, doxycycline 100 mg orally twice daily for 28 days is likely the best alternative.
    - Pregnant patients with penicillin allergies should be desensitized and treated with penicillin.[28]
- Tertiary syphilis (gummatous and cardiovascular)
  - Adults: Benzathine penicillin G 2.4 million units IM as three doses administered at 1-week intervals.
  - Pregnant patients with penicillin allergies should be desensitized and treated with penicillin.[28]
- Neurosyphilis
  - Adults: Aqueous crystalline penicillin G 18 to 24 million units per day, administered as 3 to 4 million units IV every 4 hours or continuous infusion, for 10 to 14 days.
  - In penicillin-allergic patients, desensitization should be considered. Ceftriaxone 2 g IM or IV for 10 to 14 days is an alternative regimen based on limited data.[28]
- Congenital syphilis
  - Neonate with proven or highly probable disease or born to mother with untreated early syphilis
    - Preferred treatment: Aqueous crystalline penicillin G 100,000 to 150,000 units/kg/d, administered as 50,000 units/kg/dose IV every 12 hours during the first 7 days of life and every 8 hours thereafter for a total of 10 days
    - Alternative treatment: Procaine penicillin G 50,000 units/kg/dose IM in a single daily dose for 10 days[28]
  - Neonate with no signs of disease born to mother with treated syphilis
    - Benzathine penicillin G 50,000 units/kg/dose IM in a single dose[28]

# 17. Tuberculosis

## 17.1. BACKGROUND

- Tuberculosis (TB) affects approximately a third of the world population, predominating in developing countries with high rates of poverty and malnutrition.
- Similarly to syphilis, the manifestations of TB are protean. Cutaneous manifestations of TB occur in only 1% to 4% of patients.[29]

## 17.2. CLINICAL PRESENTATION

- Cutaneous manifestations of TB occur via exogenous inoculation, endogenous spread, and hematogenous dissemination and due to hypersensitivity to the tubercle bacilli.
- Exogenous inoculation
  - Cutaneous TB can occur by exogenous inoculation. In developing countries, this typically occurs through open wounds on bare feet over grounds covered with tuberculous sputum.[30] This results in TB verrucosa cutis, a warty lesion that is typically asymptomatic. Before verrucous evolution, lesions progress through a stage of erythematous papules with a surrounding purple inflammatory halo. Differential diagnosis: warts, chromomycosis, syphilis, and hypertrophic lichen planus.[26]
  - Tuberculous chancre can also occur via exogenous inoculation, typically via trauma in previously nonsensitized patients. Lesions are reddish-brown nodules that develop into painless ulcers. Tissue culture is the main method of diagnosis. Differential diagnosis: sporotrichosis, endemic mycoses, cat scratch disease, nocardiosis, tularemia, and syphilis[26] (Fig. 4-12).
- Endogenous spread
  - Scrofuloderma results from contiguous involvement of the skin from underlying tissues such as lymph nodes, joints, or bones. Lesions initially are ulcerated purple plaques with a purulent exudate, progressing to disfiguring scars when healed. Concurrent pulmonary TB is common.[31] The face and neck are the most frequently affected. Diagnosis is made with biopsy showing caseating granulomas in the lower dermis, acid-fast bacilli, and TB on culture. Differential diagnosis: bacterial abscesses, malignancy, endemic mycoses, hidradenitis suppurativa, acne conglobata and, when the inguinal lymph nodes are involved, sexually transmitted infections such as lymphogranuloma venereum.
  - Lupus vulgaris occurs more frequently in women than men. Classically, lupus vulgaris appears as head and neck–predominant, well-demarcated, reddish-brown plaques that can reach over 10 cm. Lesions can be seen on the legs and buttocks, more commonly in tropical countries.[32] As plaques enlarge peripherally, there can be central discoloration and atrophy. Diascopy of the lesions in patients with light-toned skin reveals classic "apple jelly" quality, common to other granulomatous processes such as sarcoidosis. Biopsy reveals caseating granulomas

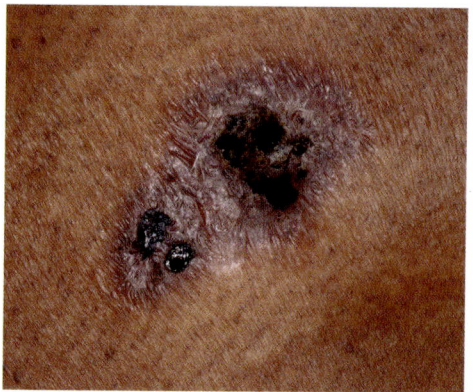

**Figure 4-12.** Cutaneous tuberculosis. (Courtesy of Arthur Eisen, MD.)

in the upper dermis. Differential diagnosis: sarcoidosis, discoid lupus, endemic mycoses, syphilis, and leishmaniasis.
- Hematogenous dissemination
  - Tuberculous gummas are the result of hematogenous dissemination and typically occur on the trunk and extremities of malnourished children and immunocompromised adults. Culture is often negative, and therefore, diagnosis is made when clinical suspicion is high, and there is a response to anti-TB therapy. Differential diagnosis: other forms of bacterial abscesses.
  - In patients with miliary TB, a sporotrichoid pattern can occur. Differential diagnosis: sporotrichosis, *Mycobacterium marinum* infection, leishmaniasis, nocardiosis, and less frequently endemic mycoses.[33]
  - The dermatologic manifestation of miliary TB is known as TB cutis miliaris disseminata.[34] Miliary TB can result in sheets of white-topped papules. Alternatively, bluish papules can be present that progress through vesiculopustules, necrosis, and ulceration.[18] Patients have severe systemic symptoms. Differential diagnosis: varicella, pityriasis lichenoides et varioliformis acuta, rickettsial pox, and enteroviral exanthems.[26]
  - Orificial TB occurs in patients with impaired cell-mediated immunity and results in painful, yellow papules on the mucosal surfaces, typically oral, nasal, anal, or vaginal. Orificial TB is a marker of severe visceral TB disease. Differential diagnosis: herpes simplex, aphthous stomatitis, pemphigus, and histoplasmosis.[26]
  - Lupus vulgaris can also occur via hematogenous dissemination.
- Hypersensitivity reactions
  - A variety of cutaneous manifestations of TB occur as a result of hypersensitivity reactions to the bacillus; these are referred to as the tuberculids. The tuberculids typically result from chronic hematogenous dissemination of the bacillus in patients with moderate to high levels of immunity. The forms include erythema induratum of Bazin (EIB), lichen scrofulosorum, papulonecrotic tuberculid, and nodular tuberculid.[29]
  - EIB predominates on the lower extremities in the form of multiple painful, indurated nodules. These nodules can ulcerate with chronicity. EIB tends to appear on the posterior surfaces of the legs and can occur in flares every 3 to 4 months.[35] Diagnosis of TB in patients with EIB is often difficult. EIB is not well understood and may also occur in infections with nontuberculous mycobacteria. Differential diagnosis: erythema nodosum. EIB differs from erythema nodosum on pathology as it is a lobular panniculitis with vasculitis, whereas erythema nodosum is a septal panniculitis without vasculitis.
  - Lichen scrofulosorum is rare and occurs mostly in children. Lesions are 1- to 2-mm skin-colored papules found on the trunk that are otherwise asymptomatic. Cultures for TB are negative, but noncaseating perifollicular granulomas can be seen in the papillary dermis.[29]
  - Nodular tuberculid appears as blue or dusky-red nodules on the shins. Histology demonstrates granulomatous inflammation at the subcutaneous fat/lower dermis junction.[36,37]
  - Papulonecrotic tuberculid presents as a symmetric eruption of dusky-red papules on the extensor surfaces of the limbs. Though typically asymptomatic, papules can progress to ulcers and scarring.[31] Lesions frequently recur without TB treatment.
  - All forms of tuberculid respond quickly to antituberculous therapy.
  - TB can manifest with erythema nodosum, particularly in young females. The differential diagnosis for erythema nodosum is broad but includes streptococcal infection, sarcoidosis, endemic mycoses, and irritable bowel disease.

### 17.3. EVALUATION

- TB is suggested by history, physical examination, and imaging findings.
- In addition to the use of tuberculin skin tests, *Mycobacterium tuberculosis* infection can be diagnosed with interferon gamma (IFN-γ) release assays (eg, QuantiFERON TB Gold, T-SPOT). In general, the IFN-γ release assays have greater specificity and similar sensitivity compared to tuberculin skin tests.
- TB can cause a false positive on RPR testing.
- Dermal biopsy can demonstrate acid-fast bacilli or caseating granulomas, but not universally.
- PCR is becoming more widely available but is still not sensitive enough to preclude diagnosis of cutaneous TB when there is high suspicion.
- Definitive diagnosis sometimes cannot be achieved. When clinical suspicion is high, response to antituberculous treatment can confirm the diagnosis.

### 17.4. TREATMENT

- The mainstay of treatment is four-drug RIPE therapy (rifampin, isoniazid, pyrazinamide, ethambutol) for 8 weeks followed by two drug therapy (based on sensitivities), typically isoniazid and rifampin, for 6 to 9 months in most cases.
- Bone or joint involvement requires 9 to 12 months of treatment.
- In cases of drug resistance, treatment should be tailored to the resistance pattern of the organism. Consultation with an infectious diseases specialist is advised.
- All patients with a diagnosis of TB should be reported to the state health department as they require directly observed therapy.
- Treatment of patients with multidrug-resistant TB or those who are coinfected with HIV should be left to experts in those areas.

## Tick-Borne Illnesses

- Ticks are second only to mosquitoes as vectors of bacterial, viral, and protozoal diseases.
- In the United States, a number of tick-borne illnesses are recognized including Lyme disease, Rocky Mountain spotted fever (RMSF), human monocytic ehrlichiosis, and babesiosis. Ticks may also bite without transmitting disease.

## 18. Lyme Disease

### 18.1. BACKGROUND

- Lyme disease is the most commonly reported vector-borne disease in the United States. The number of reported cases have increased from 10,000 in 1992 to 30,000 currently, with the true number of annual cases estimated to be as high as 300,000.[38]
- Multisystem disease caused by *Borrelia* species of spirochetes, a gram-negative organism transmitted by the *Ixodes* tick.
- *Borrelia burgdorferi* is the predominant etiologic organism in the United States with white-footed mice and white-tailed deer being the natural hosts.[39]
- Factors associated with transmission of *B burgdorferi* from ticks to humans: duration of tick feeding and geographic proportion of infected ticks. The rate of

transmission of microbe to human via tick saliva is low in the first 24 hours of attachment and increases dramatically after 48 hours.[40]
- The species of *Ixodes* tick vector varies by geographical location with *Ixodes scapularis* (also known as *Ixodes dammini*) predominant in the Eastern United States and Great Lakes region and *Ixodes pacificus* in the Western United States. In the Northeast and Midwest United States, approximately 10% to 20% of nymphal stage *I scapularis* and 30% to 40% of adult ticks are infested with *B burgdorferi*.[38]
- The incidence of Lyme disease parallels the emergence of the *Ixodes* tick, with most cases reported between May and November.

## 18.2. CLINICAL FEATURES

- Lyme disease has been classically divided into three stages of disease: early localized disease, early disseminated disease, and chronic disease.
- The most common manifestation of early localized diseases is erythema migrans that develops at the site of the tick bite within 4 to 20 days (Fig. 4-13).
  - The lesion begins as an erythematous macule and gradually expands over the course of days to weeks, and while the most common description is a targetoid

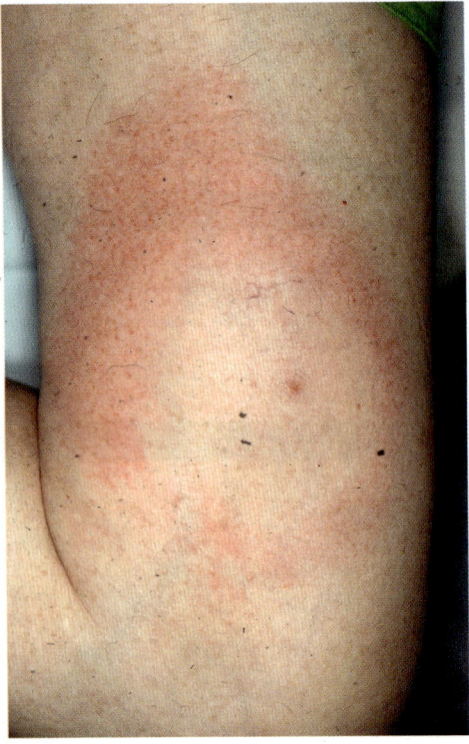

**Figure 4-13.** Lyme disease. (Courtesy of Arthur Eisen, MD.)

lesion, in approximately two-thirds of patients, the lesions either are uniformly erythematous or have enhanced central erythema.[40,41]
  - Lesions of erythema migrans favor the trunk, axilla, groin, and popliteal fossa and are seen in approximately 60% to 90% of diagnosed individuals.
- Systemic manifestations of the initial stage include flulike illness, fatigue, headache, and malaise.
- In approximately 20% of patients, erythema migrans will be the only manifestation of Lyme disease even if left untreated.
- Within the first few weeks, spirochetes disseminate hematogenously to other tissues. Secondary annular lesions develop at distant sites. This stage can also be associated with Lyme neuroborreliosis presenting as meningoradiculitis or meningitis and carditis presenting as atrioventricular conduction disturbances or rarely myocarditis or pancarditis.[42]
- Late manifestations of untreated infection include arthritis, encephalopathy, peripheral neuropathy, and encephalomyelitis.[43]

## 18.3. DIAGNOSIS

- There are no standardized diagnostic criteria for Lyme disease.
- The diagnostic gold standard is the isolation of *Borrelia* by culture with subsequent PCR-based or other confirmation of its identity. Culture is expensive and requires special media and laboratory techniques, and results require several weeks. Therefore, culture is not useful for clinical decision making.
- PCR from tissue or fluid specimens can be used to confirm infection but is generally performed only for research purposes.
- For serologic testing, the CDC recommends a two-tier approach consisting of a sensitivity enzyme immunoassay (usually ELISA), followed by immunoblotting for positive or indeterminate tests.
  - In patients with erythema migrans, serologic testing is often of little use due to poor sensitivity, with only 29% of patients with a positive IgM or IgG antibody response.[44] Of patients tested during the acute erythema migrans (EM) phase, those with evidence of disseminated disease had a higher percentage test positive for an antibody response versus those without dissemination (43% vs 17%).[44]
  - Serologic testing is most sensitive in patients with early disseminated disease with neurologic or cardiac manifestations or in those with late manifestations including arthritis (nearly 100%). Serologic tests should not be used to screen patients with nonspecific symptoms and a low probability of infection due to the poor positive predictive value.[45]
- More recently, an enzyme-linked immunoassay that detects antibodies against the C6 peptide of the variable major proteinlike sequence expressed lipoprotein has been introduced. As a single test, it is less specific than the traditional two-test approach.[46]

## 18.4. DIFFERENTIAL DIAGNOSIS

- Southern tick–associated rash illness (STARI) is a Lyme-like illness, transmitted by the lone star tick, and causes skin lesions indistinguishable from erythema migrans. Other entities that can be confused with EM include tinea, nummular eczema, granuloma annulare, contact dermatitis, fixed drug eruption, and erythema multiforme.

## 18.5. TREATMENT

- Cure rates exceed 90% when early-stage disease is treated with appropriate antibiotics. The Infectious Diseases Society of America provides treatment recommendations based upon where in the spectrum of disease activity patients fall and should be consulted prior to initiating treatment. Patients with early-stage disease with erythema migrans can be treated with doxycycline or amoxicillin for 14 days in the absence of neurologic or cardiac manifestations.
- Areas of uncertainty
  - In a minority of patients who receive appropriate antibiotics for Lyme disease and have resolution of objective signs of infection, subjective symptoms persist. These patients are classified as having post–Lyme disease symptoms if they persist for less than 6 months and as post–Lyme disease syndrome if they persist for more than 6 months.[43] The etiology of this syndrome is unknown. Randomized, placebo-controlled trial of prolonged antibiotic therapy for patients with persistent subjective symptoms after appropriate initial treatment for Lyme disease has shown minimal or no benefit and increased risk of adverse effects.[45,47] As such, prolonged antibiotics for subjective symptoms are not recommended in patients whose objective signs of Lyme disease have resolved.

# 19. Southern Tick–Associated Rash Illness

## 19.1. BACKGROUND

- A Lyme disease–like illness observed since the mid-1980s with a rash indistinguishable from the rash of early Lyme disease.[48]
- This Lyme-like disease has been described in the Southeastern United States in association with *Amblyomma americanum*, or the Lone Star tick; however, the exact etiologic organism remains uncertain.

## 19.2. CLINICAL FEATURES

- Erythema migrans–like lesions due to STARI versus those due to *B burgdorferi* infection have many clinical differences:
  - STARI skin lesions tend to be smaller, more circular, with greater likelihood of central clearing and less commonly seen in multiples.[49]
  - Less likely to have regional lymphadenopathy and tender or pruritic rashes.
  - Fewer symptoms at the time of rash onset.
- As the etiology remains uncertain with no definitive tests available, the clinical sequelae have not been definitively established.
- It is likely that the arthritis associated with STARI is less severe than that seen with Lyme disease.

## 19.3. DIAGNOSIS

- Diagnosis must be made on clinical evidence.
- Patients with STARI do not seroconvert with serologic testing for Lyme disease.

### 19.4. TREATMENT

- Treatment of STARI is similar to treatment of early Lyme disease, with doxycycline 100 mg orally twice daily.

## 20. Rocky Mountain Spotted Fever

### 20.1. BACKGROUND

- *Rickettsia rickettsii* is the etiologic agent of RMSF.
- Rickettsiae are small, obligately intracellular, gram-negative bacteria.
- Epidemiologically important vectors of *R rickettsii* in North America and Central America include the Rocky Mountain wood tick (*Dermacentor andersoni*), the American dog tick (*Dermacentor variabilis*), the Cayenne tick (*Amblyomma cajennense*), and the brown dog tick (*Rhipicephalus sanguineus*).[50]
- In the United States, RMSF still occurs predominantly in the Midwestern and Southeastern states including Oklahoma, Missouri, Arkansas, Tennessee, and North Carolina.

### 20.2. CLINICAL FEATURES

- Abrupt onset of high fever often accompanied by headache, nausea, vomiting, anorexia, and malaise.
- A rash begins on the 2nd to 4th day following appearance of fever. Only rarely is an eschar identified at the infection site (Fig. 4-14A and B).
  - Rash appears as small pink macules, typically on wrists, ankles, and forearms. Evolves into maculopapules.
  - Lesions evolve into petechiae or purpura in 50% to 60% of patients.
- Severe manifestations may include pulmonary edema, cerebral edema, myocarditis, renal failure, disseminated intravascular coagulopathy, and gangrene.
- Cutaneous findings are absent in 10% to 15% of patients.

### 20.3. DIAGNOSIS

- Diagnosis is based on clinical and epidemiologic criteria such as signs, symptoms, and exposure history.
- Empiric treatment is given based on clinical suspicion rather than waiting for confirmatory test results.
- Serologic diagnosis is usually retrospective because antibodies do not develop until at least day 7 of illness.
- Rickettsiae can be identified by immunofluorescence or immunohistochemistry in a biopsy specimen of a maculopapular lesion.

### 20.4. TREATMENT

- Drug of choice is doxycycline. Chloramphenicol is a less effective alternative, having a higher rate of fatal outcomes.
  - Chloramphenicol is recommended for treatment of RMSF during pregnancy.
  - Despite currently available effective treatment and advances in medical care, an estimated 5% to 10% of U.S. patients die.

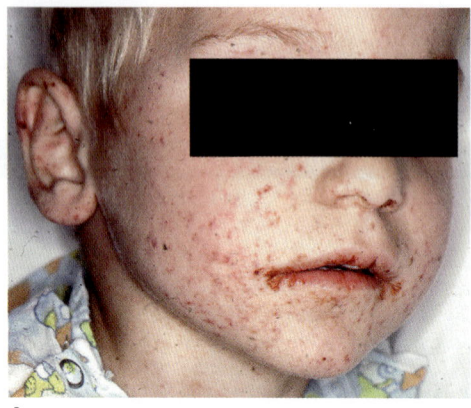

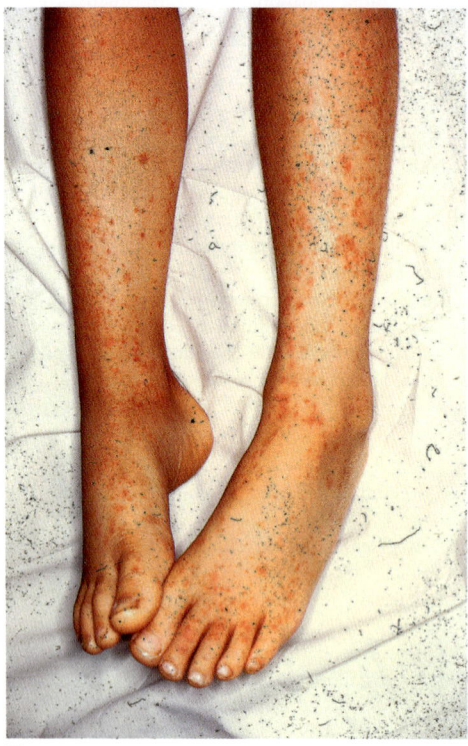

Figure 4-14. **A, B.** Rocky Mountain spotted fever. (Courtesy of Arthur Eisen, MD.)

# REFERENCES

1. Howley PM, Douglas RL. Papillomaviruses. In: Knipe DM, Howley PM, eds. *Fields Virology*. 5th ed. Lippincott Williams & Wilkins; 2001:2299-2354.
2. Rubben A, Kalka K, Spelten B, Grussendorf-Conen EI. Clinical features and age distribution of patients with HPV 2/27/57-induced common warts. *Arch Dermatol Res*. 1997;289(6):337-340.
3. Rinaldi MG. Dermatophytosis: epidemiological and microbiological update. *J Am Acad Dermatol*. 2000;43(5 suppl):S120-S124.
4. Abdel-Rahman SM, Farrand N, Schuenemann E, et al. The prevalence of infections with *Trichophyton tonsurans* in schoolchildren: the CAPITIS study. *Pediatrics*. 2010;125(5):966-973.
5. Masri-Fridling GD. Dermatophytosis of the feet. *Dermatol Clin*. 1996;14(1):33-40.
6. Miller MA, Hodgson Y. Sensitivity and specificity of potassium hydroxide smears of skin scrapings for the diagnosis of tinea pedis. *Arch Dermatol*. 1993;129(4):510-511.
7. Gupta R, Warren T, Wald A. Genital herpes. *Lancet*. 2007;370(9605):2127-2137.
8. Xu F, Sternberg MR, Kottiri BJ, et al. Trends in herpes simplex virus type 1 and type 2 seroprevalence in the United States. *JAMA*. 2006;296(8):964-973.
9. Roberts CM, Pfister JR, Spear SJ. Increasing proportion of herpes simplex virus type 1 as a cause of genital herpes infection in college students. *Sex Transm Dis*. 2003;30(10):797-800.
10. Freeman EE, Weiss HA, Glynn JR, Cross PL, Whitworth JA, Hayes RJ. Herpes simplex virus 2 infection increases HIV acquisition in men and women: systematic review and meta-analysis of longitudinal studies. *AIDS (London, England)*. 2006;20(1):73-83.
11. Corey L, Wald A, Patel R, et al. Once-daily valacyclovir to reduce the risk of transmission of genital herpes. *N Engl J Med*. 2004;350(1):11-20.
12. Hope-Simpson RE. The nature of herpes zoster: a long-term study and a new hypothesis. *Proc R Soc Med*. 1965;58:9-20.
13. Brown GR. Herpes zoster: correlation of age, sex, distribution, neuralgia, and associated disorders. *South Med J*. 1976;69(5):576-578.
14. Stevens DL, Bisno AL, Chambers HF, et al. Practice guidelines for the diagnosis and management of skin and soft tissue infections: 2014 update by the Infectious Diseases Society of America. *Clin Infect Dis*. 2014;59(2):e10-e52.
15. Crawford SE, Boyle-Vavra S, Daum RS. Community associated methicillin-resistant *Staphylococcus aureus*. In: Hooper D, Scheld M, eds. *Emerging Infections*. Vol. 7. ASM Press; 2007:153-179.
16. Herold BC, Immergluck LC, Maranan MC, et al. Community-acquired methicillin-resistant *Staphylococcus aureus* in children with no identified predisposing risk. *JAMA*. 1998;279(8):593-598.
17. Liu C, Bayer A, Cosgrove SE, et al. Clinical practice guidelines by the Infectious Diseases Society of America for the treatment of methicillin-resistant *Staphylococcus aureus* infections in adults and children: executive summary. *Clin Infect Dis*. 2011;52(3):285-292.
18. Cohen J, Opal SM, Powderly WG, eds. *Cohen & Powderly: Infectious Diseases*. 3rd ed. Elsevier Limited; 2010.
19. Andreasen TJ, Green SD, Childers BJ. Massive infectious soft-tissue injury: diagnosis and management of necrotizing fasciitis and purpura fulminans. *Plast Reconstr Surg*. 2001;107(4):1025-1035.
20. Prevention of Invasive Group A Streptococcal Infections Workshop Participants. Prevention of invasive group A streptococcal disease among household contacts of case patients and among postpartum and postsurgical patients: recommendations from the Centers for Disease Control and Prevention. *Clin Infect Dis*. 2002;35(8):950-959.
21. Linner A, Darenberg J, Sjolin J, Henriques-Normark B, Norrby-Teglund A. Clinical efficacy of polyspecific intravenous immunoglobulin therapy in patients with streptococcal toxic shock syndrome: a comparative observational study. *Clin Infect Dis*. 2014;59(6):851-857.
22. Gjestland T. The Oslo study of untreated syphilis; an epidemiologic investigation of the natural course of the syphilitic infection based upon a re-study of the Boeck-Bruusgaard material. *Acta Derm Venereol Suppl (Stockh)*. 1955;35(suppl 34):3-368. Annex I-LVI.
23. Buchacz K, Patel P, Taylor M, et al. Syphilis increases HIV viral load and decreases CD4 cell counts in HIV-infected patients with new syphilis infections. *AIDS (London, England)*. 2004;18(15):2075-2079.
24. Sellati TJ, Wilkinson DA, Sheffield JS, Koup RA, Radolf JD, Norgard MV. Virulent *Treponema pallidum*, lipoprotein, and synthetic lipopeptides induce CCR5 on human monocytes and enhance their susceptibility to infection by human immunodeficiency virus type 1. *J Infect Dis*. 2000;181(1):283-293.
25. Fleming DT, Wasserheit JN. From epidemiological synergy to public health policy and practice: the contribution of other sexually transmitted diseases to sexual transmission of HIV infection. *Sex Transm Infect*. 1999;75(1):3-17.
26. Bolognia JL, Jorizzo JL, Schaffer JV, eds. *Dermatology*. 3rd ed. Elsevier; 2012.
27. Larsen SA, Steiner BM, Rudolph AH. Laboratory diagnosis and interpretation of tests for syphilis. *Clin Microbiol Rev*. 1995;8(1):1-21.

28. Workowski K; CDC DoSTDPTG. *2010 Sexually Transmitted Diseases Treatment Guidelines*. CDC; 2010 http://www.cdc.gov/std/treatment/2010/genital-ulcers.htm#a5
29. Lai-Cheong JE, Perez A, Tang V, et al. Cutaneous manifestations of tuberculosis. *Clin Exp Dermatol.* 2007;32(4):461-466.
30. Gruber PC, Whittam LR, du Vivier A. Tuberculosis verrucosa cutis on the sole of the foot. *Clin Exp Dermatol.* 2002;27(3):188-191.
31. Barbagallo J, Tager P, Ingleton R, Hirsch RJ, Weinberg JM. Cutaneous tuberculosis: diagnosis and treatment. *Am J Clin Dermatol.* 2002;3(5):319-328.
32. Frankel A, Penrose C, Emer J. Cutaneous tuberculosis: a practical case report and review for the dermatologist. *J Clin Aesthet Dermatol.* 2009;2(10):19-27.
33. Premalatha S, Rao NR, Somasundaram V, Abdul Razack EM, Muthuswami TC. Tuberculous gumma in sporotrichoid pattern. *Int J Dermatol.* 1987;26(9):600-601.
34. Rietbroek RC, Dahlmans RP, Smedts F, Frantzen PJ, Koopman RJ, van der Meer JW. Tuberculosis cutis miliaris disseminata as a manifestation of miliary tuberculosis: literature review and report of a case of recurrent skin lesions. *Rev Infect Dis.* 1991;13(2):265-269.
35. Mascaro JM Jr, Baselga E. Erythema induratum of Bazin. *Dermatol Clin.* 2008;26(4):439-445. v.
36. Friedman PC, Husain S, Grossman ME. Nodular tuberculid in a patient with HIV. *J Am Acad Dermatol.* 2005;53(2 suppl 1):S154-S156.
37. Jordaan HF, Schneider JW, Abdulla EA. Nodular tuberculid: a report of four patients. *Pediatr Dermatol.* 2000;17(3):183-188.
38. Lyme Disease Data. http://www.cdc.gov/lyme/stats/
39. Hengge UR, Tannapfel A, Tyring SK, et al. Lyme borreliosis. *Lancet Infect Dis.* 2003;3(8):489-500.
40. Piesman J. Dynamics of *Borrelia burgdorferi* transmission by nymphal *Ixodes dammini* ticks. *J Infect Dis.* 1993;167(5):1082-1085.
41. Nadelman RB, Nowakowski J, Forseter G, et al. The clinical spectrum of early Lyme borreliosis in patients with culture-confirmed erythema migrans. *Am J Med.* 1996;100(5):502-508.
42. Borchers AT, Keen CL, Huntley AC, Gershwin ME. Lyme disease: a rigorous review of diagnostic criteria and treatment. *J Autoimmun.* 2015;57:82-115.
43. Feder HM Jr, Johnson BJ, O'Connell S, et al. A critical appraisal of "chronic Lyme disease". *N Engl J Med.* 2007;357(14):1422-1430.
44. Steere AC, McHugh G, Damle N, Sikand VK. Prospective study of serologic tests for Lyme disease. *Clin Infect Dis.* 2008;47(2):188-195.
45. Wormser GP, Dattwyler RJ, Shapiro ED, et al. The clinical assessment, treatment, and prevention of Lyme disease, human granulocytic anaplasmosis, and babesiosis: clinical practice guidelines by the Infectious Diseases Society of America. *Clin Infect Dis.* 2006;43(9):1089-1134.
46. Shapiro ED. Lyme disease. *N Engl J Med.* 2014;370:1724-1731.
47. Klempner MS, Hu LT, Evans J, et al. Two controlled trials of antibiotic treatment in patients with persistent symptoms and a history of Lyme disease. *N Engl J Med.* 2001;345(2):85-92.
48. Blanton L, Keith B, Brzezinski W. Southern tick-associated rash illness: erythema migrans is not always Lyme disease. *South Med J.* 2008;101(7):759-760.
49. Feder HM Jr, Hoss DM, Zemel L, Telford SR III, Dias F, Wormser GP. Southern Tick-Associated Rash Illness (STARI) in the North: STARI following a tick bite in Long Island, New York. *Clin Infect Dis.* 2011;53(10):e142-e146.
50. Parola P, Paddock CD, Socolovschi C, et al. Update on tick-borne rickettsioses around the world: a geographic approach. *Clin Microbiol Rev.* 2013;26(4):657-702.

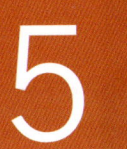

# Reactive Disorders and Drug Eruptions

Yuliya Kozina, BSc and Milan Anadkat, MD

Reactive disorders and drug eruptions encompass a broad range of dermatologic conditions in which a systemic insult manifests in the skin. While some of the clinical findings are specific, others are not and require clinicopathologic correlation.

## 1. Stasis Dermatitis

- Stasis dermatitis is considered part of the clinical spectrum of chronic venous insufficiency.
  - *Chronic venous insufficiency + eczematous dermatitis = stasis dermatitis*
- Typically seen on lower extremities. However, stasis dermatitis may rarely involve the upper limbs in patients with congenital arteriovenous malformations or in patients with arteriovenous fistulas for dialysis.[1]

### 1.1. BACKGROUND

- Epidemiology:
  - Chronic venous insufficiency is reported in 1% to 40% of women and 1% to 17% of men.[2] Stasis dermatitis develops after presentation of chronic venous insufficiency and is more common with increasing age (estimates about 6% of adults age 65+ have stasis dermatitis).[3]
- Risk factors for venous insufficiency include pregnancy, increased age, family history of venous disease, obesity, heart failure, and professions that require continuous periods of standing.[4]
- Venous valve insufficiency in venous hypertension along with eczematous changes leads to the chronic condition of stasis dermatitis. Venous hypertension can be the result of venous pump failure, poor valve function, and valve obstruction.

### 1.2. CLINICAL PRESENTATION

- Stasis dermatitis is a late manifestation of chronic venous disease. Other manifestations of chronic venous insufficiency may include the following physical examination findings (Fig. 5-1):
  - **Dependent edema** of ankles and calves, progressing proximately with worsening disease.
  - **Varicosities** may be present in the lower legs.
  - **Hyperpigmentation** develops with intermittent episodes of hemosiderin deposits present on the skin, called stasis purpura.
  - **Atrophie blanche** (pale atrophic scar) can develop in severe cases of vascular insufficiency. It is not specific to venous insufficiency. The examination finding is an ivory-white depressed atrophic plaque that can be star shaped or polyangular.[5]

---

*The authors would like to acknowledge the first edition author Shivani Tripathi.*

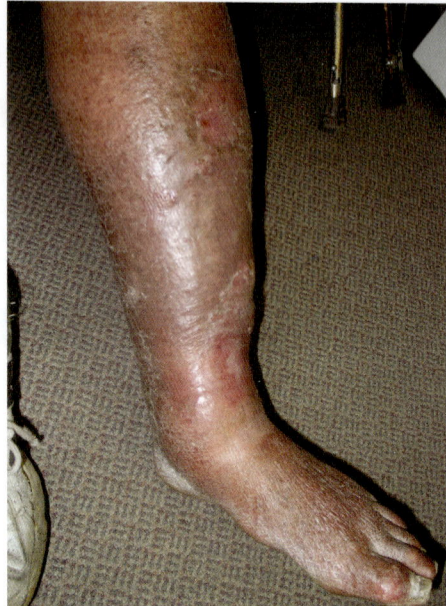

**Figure 5-1.** Venous stasis. (Reprinted with permission from *Stedman's Medical Dictionary for the Health Professions and Nursing: Illustrated.* 7th ed. Wolters Kluwer; 2012:1587.)

- ○ **Lichenification** caused by a thickening of the skin secondary to chronic rubbing or scratching of the affected area.
- ○ **Lipodermatosclerosis** or an "inverted wine bottle appearance" may also develop as the adipose tissue and deep dermis become sclerotic and adherent with a circular cuff around the distal calf.
- Stasis dermatitis is the most frequent condition that is mistaken for cellulitis, leading to unnecessary hospital admission.[6] However, unlike cellulitis, the skin findings related to stasis dermatitis develop slowly and are more likely to be bilateral. Scaling and itching are common in stasis dermatitis but are rarely seen in cellulitis.
- Vascular papules that develop from the edema can present over the changes of stasis dermatitis, called **acroangiodermatitis** or pseudo-Kaposi sarcoma (KS). These may be mistaken for classic KS on clinical examination but lack the histopathologic findings of KS.
- In acute exacerbations of the dermatitis, eczematous changes with scaly, exudative, and weeping plaques can develop.
- Complications:
  - ○ Contact sensitization, possibly due to repeated application of various topical treatments at the affected site.
    - Common culprits—balsam of Peru, lanolin, rubber or latex products, bandages, topical antibiotics (Neomycin)

- Venous leg ulcers.
- **Autoeczematization**—an acute, pruritic, papulovesicular eruption that develops at sites distant from the primary cutaneous findings. It typically involves the forearms, thighs, trunk, and face. Also called an "id reaction."
- **Superinfection**—due to the disrupted skin barrier, bacteria and fungi can colonize the areas affected by stasis dermatitis leading to impetiginized skin, cellulitis, or erysipelas with common pathogens such as *Staphylococcus aureus* and *Streptococcus pyogenes*.

## 1.3. EVALUATION

- **Skin examination**—edema, erythema, scaling, hyperpigmentation, and varicosities typically present. Consider other findings including atrophie blanche, lichenification, lipodermatosclerosis, or acroangiodermatitis, which are less common findings mentioned in previous section.
  - Edema is dependent and may be pitting or nonpitting. Unlike cellulitis, the presentation is typically chronic, bilateral, and nontender.[7]
- Doppler ultrasound can be helpful to demonstrate venous incompetency and diagnose deep venous thrombosis if present.
- If the diagnosis is uncertain, skin biopsy can be considered. However, diagnosis is typically clinical. Poor wound healing after biopsy is likely due to already compromised circulation.
  - Histopathology will demonstrate a superficial perivascular lymphocytic infiltrate, epidermal spongiosis, serous exudate, scale, and crust, in the acute setting. The more chronic lesions may show epidermal acanthosis with hyperkeratosis, hemosiderin deposits, and dilated capillaries.
- Bacterial culture and/or potassium hydroxide preparation can be useful when superinfection of the area is suspected.
- Patch testing for contact sensitization can be useful in patients who develop worsening of disease despite skin care and topical therapy.

## 1.4. TREATMENT

- Improving stasis dermatitis begins with treating underlying venous insufficiency and symptomatic management including:
  - Leg elevation, weight loss, exercise, avoiding prolonged standing, compression therapy,[8] medical and surgical management of venous disease[9]
- Symptomatic treatment of dermatitis involves addressing pruritus, dryness, and inflammation.
  - Gentle skin care is recommended with lukewarm showers and mild soaps, avoiding washcloth use, and regular application of emollients to damp skin after bathing (petrolatum jelly).
  - Mid- to high-potency topical steroids, including triamcinolone 0.1% ointment or clobetasol 0.05% ointment, should be applied twice daily during an acute flare.

# 2. Petechiae, Purpura, and Cutaneous Vasculitis

- Cutaneous vasculitis results almost exclusively from inflammation of the small- or medium-sized blood vessels in the skin. Vasculitis is a histopathologic finding with a range of clinical manifestations and associations, and presentation is determined by the size of the vessel involved.[10,11]

- Vascular injury presents as visible red or purple lesions, which is evidence of hemorrhage into the skin and mucous membranes.[12]
- Vasculitis is different from vasculopathy.
  - *Vasculitis* is defined by an inflammatory injury to the vasculature, while *vasculopathy* is a noninflammatory occlusive injury to the vessel.

## 2.1. BACKGROUND

### 2.1.1. Petechiae (Size <4 mm)[13]

- Nonblanchable and nonpalpable pinpoint macules. Result from capillary inflammation and extravasation of red blood cells (Fig. 5-2A).
- Caused by thrombocytopenia, abnormal platelet function, other nonplatelet etiologies:
  - Thrombocytopenia can be idiopathic, drug-induced, thrombotic, or secondary to disseminated intravascular coagulation.
  - Abnormal platelet function can be caused by congenital or hereditary platelet function defects. Alternatively, acquired platelet dysfunction includes secondary to medications (aspirin, nonsteroidal anti-inflammatory drugs [NSAIDs]), renal insufficiency, monoclonal gammopathy, and thrombocytosis due to myeloproliferative disorders.
  - Nonplatelet etiologies—elevations in intravascular pressures (Valsalva, etc.), fixed increase in pressure (stasis) or intermittent pressure (blood pressure cuff), trauma (often linear), scurvy/vitamin C deficiency (perifollicular), mild inflammatory conditions (pigmented purpuric eruptions, hypergammaglobulinemic purpura of Waldenström).

### 2.1.2. Ecchymosis (Size ≥1 cm)[13]

- Nonblanchable and nonpalpable patches
- Caused by a coagulant abnormality, poor dermal support, or platelet dysfunction + minor trauma
  - Coagulation abnormalities—anticoagulant use, hepatic insufficiency, vitamin K deficiency, disseminated intravascular coagulation
  - Poor dermal support—actinic purpura, corticosteroid therapy (topical or systemic), vitamin C deficiency (scurvy), systemic amyloidosis (light chain related, some familial), Ehlers-Danlos syndrome
  - Platelet dysfunction—von Willebrand disease, medication induced, metabolic disease, acquired or congenital thrombocytopenia

### 2.1.3. Purpura (Any Size)

- Nonblanchable lesions of any size. Initial presentation can appear as erythematous macules or papules progressing to purpura (Fig. 5-2B).
- Two major causes of purpura are microvascular occlusion syndromes ("vasculopathy") and vasculitis.
- Retiform purpura has a more geometric, netlike presentation. Retiform purpura can occur from both vasculitis and vasculopathy.
- **Vasculitis**, inflammation of the vessel wall, is defined by the size of the affected vessel (small, medium, mixed, or large).
  - **Small vessel (leukocytoclastic vasculitis)**—IgA vasculitis (previously called Henoch-Schönlein purpura), acute hemorrhagic edema of infancy, urticarial vasculitis, erythema elevatum diutinum, Sweet syndrome, malignancy-related, infection (group

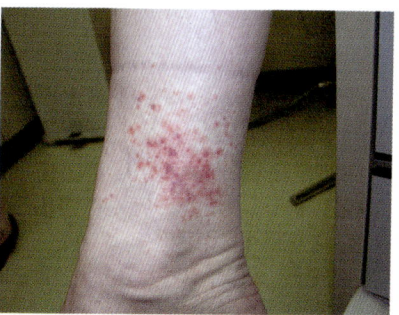

**A**

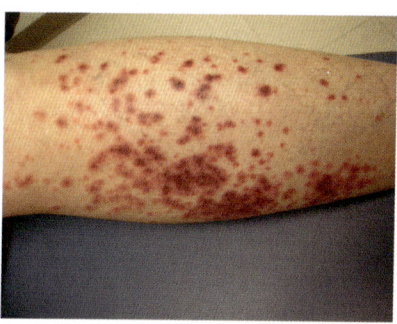

**B**

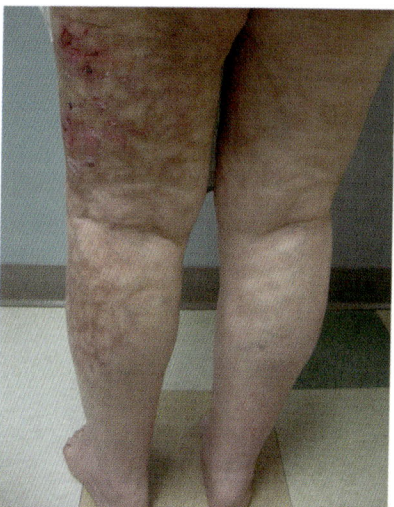

**C**

**Figure 5-2. A.** Petechiae. **B.** Vasculitis. **C.** Vasculopathy.

A strep, *Neisseria meningococcus*, human immunodeficiency virus, hepatitis C), medication (anti–tumor necrosis factor, hydralazine, minocycline, NSAIDs, quinolones), autoimmune connective tissue disease (systemic lupus erythematosus, rheumatoid arthritis, Sjögren syndrome), inflammatory bowel disease.
- **Small- to medium-sized vessels**—antineutrophil cytoplasmic antibody (ANCA)-associated vasculitides (eosinophilic granulomatosis with polyangiitis, granulomatosis with polyangiitis, microscopic polyarteritis), essential cryoglobulinemic vasculitis.
- **Medium-sized vessel vasculitis**—polyarteritis nodosa.
- **Large-vessel vasculitis**—Takayasu arteritis, giant cell arteritis.
- Vessel inflammation results in vessel wall damage and extravasation of erythrocytes seen on examination. Vasculitis may be a primary process or may be secondary to an underlying disease.
  - Secondary causes—infections, inflammatory disorders (autoimmune connective tissue disease), drug exposure, neoplasms
- **Vasculopathy** refers to vascular damage due to microvascular occlusion. Etiology of thrombosis includes disseminated intravascular coagulation, heparin-induced skin necrosis, cryoglobulinemia, antiphospholipid antibody syndrome, or inherited hypercoagulability disorders.[14]

## 2.2. CLINICAL PRESENTATION

- All forms of purpura do not blanch when pressed, as there exists vascular extravasation.
- **Small- to medium-sized vessel involvement**—subcutaneous nodules, purpura, and livedo racemosa (fixed livedo reticularis which does not resolve with warming).[15]
  - Typically presents 7 to 10 days after exposure to an inciting agent with a single group of lesions made up of palpable purpura, erythematous papules, vesicles, or urticarial lesions.
  - Initial lesion is a purpuric macule or partially blanching urticarial papule.
  - Diameter can range from 1 mm to multiple centimeters.
  - Lesions of cutaneous small-vessel vasculitis favor dependent areas as well as areas affected by trauma (pathergy) or under tight-fitting clothing.
  - Typically asymptomatic, but can be associated with pain, burning, and pruritus.
  - Residual postinflammatory hyperpigmentation can persist for months or more.
  - Constitutional symptoms may accompany episodes of cutaneous small-vessel vasculitis.[16]
- **Medium-sized vessel disease** presents with livedo reticularis, retiform purpura, subcutaneous nodules, claudication, ulceration, and necrosis.
  - Lesions favor dependent sites as well as areas under tight-fitting clothing.
  - Lesions are typically asymptomatic but may be associated with burning, pain, and pruritus.

## 2.3. EVALUATION

- Leukocytoclastic vasculitis secondary to drug and infectious disorders accounts for many cases of cutaneous vasculitis, and a history should be obtained of new medications and constitutional symptoms in relation to the onset cutaneous findings.[16]
- **Targeted history and physical examination assessment:**
  - Drug-induced vasculitis typically occurs 7 to 10 days after the introduction of the medication at fault.

- Associated symptoms can suggest an underlying connective tissue disease. These include weight loss, joint pain, photosensitivity, mucosal ulcerations, Raynaud phenomenon, xerostomia, and xerophthalmia.
- Similar symptoms including weight loss, night sweats, and fevers can suggest malignancy.
- Patients should be asked whether they have experienced a change in urinary symptoms to determine renal function, or new-onset pulmonary symptoms to determine if vasculitis could be associated with systemic findings.
- Levamisole-tainted cocaine can lead to retiform purpura[17]; patients with this finding should be asked about recreational drug use.
- Other examination findings can include polyneuropathy, bruits, and abnormal pulses.
- A **punch biopsy** can be particularly helpful in diagnosing leukocytoclastic vasculitis. In addition to a biopsy for hematoxylin and eosin, a biopsy for direct immunofluorescence can be particularly important in the diagnosis of IgA vasculitis, vasculitis related to cryoglobulinemia, and hypocomplementemic vasculitis.[18,19]
  - Lesions between 24 and 48 hours old are most likely to be diagnostic.
  - Location of skin biopsy—in livedo racemosa, a biopsy should be taken from the pale center of the lesion. If an ulcer is present, a biopsy for hematoxylin and eosin staining should be taken from the edge of the ulcer. A biopsy for direct immunofluorescence should be taken from within the purpuric lesion.
  - Findings for small-vessel disease include involvement of venules and arterioles—angiocentric and/or angioinvasive inflammatory infiltrates, disruption of the vessel walls by inflammatory infiltrates, and fibrinoid necrosis.
  - Findings for medium-sized vessel disease include involvement of small arteries and veins—inflammatory infiltrate of the muscular vessel wall and fibrinoid necrosis.
- **Laboratory testing** primary studies include CBC with differential, liver function tests, BUN/Cr level, and urinalysis with microscopy for kidney function. These are nonspecific tests to evaluate systemic involvement.
  - Secondary studies—hepatitis B and C serologies, serum complement levels (CH50, C3, C4), antinuclear antibody, anti-dsDNA, anti-Ro, anti-La, anti-RNP, anti-Sm, rheumatoid factor, serum cryoglobulins, ANCAs, serum and urine protein electrophoresis and immunofixation, and human immunodeficiency virus
  - Chest radiograph in patients with cutaneous vasculitis and pulmonary symptoms, as ANCA-associated vasculitis can affect small and medium vessels of the lungs

## 2.4. TREATMENT

- Treatment of vasculitis depends on the underlying etiology. As most cases of leukocytoclastic vasculitis can be attributed to underlying infection or drug, removing the eliciting agent is the first step.
- Prednisone, colchicine, and dapsone are indicated in idiopathic or persistent disease.[20]

# 3. Urticaria

- **Definition**—typically pruritic, pink, red, pale or skin-tone edema of the superficial dermis ranging in size from a few millimeters in diameter to multiple centimeters (wheal). Lesions can be numerous or single. The hallmark of a wheal is that it appears and disappears rapidly—within 24 hours. Urticaria can also present with angioedema,

in which swelling occurs deeper in the dermis and subcutaneous or submucosal tissue. Angioedema can affect the mouth and, rarely, the bowel. Angioedema tends to be painful rather than itchy, and lesions can often last for 2 to 3 days.[21]
- Urticaria is typically categorized as **acute** (present for <6 weeks) or **chronic** (recurrent, with signs and symptoms recurring most days of the week for 6 weeks or longer).

## 3.1. BACKGROUND

- Epidemiology—approximately 20% of the general population will experience hives during their lifetime.[22]
- Clinical classifications of urticaria and angioedema include classic urticaria, physical or inducible urticarias, contact urticaria, urticarial vasculitis, angioedema (without urticaria), and distinctive urticarial syndromes.
- Common causes of urticaria include infection, allergic reactions (medications, foods, or insect stings and bites), nonallergic mast cell activation secondary to medications (eg, narcotics), autoimmunity, NSAIDs.
  - Note—C1 esterase inhibitor deficiency should be considered a cause of recurrent angioedema without wheals.
  - Infections—acute urticaria may develop during or following viral or bacterial infection. Over 80% of cases of acute urticaria in children are associated with an infectious process.[23]
- Urticaria develops as cutaneous mast cells, located in the superficial dermis, release preformed granules containing histamines and cytokines.[24]
- Classic immediate hypersensitivity reactions occur as an allergen binds to mast cell receptor–bound immunoglobulin E (IgE). Other nonimmunologic stimuli, such as opiates and neuropeptides (eg, substance P), can activate mast cell degranulation independent of the high-affinity IgE receptor.

## 3.2. CLINICAL PRESENTATION (FIG. 5-3)

- The individual lesions of classic urticaria last for ≤24 hours and resolve without sequelae, but often return episodically.
- Acute urticaria is common in young children with atopic dermatitis.

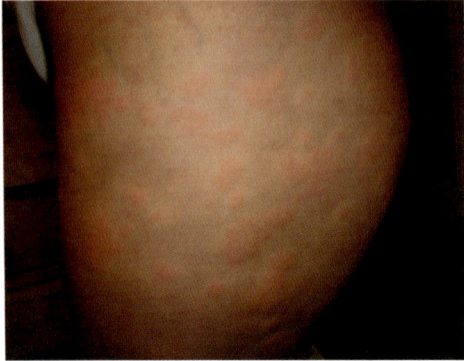

**Figure 5-3.** Urticaria (hives).

- Chronic urticaria (CU)—symptoms last for 6 or more weeks. CU is applied to continuous bouts of urticaria occurring at least twice a week off treatment. CU incidence peaks in the fourth decade, is more common in the evening or upon waking, can significantly affect quality-of-life measures, and can have premenstrual exacerbations in women.
  - CU has been associated with autoimmune thyroid disease, rheumatoid arthritis, celiac disease, and other autoimmune disorders.[25]
  - An association with *Helicobacter pylori* gastritis and urticaria has been shown, with studies showing higher frequency of remission when the infection was eradicated than when it was not.[26]
- Urticaria occurring less than twice per week is termed recurrent or episodic urticaria.
- Genetic susceptibility to CU has a very strong association with HLA-DR4 and associated alleles HLA-DQ8 (common in patients with histamine-releasing autoantibodies).[22,27]
- Physical urticarias are induced by exogenous physical stimuli and may severely affect quality of life.
  - Classification:
    - Induced by mechanical stimuli: dermatographism (Fig. 5-4) and delayed pressure urticaria (including vibratory angioedema, inherited, and acquired)
    - Induced by temperature changes and stress
      - Cholinergic, adrenergic, cold (including cold contact and secondary to cryoglobulins), solar, aquagenic
- **Dermatographism**
  - Immediate dermatographism is divided into simple and symptomatic.
    - Simple immediate dermatographism occurs in about 5% of normal people in response to moderate friction on the skin and may be regarded as an exaggerated physiologic response.
    - Symptomatic dermatographism is the most common of the physical urticarias and differs from simple dermatographism due to significant associated itch and symptom induction by light pressure.
  - Linear wheals at sites of scratching and at other sites of friction.
  - Most commonly occurs in young adults.
  - Pruritus can coexist and present concurrently with wheals.
  - Worst in the evening and usually resolves within an hour.

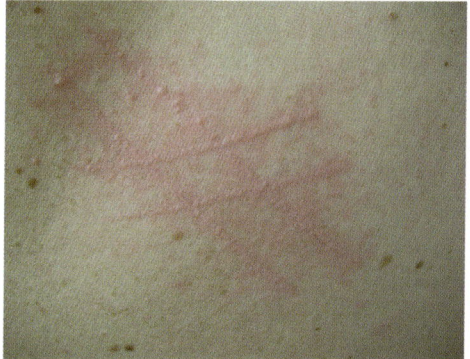

**Figure 5-4.** Dermatographism.

- **Delayed pressure urticaria**
  - Development of deep erythematous edema at sites of sustained pressure to the skin, after a delay of 30 minutes to 12 hours.
  - Swelling can be pruritic, painful, or both and may persist for days.
  - Most commonly found at the waistline, below the elastic of socks, feet in tight shoes, palms after manual work, and genitalia after intercourse.
  - Systemic features like fatigue, arthralgias, etc., may be present.
  - Mean duration is 6 to 9 years.
- **Vibratory angioedema**
  - Vibratory stimulus (such as jogging, rubbing with a towel, or using machinery such as a lawnmower) induces localized swelling and erythema within minutes.
  - Familial form with autosomal dominant inheritance.
- **Stress exposure**
  - **Cholinergic** urticaria—transient papular wheals measuring 2 to 3 mm in size and surrounded by an obvious flare, occurring within 15 minutes of sweat-inducing stimuli (physical activity, hot baths, emotional stress), moving from a hot to cold room, eating spicy food. Pruritus can follow the development of the monomorphic wheals. Cold urticaria, symptomatic dermatographism, or aquagenic urticaria may be associated with cholinergic urticaria.
  - **Adrenergic** urticaria—sudden stress induces small pink wheals surrounded by blanched vasoconstricted skin.
  - **Local heat contact urticaria**—one of the rarest forms of urticaria. Within minutes of contact with heat from any source, itching begins and wheals form at the precise location of contact. Symptoms can last for an hour.
  - **Cold urticaria**—includes primary cold urticaria and secondary cold urticaria.
    - Primary cold urticaria—itching, burning, hives occur minutes after the exposure to cold temperatures. Can also follow respiratory infection, arthropod bites, and be associated with HIV.
    - Secondary cold urticaria—seen with serum abnormalities such as cryoglobulinemia, cryofibrinogenemia, or with hepatitis B or C, lymphoproliferative diseases, infectious mononucleosis, Raynaud phenomenon. Wheals can last 24+ hours, and cryoglobulins and cryofibrinogens should be measured.
  - **Solar urticaria**—itching and whealing begin within minutes of UV exposure (UV rays may penetrate light clothing), and systemic symptoms may also be present.
    - Primary solar urticaria—mediated by an immediate type I hypersensitivity reaction to a cutaneous or circulating irradiation-induced neoantigen.
    - Secondary solar urticaria is seen in patients with certain types of porphyria.
  - **Aquagenic urticaria**—contact with water of any temperature induces an urticarial eruption resembling cholinergic urticaria. Lesions occur most frequently on the upper part of the body and last for an hour or less. Other physical urticarias, as well as aquagenic pruritus, must be excluded.
  - **Contact urticaria** presents after exposure to a specific trigger and can be immune or nonimmune mediated. The immunogenic form is a type 1 hypersensitivity reaction. The nonimmunogenic is prostaglandin mediated and may not have the typical wheal presentation and is instead treated with NSAIDs; examples of exposure sources include caterpillar toxin, cinnamic acid, nettles. Nonimmunogenic contact urticaria can be differentiated from contact dermatitis by brevity of symptoms and absence of blistering or scaling.[28]
    - Muckle-Wells syndrome—rare autosomal dominant condition characterized by mutation in the NALP3 (CIAS1) gene that produces the protein cryopyrin. Burning and itching urticarial plaques can last up to 2 days and develop because

of drop in body temperature. Fever, headaches, and leukocytosis may also be present. The spectrum can also include chronic infantile neurologic cutaneous and articular syndrome, associated with sensorineural deafness and amyloidosis.
  □ Muckle-Wells is one of three cryopyrin-associated periodic syndromes (CAPS). Others include familial cold autoinflammatory syndrome and neonatal-onset multisystem inflammatory disease.
- Familial Mediterranean fever—autosomal recessive, eastern European and Middle Eastern descent. Patients may present with peritonitis, pleurisy, or synovitis. Urticaria is a rare symptom of the disorder.
- Schnitzler syndrome—nonpruritic urticarial eruption, recurrent fevers, bone pain, arthritis and arthralgias, as well as monoclonal gammopathy, which can progress to a lymphoproliferative disorder.[29] Absence of angioedema is a distinguishing characteristic of this disorder.

## 3.3. EVALUATION

- **Differential diagnosis**—arthropod bites, febrile neutrophilic dermatosis (Sweet syndrome), prebullous pemphigoid (urticarial bullous pemphigoid), acute facial contact dermatitis, urticarial drug reactions, and mastocytosis.
  ○ It is important to differentiate allergic or contact dermatitis from urticaria by considering timing and duration of skin findings, symptom onset, and absence of blisters or scaling in urticaria.
  ○ **Urticarial vasculitis** (Fig. 5-5)—cutaneous lesions resemble urticaria clinically, but last longer than 24 hours, are painful instead of itchy, and show evidence of small vessel vasculitis/leukocytoclastic vasculitis on histopathology. Involves

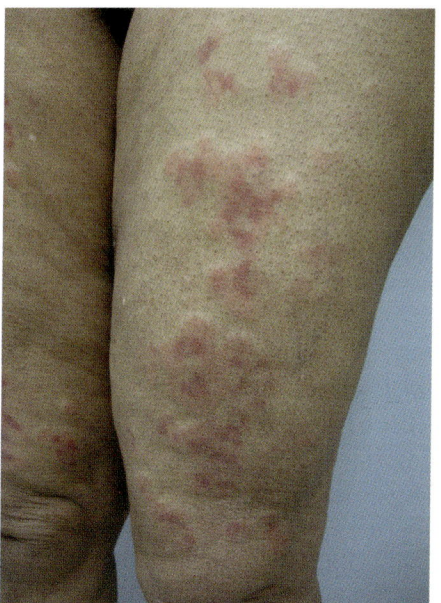

**Figure 5-5.** Urticarial vasculitis.

circulating immune complexes (type III hypersensitivity reaction). The complexes embed in vessel walls leading to urticarialike lesions, which histologically are consistent with small vessel vasculitis.[30]
  - In urticarial-like dermatoses (ie, bullous pemphigoid), the lesions can last many days and may present with other cutaneous findings, such as blistering, to help differentiate from classic urticaria.
- **Comprehensive history**—duration of disease, frequency of attacks, duration of individual lesions, presence or absence of angioedema, associated symptoms (joint pain, fever), associated illness, previous treatments, known allergies or adverse reactions, personal and familial medical history, occupation and leisure activities, and quality of life measures.
  - Constitutional symptoms such as fatigue may be present in urticaria, but recurrent fevers and arthritis warrant an additional workup to rule out urticarial vasculitis or urticarial syndromes, such as CAPS or Schnitzler syndrome.
- **Labs**—urticaria that is responsive to antihistamines does not typically necessitate an extensive work-up. In complicated cases, basic laboratory tests (CBC, CMP, etc.), skin biopsy for lesions lasting more than 24 hours, question of food additives and drugs, and occasionally skin tests for allergies might be indicated.[29,31]
- **Acute urticaria** work-up—IgE-mediated reactions to environmental allergens related to acute and contact urticaria can be confirmed by skin prick testing and radioallergosorbent test of the blood.
- **Chronic urticaria**—complete blood count and white cell differential (to detect eosinophilia related to intestinal parasitosis) and erythrocyte sedimentation rate (typically normal in CU, but may be raised in urticarial vasculitis or other associated diseases). Thyroid function, thyroid stimulating hormone, and free T4 (the presence of thyroid autoantibodies is higher in patients with CU and could be an indicator of autoimmune urticaria).
- **Physical urticarias**—symptomatic dermatographism can be tested by stroking the skin of the back lightly with the rounded edge of a wooden spatula. Provocation tests for cholinergic urticaria include exercise to the point of sweating in an overheated environment or partial immersion in a hot bath at 42 °C for 10 minutes. Cold contact urticaria is confirmed by the development of whealing at the site of application of an ice cube in a glove for 20 minutes. Phototesting confirms the diagnosis of solar urticaria, with development of wheals within minutes of exposure to sunlight.
- **Urticarial vasculitis**—lesional skin biopsy is essential and should be done on lesions that last more than 24 hours to confirm the histologic presence of leukocytoclastic vasculitis.
- **Test for associated diseases**—serum antibodies for systemic lupus erythematosus and celiac disease, Sjögren syndrome, serum protein and immunofixation electrophoreses, cryoglobulins, hepatitis B and C and Epstein-Barr viral serologies, breath test for *H pylori*, and *Borrelia* antibody tests.
- **Wheals without angioedema**—consider CAPS, Schnitzler, Familial Mediterranean fever.
- **Angioedema without wheals**—the types of angioedema can be differentiated with complement and, in some cases, genetic testing. Consider angiotensin-converting enzyme (ACE) inhibitor–induced angioedema.[29]

## 3.4. TREATMENT

- Any life-threatening symptoms of airway obstruction from angioedema are considered a medical emergency and should be treated appropriately with subcutaneous epinephrine.

- A majority of urticaria is nonemergent, and two-thirds of new-onset urticaria will be self-limited and resolve spontaneously. Initial treatment of new-onset urticaria should focus on short-term relief. An antihistamine can help to address the short-term discomfort and prevent recurrent episodes of urticaria.
  - Treatment should begin with eliminating underlying causes, followed by symptomatic management.
  - **H$_1$ antihistamines**: Second-generation H$_1$ antihistamines are preferred (cetirizine, loratadine, and fexofenadine). Older, first-generation H$_1$ antihistamines (diphenhydramine, chlorpheniramine, and hydroxyzine) are lipophilic and cross the blood-brain barrier, leading to more sedation when compared with second-generation H$_1$ antihistamines.[32] For some individuals, higher dosage of second-generation H$_1$ antihistamines (up to fourfold) can be effective.[29]
  - **H$_2$ antihistamines**: Some data suggest a synergistic effect with the combination of H$_1$ antihistamines with H$_2$ antihistamines (ranitidine, famotidine, cimetidine) in treating acute urticaria.[33] This combination is not currently the standard treatment for acute urticaria.
- **Chronic urticaria (CU)** may require additional treatment when it is refractory to antihistamines. Additionally, patients who require repeated courses of oral glucocorticoids are also candidates for additional therapies as steroids are not suitable for long-term therapy. In patients with autoinflammatory syndromes (ie, Muckle-Wells, familial cold autoinflammatory syndrome, and neonatal-onset multisystem inflammatory disease), therapies will differ.
  - Omalizumab, a monoclonal antibody against IgE, is safe and effective and is typically recommended over immunosuppressive (cyclosporine, tacrolimus, or methotrexate) treatments and other anti-inflammatory agents (dapsone, sulfasalazine, or hydroxychloroquine).[34,35]
  - Cyclosporin can be added as a fourth-line medication after H$_1$ antihistamines, four times dose H$_1$ antihistamines, and omalizumab.[22,29]
  - Leukotriene receptor antagonists have low evidence, but some randomized clinical trials have demonstrated benefit for montelukast.[29]
- **Nonimmune contact urticaria**—NSAIDs may be beneficial after antihistamine options have been tried.[19]
- **Adrenergic urticaria**—identification and avoidance of triggers is the first-line treatment.
- **Cold, cholinergic, and solar urticaria**—tolerance induction has been shown to be beneficial, but maintenance can be challenging for patients requiring daily exposures.

## 4. Viral Exanthems

- An exanthem is an acutely appearing rash that affects many locations on the skin simultaneously and may be associated with fever or other systemic symptoms (Table 5-1). Viral infection is the most common etiology for exanthems.
- The Greek word *exanthema* means "a breaking out."
- *Enanthem* is an eruption on the mucous membranes ("a breaking in").
- Various viruses cause common morbilliform eruptions. A morbilliform eruption is a group of macules and papules resembling a measles rash. With characteristic lesions and distinctive prodromes, the diagnosis can be straightforward. However, a nonspecific rash may keep the differential broad.[36]
- Common culprits of exanthem.

### TABLE 5-1 Viral Exanthems

| Name | Etiology | Incubation | Presentation | Associations Treatment/Prevention |
|---|---|---|---|---|
| **Measles**, Rubeola, first disease | Paramyxovirus, measles virus | 8-12 d | Prodrome: fever, irritability, malaise, coryza, conjunctivitis, and Koplik spots. Morbilliform eruption that is cranial to caudal, starting at the hairline and involving the rest of the body by day 3 | Cough, coryza, conjunctivitis. Patients should be isolated for 4 d after the onset of eruption, and for the immunocompromised, for the entire duration of the disease. MMR (measles, mumps, rubella) vaccination |
| **Rubella**, German measles, third disease | Togavirus/rubella virus | Spread by respiratory droplets 14-21 d | Mild exanthema in children, starts on face then generalizes. Associated with cervical lymphadenopathy, Forchheimer spots | If contracted in the first trimester of pregnancy, fetus can have severe ocular, cardiac, and pulmonary abnormalities. |
| **Erythema infectiosum**, slapped cheek disease, fifth disease | Parvovirus B19 | Spread by respiratory secretions, blood products, and vertical transmission 4- to 14-d incubation | Bright erythematous patches on cheeks; tends to avoid trunk, and can also present with purpuric papules on hands/feet of young adults (papular purpuric gloves and socks syndrome) | If infected during pregnancy, can lead to complications and aplastic crisis in those with sickle cell disease |

| | | | | |
|---|---|---|---|---|
| **Roseola infantum** | HHV-6 | Present in most individuals after 6 mo | 9- to 12-mo-old infant, onset of high fever (40 °C) lasting for 3 d<br>Defervescence and appearance of morbilliform exanthema | Erythematous papules on mucosa of soft palate and uvula |
| **Pityriasis rosea** | HHV-6 and HHV-7 suspected | | Begins with a salmon-colored "herald patch"<br>Evolves into a generalized eruption after 1-2 wk with a duration of 6-8 wk<br>Bilateral and symmetric macules with a collarette of scale along the cleavage lines | Self-resolving |
| **Hand, foot, and mouth** | Coxsackie A16 | 1 wk | Macular lesions → blisters, vesicles on buccal mucosa, tongue, hard palate<br>Tender macules and vesicles on palms and soles | |

- **Varicella** (aka chickenpox)
- **Measles** (aka first disease, rubeola)
- **Rubella** (aka third disease, German measles, 3-day measles)
- **Erythema infectiosum** (fifth disease)—parvovirus B19
- **Roseola infantum (sixth disease)**—human herpesvirus (HHV)-6 and HHV-7
- **Pityriasis rosea (PR)**—HHV-7
- **Hand, foot, and mouth disease**—coxsackievirus A type 16, but also associated with other strains of coxsackievirus (A5, A7, A9, A10, B2, B5) and enterovirus 71

## 4.1. BACKGROUND

- **Varicella**
  - Caused by the varicella zoster virus (VZV), a deoxyribonucleic acid (DNA) virus in the herpes family.
  - Vaccination for VZV was introduced in 1995. There has been a decline in primary varicella infection since that time.
  - Two doses of the vaccination are recommended for all individuals who are not already immune.[37]
  - Spread by airborne respiratory droplets or contact with blister fluid, the virus first colonizes the upper respiratory tract. Replication takes place in the regional lymph nodes over 2 to 4 days before the virus spreads to the liver and spleen. After 1 week, secondary viremia disseminates, producing the typical skin lesions.[38]
  - Incubation period is 10 to 21 days, average of about 2 weeks.
  - There is a greater possibility of severe side effects with exposure during pregnancy for the affected mother and fetus.
- **Measles**
  - Caused by the measles virus, a single-stranded, negative-sense enveloped ribonucleic acid (RNA) virus in the Paramyxoviridae family.
  - Incubation period—8 to 12 days from exposure to onset of symptoms.
  - Contagious for 3 to 5 days prior to rash onset and 4 days after the appearance of rash.
    - Spreads by respiratory droplets and is highly contagious
  - Most common in children ages 3 to 5 years old.
  - Children/adolescents who were never vaccinated are highly susceptible; common in developing countries with 50 to 1,500 yearly cases in the United States.
  - Presents in late winter/spring.
- **Rubella**
  - Caused by the rubella virus, a single stranded, positive-sense, RNA virus in the Matonaviridae family.
  - School-age children, adolescents, and young adults.
  - Outbreaks occur most frequently in late winter and early spring.
  - Spreads through direct or droplet contact from nasopharyngeal secretions.
  - Noncongenital rubella can be subclinical, and incidence has decreased with vaccination.
- **Erythema infectiosum**
  - Erythema infectiosum is only one of the clinical presentations of parvovirus B19, ranging from asymptomatic and benign to life threatening.
    - Caused by the nonenveloped, single-stranded, DNA virus in the Parvoviridae family
  - Most common in children 4 to 10 years old but can affect all ages.
  - Outbreaks late winter to early spring.

- Increasing prevalence of antibodies with age (50% of young adults and 90% of older adult population).
- Transmission via contact with respiratory tract secretions, percutaneous exposure to blood or blood products, and vertical transmission from mother to fetus.
- Incubation period from exposure to onset of rash, usually between 1 and 2 weeks.
- Individuals are most infectious prior to the onset of rash.
- **Roseola infantum (sixth disease, exanthem subitum)**
  - Has a multivirus etiology and is most commonly caused by the HHV-6 and less commonly by HHV-7.[39,40]
  - Called roseola infantum because it affects infant and older babies and is the most common exanthema before age 2.
  - The infection results in immunity, and there is no vaccination for roseola.
  - Seroprevalence of HHV-6 in the adult population is 95%.
- **Pityriasis rosea**
  - Exact cause is unknown but often follows upper respiratory tract infections, suggesting role of *Streptococcus*.[41]
    - A viral etiology is also suggested, particularly for HHV-6 and HHV-7, but has not been confirmatory.[42,43]
  - Most common in children and young adults.
  - Most cases occur in the spring.
  - Acute self-limiting eruption of fine scaling lesions.
  - Duration of 6 to 8 weeks.
  - Usually begins with a single, larger, "herald patch," which is seen in 50% to 90% of cases a week or more before the numerous smaller lesions, which are distributed in a "Christmas tree"-like pattern on the back and torso following Langer lines of cleavage.
  - Recurrence of PR is rare, and the disease is not considered transmissible.
  - During pregnancy, it can be associated with miscarriage during the first 15 weeks, or premature delivery.[44]
- **Hand, foot, and mouth disease**
  - Caused by the coxsackievirus or A16 or enterovirus A71, nonenveloped, positive-sense, single-stranded RNA viruses in the Picornaviridae family.
  - Presents with sore mouth, malaise, and fever.
  - Macular lesions may also be present on buccal mucosa, tongue, and hard palate, which develop into vesicles that erode and have an erythematous halo.
  - Uncommonly, patient may develop an aseptic meningitis. This is more likely with enterovirus-71.

## 4.2. CLINICAL PRESENTATION

- **Varicella (chickenpox; see Chapter 4, Fig. 4-6A)**
  - **Prodrome**—mild coldlike symptoms present 1 to 2 days before rash. Alternatively, systemic symptoms present with the rash, including fever, headache, decreased appetite, arthralgia, myalgias, gastrointestinal disturbance, and URI symptoms.
  - **Exanthem**—pruritic and erythematous eruption that develops into small blisters on the torso, face, scalp, axilla, and extremities. May start on the trunk and back and spread to extremities. Individuals are infectious 1 to 2 days prior to the appearance of the rash and until the blisters have dried and become scabs. Though blisters usually dry and become scabs within 4 to 5 days, there are typically several crops of blisters in different stages of healing, so infected individuals should stay home and away from others until ALL blisters have crusted over.

- **Enanthem**—in the oral mucosa.
- **Recovery**—generally self-resolving within 2 to 4 weeks.
- **Complications**—superimposed bacterial infections may occur with the rash, systemic risk includes encephalitis, cerebellar ataxia, transverse myelitis, pneumonia, Reye syndrome, and hemorrhagic complications. Adults can have more severe systemic complications (central nervous system infection/encephalitis, pneumonia, and hepatitis).

  Immunocompromised patients have high risk of mortality from disseminated varicella. Varicella congenital syndrome is a potential complication of infection of pregnant individuals.[45]

- **Measles (first disease; see Fig. 5-6)**
  - **Prodrome**—fever, malaise, conjunctivitis, cough, coryza (head cold with nasal congestion, rhinorrhea sore throat), Koplik spots (enanthem that consists of punctate blue-white lesions with an erythematous rim on the buccal mucosa that manifests 2 to 3 days before full body rash).
  - **Exanthem**—erythematous macules and papules that start on the face and spread cranial to caudal. Also move centrifugally, starting centrally and moving outward to cover the entire body in 2 to 3 days.
  - **Recovery**—constitutional symptoms begin to improve 2 days after the rash presents, with rash progressively improving and lasting about a week.
  - **Complications**—otitis media, pneumonia (most common fatal complication in children and most common overall in adults), laryngotracheobronchitis (croup), and diarrhea.
- **Rubella**
  - **Prodrome**—low-grade fever, headache, sore throat, conjunctivitis, rhinorrhea, cough, and lymphadenopathy, occasionally with arthritis.
  - **Exanthem**—pruritic pink to red macules and papules that start on the face and then spread to trunk and extremities within 24 hours. Within 2 to 3 days, the rash clears, starting at the head and neck first.
  - **Enanthem**—petechial lesions on the soft palate and uvula (Forchheimer sign).
  - **Complications**—encephalitis, thrombocytopenia, peripheral neuritis, optic neuritis, myocarditis, pericarditis, hepatitis, orchitis, and hemolytic anemia.
- **Erythema infectiosum (fifth disease); see Figure 5-7**
  - **Prodrome**—low-grade fever, malaise, headache, pruritus, coryza, myalgias, and joint pain.
  - **Exanthem**—bright red cheeks (slapped cheeks), and, as the facial rash fades over 1 to 4 days, a symmetric, erythematous, reticular (lacelike) rash appears on the torso and extremities, lasting 5 to 9 days. Patients with the rash are viremic and contagious.
  - **Papular purpuric gloves and socks syndrome**—painful, pruritic papules, petechiae, and purpura of the hands and feet.
    - **Enanthem**—oral erosions
  - **Complications**—hydrops fetalis and fetal death in pregnancy, aplastic crisis in patients with sickle cell disease.
- **Roseola infantum**
  - HHV-6 infection in children can present as either (a) subclinical infection, (b) acute febrile illness without rash, or (c) sudden rash/exanthema subitum.
  - **Prodrome**—high fever (39 °C-40 °C), palpebral edema, cervical lymphadenopathy, and mild upper respiratory tract symptoms. As fever subsides, exanthem appears.
  - **Exanthem**—macules and papules with a surrounding white halo, beginning on the trunk and spreading to the neck and proximal extremities.

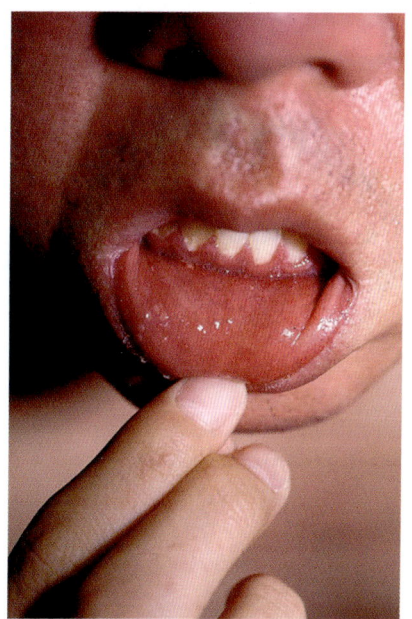

A

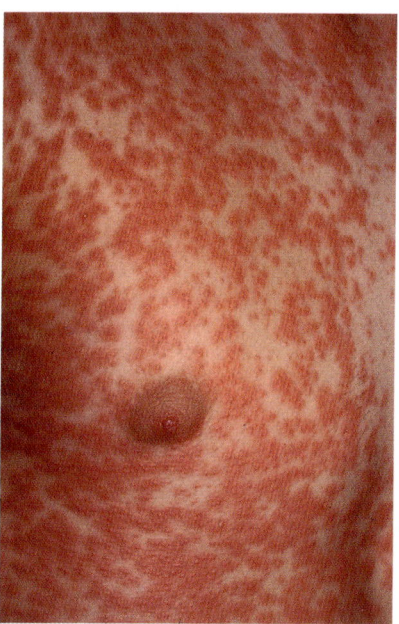

B

**Figure 5-6. A, B.** Measles. (Reprinted with permission from Mallory SB, Bree A, Chern P. *Illustrated Manual of Pediatric Dermatology.* Taylor and Francis Publishing; 2005:119-120. Figures 8.1 and 8.2.)

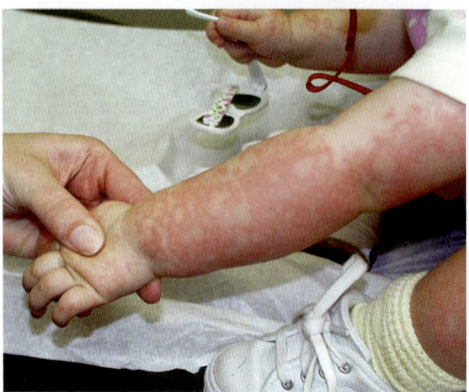

**Figure 5-7.** Erythema infectiosum.

- **Pityriasis rosea**
  - Initially a pink patch develops and expands becoming well-demarcated with a collarette of "trailing" scale, known as the herald patch typically on the back though can be anywhere on the body.
  - **Exanthem**—a generalized eruption of ovoid patches with trailing scale develops over 1 to 2 weeks with long axis of patch parallel to skin tension lines in a symmetric distribution on neck, torso and extremities sparing face, hands, and feet known as the "Christmas tree" pattern; lasting approximately 2 months.
    - Atypical variants are seen as well (inverse PR, nonsymmetric distribution, etc.).
- **Hand, foot, mouth disease**
  - **Prodrome**—1 to 3 days including low-grade fever, anorexia, malaise, cough, sore throat, abdominal pain.
  - **Enanthem**—can precede the exanthem. Oral lesions begin as red macules evolving into blisters that can be painful and tender.
  - Skin findings are located on the hands, feet, and buttock as red macules that develop central grey vesicles. Unlike oral lesions, cutaneous lesions are typically asymptomatic.
  - **Recovery**—generally uncomplicated recovery within 10 to 14 days.
  - **Complications**—persistent painful stomatitis. Rarely, aseptic meningitis, myocarditis, and pneumonia.[46]

## 4.3. EVALUATION

- Diagnosis relies on clinical findings, viral cultures, or serologic cultures.
- **Varicella**
  - Diagnosis suspected based on history and physical examination.
  - Tzanck smear (scraping of base of vesicle for Giemsa staining) shows multinucleated giant cells and epithelial cells with eosinophilic intranuclear inclusion bodies.
  - A vesicular fluid culture can be helpful but is positive less than 40% of the time.
  - Varicella zoster virus (VZV) PCR testing is highly specific, readily available, and can be done using samples from skin lesions, plasma, or other fluids. The most sensitive testing for VZV antibodies is the flow cytometry-adapted fluorescent sntibody to membrane antigen (FAMA) test.[47]

- **Measles**
  - Diagnosis is suspected from presence of high fever, Koplik spots, conjunctivitis, upper respiratory tract infectious symptoms, and typical exanthem.
  - If suspected, serologically confirm with antimeasles IgM and IgG, isolation of measles virus, or identification of measles RNA.
  - Report immediately to local or state health department without waiting for diagnostic test results.
- **Rubella**
  - Suspected from clinical examination
  - Diagnosis confirmed with serology: rubella-specific IgM antibody or a fourfold rise in antibody titer in acute and convalescent-phase serum
- **Erythema infectiosum**
  - Detection of serum parvovirus B19–specific IgM antibody indicates that infection has likely occurred within the previous 2 to 4 months.

## 4.4. TREATMENT

- **Varicella**
  - Vaccination is available and was approved by the U.S. Food and Drug Administration in 1995 for prophylactic use in healthy children and adults: 1 dose for children 12 to 18 months and 2 doses in a 4- to 8-week interval in those over 13 years.[48]
  - Treatment for a healthy child is supportive, while an adult or an immunocompromised individual typically requires systemic therapy.[49]
  - **Supportive care for a healthy child (<12 years)**
    - Acetaminophen for fever.
    - Do not give aspirin as this can lead to Reye syndrome (fatal multiorgan failure, specifically brain and liver).
    - Calamine lotion to relieve pruritus.
    - Antiviral treatment, acyclovir, for severe cases.
    - Cool oatmeal baths.
    - Rest and hydration.
    - Keep nails short to prevent excessive itching, which can lead to scarring and bacterial superinfection.
  - The virus remains dormant in nerves and can reactivate as herpes zoster (shingles).
  - *Treatment in immunocompetent adults*
    - Since individuals greater than 12 years are likely to have more severe reactions, oral acyclovir, 800 mg 5 times daily for 1 week, has been shown to decrease the duration of lesions, if started within 24 hours of the appearance of symptoms.
  - *Treatment in immunocompromised individuals*
    - IV acyclovir therapy is indicated in these patients because of the possible life-threatening complications.
    - Foscarnet can be used in individuals with acyclovir-resistant VZV.
- **Measles**
  - Uncomplicated measles is self-limiting, lasting 10 to 12 days.
  - In majority of cases, treatment is supportive.
  - Malnutrition, immunosuppression, and lack of substantial supportive care worsen prognosis.
  - Vitamin A supplementation has been shown to reduce mortality.

- **Rubella**
  - Report suspected cases to the local health department.
  - Droplet precautions and minimal to no contact (especially school/daycare) for 1 week AFTER the onset of rash.
  - Treatment is supportive, no specific therapy.
- **Erythema infectiosum (fifth disease)**
  - No specific treatment for uncomplicated Parvovirus B19 infection and supportive therapy for fatigue, malaise, pruritus, and arthralgias
  - Typically resolves within 5 to 10 days but can last for months depending on environmental exposures

## 5. Drug Eruptions

- Adverse drug reactions can commonly present with cutaneous manifestations, and determining the cause of a drug eruption depends on the chronicity of the offending agent and the clinical manifestations. Below is the list of some of the most commonly encountered drug eruptions that will be reviewed in this section.
  - Exanthematous eruption
  - Urticaria, angioedema, anaphylaxis
  - Photosensitivity
  - Fixed drug eruption
  - Acute generalized exanthematous pustulosis (AGEP)
  - Drug-induced hypersensitivity syndrome (DIHS), also referred to as drug reaction with eosinophilia and systemic symptoms (DRESS)
  - Anticoagulant-induced skin necrosis
  - Reactions to chemotherapy
  - Stevens-Johnson syndrome (SJS)
  - Toxic epidermal necrolysis (TEN)
- DIHS, AGEP, SJS, and TEN include some of the more severe drug reaction. Though rare, these are associated with the greatest morbidity and mortality.

### 5.1. BACKGROUND

- Skin is one of the most common targets for adverse drug eruptions, and antibiotic and anticonvulsants are reported to produce adverse events in 1% to 5% of patients.
- Women, the older adult, and those who are immunosuppressed from human immunodeficiency virus have a greater risk of developing adverse drug reactions.
  - Those with a CD4+ less than 200 have a 10- to 50-fold greater chance of developing an adverse eruption compared to the general population.

### 5.2. CLINICAL PRESENTATION

- **Exanthematous eruption or morbilliform drug eruptions**
  - Most common adverse drug reaction affecting the skin; very commonly seen in hospitalized patients.
  - Type IV delayed type hypersensitivity reaction.
  - Classically begins 7 to 14 days after the start of a new medication, but can also occur earlier, or even after the drug is discontinued.
  - Begin as erythematous macules that evolve into confluent papules on the trunk and upper extremities; face, palms, soles, and mucous membranes are typically spared. The eruption resolves without sequelae in 1 to 2 weeks.

- Commonly associated drugs: aminopenicillins, sulfonamides, cephalosporins, and anticonvulsants.
- **Urticaria and angioedema**
  - Urticaria presents with transient, pruritic, edematous, and erythematous plaques. Lesions may appear anywhere on the body and typically last several hours.
  - Type I IgE-mediated hypersensitivity reaction.
  - Drugs are responsible for fewer than 10% of cases.
  - Medications may cause an immunologically based urticaria, especially antibiotics (most commonly penicillins or cephalosporins) and monoclonal antibodies used in treatment for neoplastic or inflammatory diseases.
  - Angioedema is a transient edema of the deep subcutaneous and submucosal tissue, and about 50% of cases are associated with urticaria. New users of ACE can experience angioedema, at a rate of 1 to 2 per 1,000.
  - Angioedema presents with acute subcutaneous swelling of the face (eyelids, lips, ears, nose), and buccal mucosa and tongue may also occur. Edema of the larynx, epiglottis, and surrounding tissue may lead to impaired swallowing and upper airway obstruction.
  - Drugs implicated in angioedema: penicillins, ACE inhibitors, NSAIDs, radiographic contrast media, and monoclonal antibodies.
    - NSAID-induced angioedema and urticaria are classified into four distinct forms based on timing of onset and associated symptoms.
  - About 1 in 5,000 exposures to penicillin can progress to anaphylaxis.
- **Photosensitivity**
  - The combination of light and drug can lead to several forms of cutaneous inflammation. Photosensitivity is typically divided into two major types: **phototoxic** (more common) and **photoallergic**.
  - A phototoxic drug eruption presents as an exaggerated sunburn and occurs in a short exposure time. The area will heal with hyperpigmentation.
    - Common offenders include tetracyclines (doxycycline), the NSAIDs, and fluoroquinolones. Additionally, amiodarone, psoralens, phenothiazines, and oral retinoids can also lead to phototoxic eruptions.
  - Photoallergic drug eruptions are more chronic and pruritic than phototoxic drug eruptions. Lesions clinically may resemble dermatitis or lichen planus. The offending agent should be immediately removed to prevent long-term sequelae.
    - Common offenders include topical agents in soaps and fragrances. Systemic photoallergens include thiazide diuretics, sulfonamide antibiotics, and sulfonylureas. Additionally, quinine, quinidine, tricyclic antidepressants, and antimalarials are also culprits in photoallergic reactions.[50]
- **Fixed drug eruption (Fig. 5-8)**
  - Eruptions develop 1 to 2 weeks after first exposure and within 24 hours of subsequent exposures.
  - Clinically, these present as one or a few round sharply demarcated erythematous and edematous plaques with a violaceous hue, dusky color, central blister, or a detached epidermis.
  - Favored locations include the lips, hands, feet, and genitalia but can occur anywhere, and a reexposure to the offending agent leads to lesions *recurring at exactly the same location as previously affected sites*, hence the name "fixed drug." Additional sites may subsequently develop.
  - Commonly associated drugs: sulfonamides, NSAIDs, barbiturates, tetracyclines, and carbamazepines.

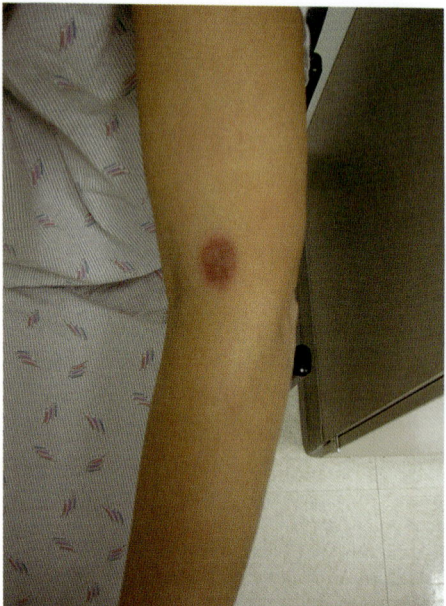

**Figure 5-8.** Fixed drug eruption.

- **Acute generalized exanthematous pustulosis (AGEP, Fig. 5-9)**
  - Rapid onset (24-48 hours) after drug exposure, characterized by multiple, nonfollicular sterile pustules, less than 5 mm in size, overlying areas of edematous erythema.
    - Common causal agents include antibiotics, particularly beta-lactams (penicillins, aminopenicillins, cephalosporins) and macrolides. Other common culprits are calcium channel blockers (diltiazem) and antimalarials. Although less common, other drugs have been implicated. Uncommon triggers include spider bites and mercury exposure.
  - May present with co-occurring or preceding high fever. The eruption begins on the face, axilla, and groin and then disseminates over the course of a few hours.
    - Rash may also present with edema of face and hands, vesicles, bullae, and purpura and can involve mucous membranes.
  - The main differential for AGEP is pustular psoriasis. A history can distinguish the two entities, with acute onset of the rash and use of a causative drug more consistent with AGEP. Additionally, skin biopsy findings are more likely to show dermal edema, keratinocyte necrosis, and exocytosis of eosinophils in AGEP versus acanthosis in pustular psoriasis.
- **Drug reaction with eosinophilia and systemic symptoms (DRESS)**
  - **Can also be referred to as drug-induced hypersensitivity syndrome (DIHS).**
    - Eosinophilia increases likelihood of DRESS/DIHS but is not required for diagnosis based on RegiSCAR Group.[51]
  - Develops 2 to 6 weeks after exposure to the drug as toxic drug metabolites are believed to be the cause. Symptoms after discontinuation of the medication, typically 2 weeks or longer.

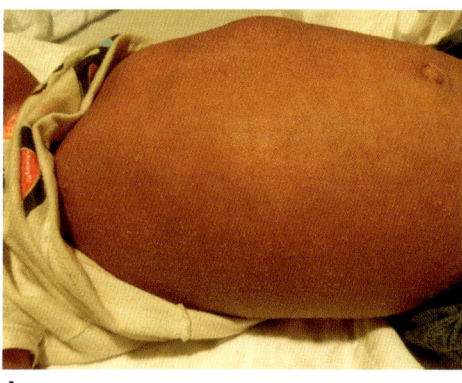

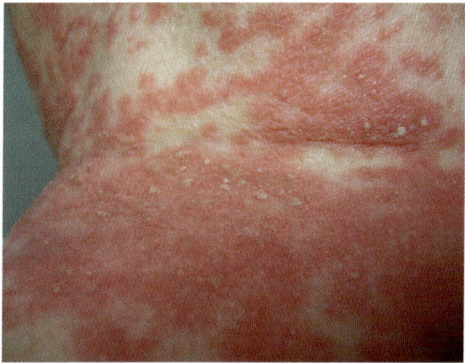

**Figure 5-9. A, B.** Acute generalized exanthematous pustulosis.

- Skin involvement begins as a morbilliform eruption, which later becomes edematous with follicular accentuation.
  - Other physical examination findings include edema affecting the face or upper extremities and lymphadenopathy.
- Systemic signs include fever greater than 38 °C, absolute eosinophilia (700-1,500+), multiorgan involvement, lymphocyte activation (lymphocytosis, atypical lymphocytes, lymphadenopathy), and viral reactivation (predominately HHV-6, but also cytomegalovirus, Epstein-Barr virus, and HHV-7).
- Severe liver involvement can occur, and this finding is associated with 10% of deaths in DIHS/DRESS.[52]
- Potential acute visceral complications of DIHS/DRESS include colitis, encephalitis, aseptic meningitis, interstitial nephritis, interstitial pneumonitis, sialadenitis, and myocarditis.
- Potential delayed complications of DIHS/DRESS include syndrome of inappropriate secretion of antidiuretic hormone, thyroiditis, diabetes mellitus, myocarditis, and rarely systemic lupus. Monitoring for these sequelae should occur during and for months after withdrawal of the offending agent.[53]

- The most common drug culprits include aromatic anticonvulsants (phenobarbital, carbamazepine, and phenytoin), lamotrigine (especially when coadministered with valproate), and sulfonamides.[54,55] However, in 10% to 20% of cases, the causal agent cannot be identified.
- Minocycline, allopurinol (especially in those with renal failure and HLA-5801), gold salts, dapsone, and abacavir (used to treat HIV) can also lead to DIHS/DRESS.
- Defects in drug metabolism (as in the detoxification of anticonvulsants and sulfonamides) have been seen in patients with DRESS. Immune mechanisms and the role of viral reactivation (HHV-6 and HHV-7) have also been implicated.

- **Anticoagulant-induced skin necrosis**
  - Warfarin necrosis begins 2 to 5 days after therapy and coincides with the expected drop in protein C function. This occurs as vitamin K-dependent anticoagulant factors (protein C) deplete more quickly than procoagulant factors (factors II, VII, IX, X) leading to a paradoxical hypercoagulable state, diffuse thrombosis with skin and potential limb necrosis.
  - Presents with erythematous, painful plaques that develop into hemorrhagic blisters and necrotic ulcers due to occlusive thrombi in the skin and subcutaneous tissues.
  - Most commonly affected areas include breasts, thighs, and buttock.
  - Patients with protein C deficiency are at higher risk of developing warfarin necrosis.
  - Heparin-induced cutaneous necrosis is due to antibodies that bind to complexes of heparin and platelet factor 4, leading to platelet aggregation and consumption, which cause thrombosis and cutaneous necrosis at site of injection and distant locations.

- **Stevens-Johnson syndrome (SJS)/toxic epidermal necrolysis (TEN) (Fig. 5-10)**
  - Rare, life-threatening, acute mucocutaneous diseases.
  - Keratinocyte cell death results in separation of significant areas of skin at the dermal-epidermal junction (denudation) and also affects the mucous membranes.
  - SJS—skin detachment is less than 10% body surface area (BSA), and SJS-TEN overlap 10% to 30% BSA, TEN greater than 30% BSA.
  - Initial symptoms can include fever, stinging eyes, and pain upon swallowing. These can occur 1 to 3 days prior to the onset of skin findings.
  - Skin findings will present initially on the trunk before spreading to the neck, face, and extremities, with palms and soles involved though distal arms are spared.

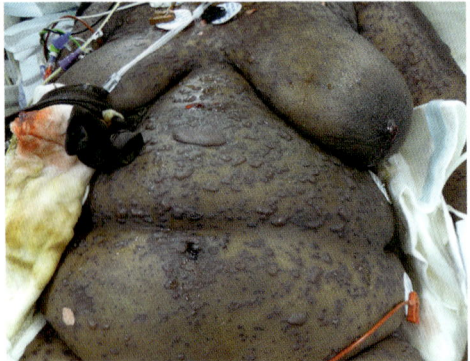

**Figure 5-10.** Toxic epidermal necrolysis. (Courtesy of Amy Musiek, MD.)

Oral, ocular, and genital mucosal involvement occurs in most patients, and 25% of TEN patients have respiratory tract involvement.
- The skin lesions are usually tender, and the mucosal erosions are painful. First, the skin lesions appear as erythematous, dusky, red, or purpuric macules of irregular size and shape. The addition of mucosal involvement, as well as tenderness, suggests progression to SJS and TEN.
- The Nikolsky sign—tangential mechanical pressure with a finger on erythematous zones, which leads to detachment of the epidermis and confirms diagnosis.
- Asboe-Hansen sign—placing pressure adjacent to the blister extends it laterally. Denudation or loss of the epidermal layer leaves a wet and bright red erosion.
- Pathology findings are similar between erythema multiforme and SJS/TEN, so clinical characteristics are what helps to distinguish the two.
- Medications most commonly associated with SJS/TEN: allopurinol, aminopenicillins, antiretroviral drugs, barbiturates, carbamazepine, chlormezanone, phenytoin antiepileptics, lamotrigine, phenylbutazone, piroxicam, sulfadiazine, sulfasalazine, and trimethoprim-sulfamethoxazole (see Table 5-2).[56,57]
- Occurs within 7 to 21 days after first exposure of the causative agent but can occur within 2 days after re-exposure. Reactions can present even if medication has been discontinued up to 2 weeks prior.

| TABLE 5-2 | Drug Eruptions | |
|---|---|---|
| Name of Drug Eruption | Onset From Medication Exposure | Responsible Medications |
| Exanthematous eruption | 4-14 d | Aminopenicillins<br>Sulfonamides<br>Cephalosporins<br>Anticonvulsants<br>Allopurinol |
| Urticaria<br>Anaphylaxis | Minutes to hours | Penicillins<br>Cephalosporins<br>NSAIDs<br>Monoclonal antibodies<br>Contrast media |
| Fixed drug eruption | First exposure: 1-2 wk<br>Reexposure: <48 h, usually 24 h | TMP-SMX<br>NSAIDs<br>Tetracyclines<br>Pseudoephedrine |
| Acute generalized exanthematous pustulosis (AGEP) | <4 d | β-Lactam antibiotics<br>Macrolides<br>Calcium channel blockers |
| Drug-induced hypersensitivity syndrome (DRESS) | 15-40 d | Anticonvulsants<br>Sulfonamides<br>Allopurinol<br>Minocycline<br>Lamotrigine |
| Stevens-Johnson syndrome (SJS)<br>Toxic epidermal necrolysis (TEN) | 7-21 d | Sulfonamides<br>Anticonvulsants<br>NSAIDs<br>Allopurinol |

## 5.3. EVALUATION

- Begin with obtaining a list of all the medications a patient is taking: prescription, nonprescription, and alternative medications. Note the dates of drug administration and the doses.
- Identify the time between initiation of the drug and onset of drug eruption (Table 5-2) (AGEP has a shorter time of onset vs DIHS).[52]
  - RegiSCAR Scoring System Predicts likelihood of DRESS diagnosis.
- The severity-of-illness score for toxic epidermal necrolysis (SCORTEN) scale is a TEN severity grading system that can help to predict mortality.[58]
  - SCORTEN—age greater than 40 years, heart rate greater than 120 beats per minute, malignancy, BSA on day 1 above 10%, serum urea level (>10 mmol/L), serum bicarbonate level (<20 mmol/L), and serum glucose level (>14 mmol/L). Each prognostic factor is a point, and 0 to 1 point portends a 3.2% mortality rate, whereas ≥5 portends a 90% mortality rate.
  - Additional marker of RDW/Hb ratio (higher ratio = worse prognosis) can be added to SCORTEN to increase predictability of mortality.

## 5.4. TREATMENT

- Depends on the severity of eruption
  - Discontinuation of inciting medication in severe eruptions—AGEP, DIHS, SJS, and TEN.
  - DRESS—systemic steroids are needed, and patients must avoid medications that cross-react. This is particularly important for aromatic anticonvulsants (phenytoin, carbamazepine, phenobarbitone).
  - AGEP—topical or systemic steroids.
  - SJS/TEN—wound care, electrolyte balance, nutritional support, short course steroids, cyclosporine, etanercept, and/or IVIG. Management of urogenital and ophthalmic complications needs to be monitored; transfer to burn unit when possible, may be beneficial. No conclusive best practices have established for management.
  - Photosensitizing eruptions—can continue treatment in phototoxic drug eruptions, but avoid UVR exposure, encourage photoprotection.

# REFERENCES

1. Deguchi E, Imafuku S, Nakayama J. Ulcerating stasis dermatitis of the forearm due to arteriovenous fistula: a case report and review of the published work. *J Dermatol.* 2010;37(6):550-553.
2. Beebe-Dimmer JL, Pfeifer JR, Engle JS, Schottenfeld D. The epidemiology of chronic venous insufficiency and varicose veins. *Ann Epidemiol.* 2005;15(3):175-184.
3. Silverberg J, Jackson JM, Kirsner RS, et al. Narrative review of the pathogenesis of stasis dermatitis: an inflammatory skin manifestation of venous hypertension. *Dermatol Ther (Heidelb).* 2023;13(4):935-950. doi:10.1007/s13555-023-00908-0. PMID: 36949275; PMCID: PMC10060486.
4. Yosipovitch G, Nedorost ST, Silverberg JI, Friedman AJ, Canosa JM, Cha A. Stasis dermatitis: an overview of its clinical presentation, pathogenesis, and management. *Am J Clin Dermatol.* 2023;24(2):275-286. doi:10.1007/s40257-022-00753-5. PMID: 36800152; PMCID: PMC9968263.
5. Barron GS, Jacob SE, Kirsner RS. Dermatologic complications of chronic venous disease: medical management and beyond. *Ann Vasc Surg.* 2007;21(5):652-662.
6. Keller EC, Tomecki KJ, Alraies MC. Distinguishing cellulitis from its mimics. *Cleve Clin J Med.* 2012;79(8):547-552.
7. David CV, Chira S, Eells SJ, et al. Diagnostic accuracy in patients admitted to hospitals with cellulitis. *Dermatol Online J.* 2011;17(3):1.

8. Partsch H. Compression therapy: clinical and experimental evidence. *Ann Vasc Dis.* 2012;5(4):416-422.
9. Word R. Medical and surgical therapy for advanced chronic venous insufficiency. *Surg Clin North Am.* 2010;90(6):1195-1214.
10. Gonzalez-Gay MA, Garcia-Porrua C, Pujol RM. Clinical approach to cutaneous vasculitis. *Curr Opin Rheumatol.* 2005;17(1):56-61.
11. Jennette JC, Falk RJ. The role of pathology in the diagnosis of systemic vasculitis. *Clin Exp Rheumatol.* 2007;25(1 suppl 44):S52-S56.
12. Jennette JC, Falk RJ, Bacon PA, et al. 2012 Revised International Chapel Hill Consensus Conference Nomenclature of Vasculitides. *Arthritis Rheum.* 2013;65(1):1-11.
13. Carlson JA, Ng BT, Chen K-R. Cutaneous vasculitis update: diagnostic criteria, classification, epidemiology, etiology, pathogenesis, evaluation and prognosis. *Am J Dermatopathol.* 2005;27(6):504-528.
14. Pickert A. An approach to vasculitis and vasculopathy. *Cutis.* 2012;89(5):E1-E3. PMID: 23967440.
15. Xu LY, Esparza EM, Anadkat MJ, Crone KG, Brasington RD. Cutaneous manifestations of vasculitis. *Semin Arthritis Rheum.* 2009;38(5):348-360.
16. Chen K-R, Carlson JA. Clinical approach to cutaneous vasculitis. *Am J Clin Dermatol.* 2008;9(2):71-92.
17. Chung C, Tumeh PC, Birnbaum R, et al. Characteristic purpura of the ears, vasculitis, and neutropenia—a potential public health epidemic associated with levamisole-adulterated cocaine. *J Am Acad Dermatol.* 2011;65(4):722-725.
18. Hoffman GS, Calabrese LH. Vasculitis: determinants of disease patterns. *Nat Rev Rheumatol.* 2014;10(8):454-462.
19. Marzano AV, Vezzoli P, Berti E. Skin involvement in cutaneous and systemic vasculitis. *Autoimmun Rev.* 2013;12(4):467-476.
20. Micheletti RG. Treatment of cutaneous vasculitis. *Front Med (Lausanne).* 2022;9:1059612. doi:10.3389/fmed.2022.1059612. PMID: 36465944; PMCID: PMC9716566.
21. Beltrani VS. Urticaria and angioedema. *Dermatol Clin.* 1996;14(1):171-198.
22. Kolkhir P, Giménez-Arnau AM, Kulthanan K, Peter J, Metz M, Maurer M. Urticaria. *Nat Rev Dis Primers.* 2022;8:61. https://doi.org/10.1038/s41572-022-00389-z
23. Sackesen C, Sekerel BE, Orhan F, Kocabas CN, Tuncer A, Adalioglu G. The etiology of different forms of urticaria in childhood. *Pediatr Dermatol.* 2004;21(2):102-108.
24. Kaplan AP, Greaves M. Pathogenesis of chronic urticaria. *Clin Exp Allergy.* 2009;39(6):777-787.
25. Dabija D, Tadi P, Danosos GN. Chronic urticaria [Updated 2023 Apr 17]. In: *StatPearls* [Internet]. StatPearls Publishing; 2024 Jan-. https://www.ncbi.nlm.nih.gov/books/NBK555910/
26. Federman DG, Kirsner RS, Moriarty JP, Concato J. The effect of antibiotic therapy for patients infected with *Helicobacter pylori* who have chronic urticaria. *J Am Acad Dermatol.* 2003;49(5):861-864.
27. Bozek A, Krajewska J, Filipowska B, et al. HLA status in patients with chronic spontaneous urticaria. *Int Arch Allergy Immunol.* 2010;153(4):419-423. doi:10.1159/000316354. PMID:20559009.
28. Vethachalam S, Persaud Y. Contact urticaria. [Updated 2023 Jul 31]. In: *StatPearls* [Internet]. StatPearls Publishing; 2024 Jan-. https://www.ncbi.nlm.nih.gov/books/NBK549890/
29. Zuberbier T, Aberer W, Asero R, et al. The EAACI/GA²LEN/EDF/WAO guideline for the definition, classification, diagnosis and management of urticaria. *Allergy.* 2018;73(7):1393-1414. doi:10.1111/all.13397 PMID:29336054.
30. Kolkhir P, Bonnekoh H, Kocatürk E, et al. Management of urticarial vasculitis: a worldwide physician perspective. *World Allergy Organ J.* 2020;13(3):100107. doi:10.1016/j.waojou.2020.100107. PMID: 32180892; PMCID: PMC7063238.
31. Joint Task Force on Practice Parameters. The diagnosis and management of urticaria: a practice parameter part I: acute urticaria/angioedema part II: chronic urticaria/angioedema. Joint Task Force on Practice Parameters. *Ann Allergy Asthma Immunol.* 2000;85(6 Pt 2):521-544.
32. Zuberbier T, Asero R, Bindslev-Jensen C, et al. EAACI/GA(2)LEN/EDF/WAO guideline: management of urticaria. *Allergy.* 2009;64(10):1427-1443.
33. Fedorowicz Z, van Zuuren EJ, Hu N. Histamine H2-receptor antagonists for urticaria. *Cochrane Database Syst Rev.* 2012;(3):CD008596.
34. Romano C, Sellitto A, De Fanis U, et al. Maintenance of remission with low-dose omalizumab in longlasting, refractory chronic urticaria. *Ann Allergy Asthma Immunol.* 2010;104(1):95-97.
35. Kaplan A, Ledford D, Ashby M, et al. Omalizumab in patients with symptomatic chronic idiopathic/spontaneous urticaria despite standard combination therapy. *J Allergy Clin Immunol.* 2013;132(1):101-109.
36. Biesbroeck L, Sidbury R. Viral exanthems: an update. *Dermatol Ther.* 2013;26(6):433-438.
37. Magel GD, Mendoza N, Digiorgio CM, Haitz KA, Lapolla WJ, Tyring SK. Vaccines in dermatological diseases. *G Ital Dermatol Venereol.* 2011;146(3):225-233.
38. Heininger U, Seward JF. Varicella. *Lancet.* 2006;368(9544):1365-1376.
39. Stone RC, Micali GA, Schwartz RA. Roseola infantum and its causal human herpesviruses. *Int J Dermatol.* 2014;53(4):397-403.
40. Yamanishi K, Okuno T, Shiraki K, et al. Identification of human herpesvirus-6 as a causal agent for exanthem subitum. *Lancet.* 1988;1(8594):1065-1067.

41. Litchman G, Nair PA, Le JK. Pityriasis rosea. [Updated 2022 Jul 18]. In: *StatPearls* [Internet]. StatPearls Publishing; 2024 Jan-. https://www.ncbi.nlm.nih.gov/books/NBK448091/
42. Drago F, Broccolo F, Rebora A. Pityriasis rosea: an update with a critical appraisal of its possible herpesviral etiology. *J Am Acad Dermatol.* 2009;61(2):303-318.
43. Wolz MM, Sciallis GF, Pittelkow MR. Human herpesviruses 6, 7, and 8 from a dermatologic perspective. *Mayo Clin Proc.* 2012;87(10):1004-1014.
44. Drago F, Broccolo F, Javor S, Drago F, Rebora A, Parodi A. Evidence of human herpesvirus-6 and -7 reactivation in miscarrying women with pityriasis rosea. *J Am Acad Dermatol.* 2014;71(1):198-199.
45. Ayoade F, Kumar S. Varicella-zoster virus (chickenpox) [Updated 2022 Oct 15]. *StatPearls [Internet].* StatPearls Publishing; 2024. https://www.ncbi.nlm.nih.gov/books/NBK448191/
46. Guerra AM, Orille E, Waseem M. Hand, foot, and mouth disease [Updated 2023 Mar 4]. *StatPearls [Internet].* StatPearls Publishing; 2024. https://www.ncbi.nlm.nih.gov/books/NBK431082/
47. Pan D, Wang W, Cheng T. Current methods for the detection of antibodies of varicella-zoster virus: a review. Microorganisms. 2023;11(2):519. doi:10.3390/microorganisms11020519. PMID: 36838484; PMCID: PMC9965970.
48. Andrei G, Snoeck R. Advances in the treatment of varicella-zoster virus infections. *Adv Pharmacol.* 2013;67:107-168.
49. Gershon AA, Gershon MD. Pathogenesis and current approaches to control of varicella-zoster virus infections. *Clin Microbiol Rev.* 2013;26(4):728-743.
50. Monteiro AF, Rato M, Martins C. Drug-induced photosensitivity: photoallergic and phototoxic reactions. *Clin Dermatol.* 2016;34(5):571-581. doi:10.1016/j.clindermatol.2016.05.006. PMID:27638435.
51. Calle AM, Aguirre N, Ardila JC, Villa RC. DRESS syndrome: a literature review and treatment algorithm. *World Allergy Organ J.* 2023;16(3):100673. doi:10.1016/j.waojou.2022.100673. PMID: 37082745; PMCID: PMC10112187.
52. Lee T, Lee YS, Yoon S-Y, et al. Characteristics of liver injury in drug-induced systemic hypersensitivity reactions. *J Am Acad Dermatol.* 2013;69(3):407-415.
53. Ushigome Y, Kano Y, Ishida T, Hirahara K, Shiohara T. Short- and long-term outcomes of 34 patients with drug-induced hypersensitivity syndrome in a single institution. *J Am Acad Dermatol.* 2013;68(5):721-728.
54. Husain Z, Reddy BY, Schwartz RA. DRESS syndrome: part I. Clinical perspectives. *J Am Acad Dermatol.* 2013;68(5):693.e1-693.e14. quiz 706-708.
55. Husain Z, Reddy BY, Schwartz RA. DRESS syndrome: part II. Management and therapeutics. *J Am Acad Dermatol.* 2013;68(5):709.e1-709.e9. quiz 718-720.
56. Schwartz RA, McDonough PH, Lee BW. Toxic epidermal necrolysis: part I. Introduction, history, classification, clinical features, systemic manifestations, etiology, and immunopathogenesis. *J Am Acad Dermatol.* 2013;69(2):173.e1-173.e13. quiz 185-186.
57. Schwartz RA, McDonough PH, Lee BW. Toxic epidermal necrolysis: part II. Prognosis, sequelae, diagnosis, differential diagnosis, prevention, and treatment. *J Am Acad Dermatol.* 2013;69(2):187.e1-187.e16. quiz 203-204.
58. Koh HK, Fook-Chong SMC, Lee HY. Improvement of mortality prognostication in patients with epidermal necrolysis: the role of novel inflammatory markers and proposed revision of SCORTEN (Re-SCORTEN). *JAMA Dermatol.* 2022;158(2):160-166. doi:10.1001/jamadermatol.2021.5119. PMID: 34935871; PMCID: PMC8696686.

# Disorders of Pigmentation

Cynthia Chen, BS, Caroline Mann, MD, and Sunaina Rengarajan, MD, PhD

Disorders of pigmentation can manifest as light or dark areas of the skin or as hyperpigmentation or depigmentation of the entire skin surface. Although not typically harmful, these changes can have a significant psychosocial impact on affected patients.

## 1. Vitiligo

- Vitiligo is an acquired condition characterized by circumscribed areas of depigmentation due to loss of epidermal melanocytes.

### 1.1. BACKGROUND

- Epidemiology
  - Can occur at any age but most commonly occurs during the second and third decades.
  - Prevalence is estimated to be 0.5% to 2% overall and equal in men and women.[1,2]
- Pathogenesis
  - There are likely multiple pathogenic mechanisms, which all lead to the loss of melanocytes. The autoimmune destruction of melanocytes is the mechanism that has the most supporting evidence.
  - Other hypotheses include melanocyte adhesion defects, genetic risk alleles, and melanocyte oxidative stress.[3-5]
    - Several genes associated with the pathogenesis of vitiligo include *XBP1*, *NLRP1*, *FOXD3*, *PDGFRA*, and many HLA genes, which are involved in regulating immune system activation, cellular response to stress, regulating melanoblast differentiation, and/or conferring risk for vitiligo and other autoimmune diseases.[6-10]
  - Recurrence of vitiligo in previously affected skin suggests a role of resident memory T cells.[11]

### 1.2. CLINICAL PRESENTATION

- Clinical Features
  Completely amelanotic (milk- or chalk-white) macules and patches with well-defined, convex borders that may be round, oval, irregular, or linear in shape and are surrounded by normal skin (Fig. 6-1).
  - Can be subtle in light-skinned individuals and is accentuated or becomes apparent with tanning.
  - Often occur in areas of trauma (Koebner phenomenon) such as surgical sites or thermal burns.

---

*The authors would like to acknowledge the first edition author Shaanan Shetty.*

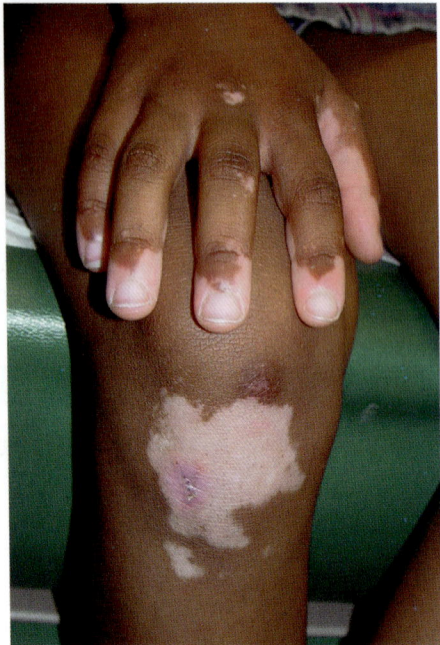

**Figure 6-1.** Depigmented vitiligo patches on knees and hands.

- Common locations include periocular skin, perioral skin, nipples, axillae, umbilicus, dorsal hands, digits, flexor wrists, elbows, knees, and sacral, inguinal, and anogenital regions.
- Loss of pigment in hairs within areas of vitiligo (leukotrichia) can also occur due to loss of follicular melanocytes.
- Classification[12,13]
  - Two main classifications: segmental and nonsegmental
  - Segmental vitiligo: characterized by unilateral segmental patches with abrupt midline demarcation (Fig. 6-2); tends to present early, stabilizes rapidly, and is often associated with leukotrichia (Fig. 6-3)
    - Nonsegmental vitiligo (NSV):
      - Acrofacial—depigmented patches limited to the face, head, and distal extremities
      - Mucosal—affects more than one mucosal site
      - Generalized (vulgaris)—scattered and widely distributed patches that do not follow a pattern (Fig. 6-4)
      - Universal—total or near-total depigmentation of skin (>80% of the body surface area involved)
    - Undetermined vitiligo
      - Focal—single depigmented macule or patch without a segmental distribution (Fig. 6-5)
      - Mucosal—when affecting *one site in isolation*
      - Mixed—combination of segmental and nonsegmental subtypes

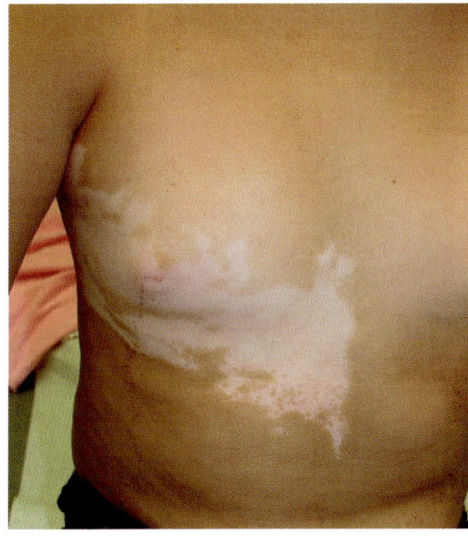

**Figure 6-2.** Segmental vitiligo depigmented patch on the chest.

- Variants
  - Follicular vitiligo—leukotrichia without depigmentation of epidermis.[14]
  - Blue vitiligo—vitiligo that develops in areas with postinflammatory hyperpigmentation. The presence of dermal melanin gives lesions a blue-gray appearance.
  - Inflammatory vitiligo—vitiligo macule with erythematous raised borders.
  - Trichrome vitiligo—an intermediate hypopigmented zone is present between normal skin and depigmented skin.
  - Vitiligo ponctué—multiple, small, discrete amelanotic macules (confetti-like) that can occur within normal or hyperpigmented skin.

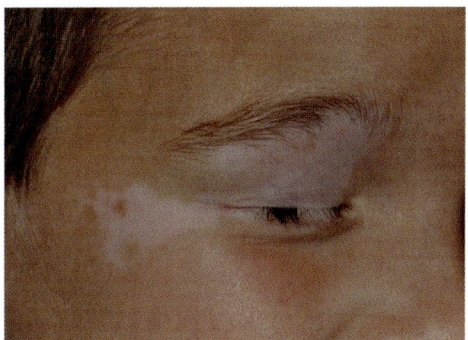

**Figure 6-3.** Segmental vitiligo depigmented patch associated with leukotrichia.

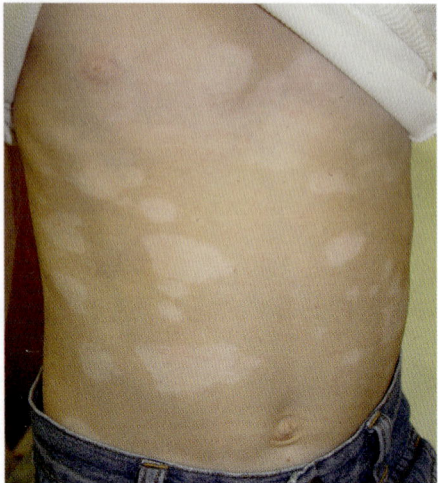

**Figure 6-4.** Scattered, generalized depigmented vitiligo patches on the chest.

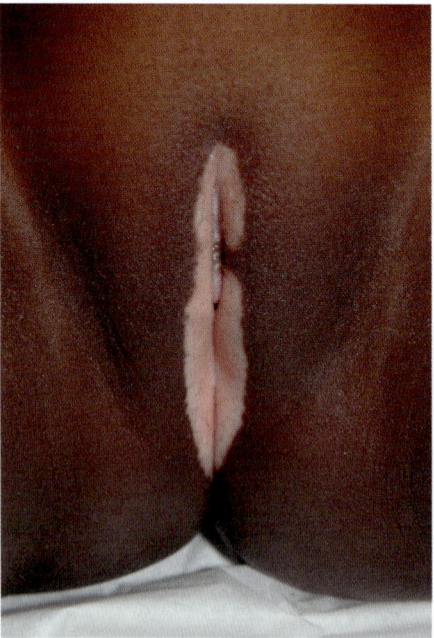

**Figure 6-5.** Focal vitiligo depigmented patch on the labia.

- Hypopigmented vitiligo—described in patients with skin phototypes V and VI[15]; persistent hypopigmented macules presenting in seborrheic distribution, with coalescing lesions on the face, neck, trunk, and scalp.
- Course
  - NSV typically presents with insidious onset and a chronic course.[16]
  - Segmental vitiligo is characterized by early onset, rapid stabilization, and reaching its full extent within 1 to 2 years and is typically less responsive to medical treatment than NSV.[17]
  - Most appreciable in summer due to the contrast between depigmented skin and uninvolved, tanned skin.
  - Course varies significantly between individuals—slow progression is most common.
  - Without treatment, complete, stable repigmentation is rare. Some degree of repigmentation can occur spontaneously or with sun exposure.

## 1.3. EVALUATION

- Diagnosis
  - Can usually be made based on physical examination and history alone.
  - A Wood lamp can help in evaluating the extent of involvement.
  - Biopsy may be useful in less obvious cases. The biopsy will reveal the absence or low presence of melanocytes, where melanocyte density can be evaluated with melanocyte-specific immunohistochemical stains.
- Associated disorders
  - Associated with higher frequency of autoimmune thyroid diseases (autoimmune thyroiditis, hypothyroidism, hyperthyroidism, Graves disease, Hashimoto thyroiditis), metabolic disease (metabolic syndrome, diabetes mellitus), and allergic and dermatologic diseases such as psoriasis and atopic dermatitis.[18]
  - Studies demonstrate a range of prevalences for each of these diseases in vitiligo patients that vary by geographic population studied[19,20]: subclinical hyperthyroidism—2% to 8%; overt hyperthyroidism—7% to 30%; subclinical hypothyroidism—1% to 13%; Graves disease—3% to 10%; Hashimoto thyroiditis—2% to 11%; diabetes mellitus—1% to 7%; psoriasis—2% to 8%; atopic dermatitis—3% to 8%.

## 1.4. TREATMENT

- Younger patients and patients with dark skin are most likely to respond to treatment.
- The face, neck, mid-extremities, and trunk are generally the most responsive areas, whereas the distal extremities and lips are often the least responsive.
- Repigmentation tends to spread from the hair follicle or the periphery of lesions or in a combined pattern.
- Generally, treatment must be trialed for at least 6 months to determine treatment efficacy.
- Treatment algorithm[21]:
  - For stabilization or repigmentation of a disease that has been active in last 12 months:
    - Topical treatment with corticosteroids or immunomodulators
    - Targeted phototherapy (narrowband UVB [NBUVB])
    - Optional for nonsegmental vitiligo: systemic treatment with oral steroid mini-pulse (most investigated), methotrexate, cyclosporine, azathioprine, minocycline, and Janus kinase (JAK) inhibitors (currently investigated)

- For management of disease that has been stable for 6 months:
  - Maintenance treatment with topical corticosteroids/immunomodulators for nonsegmental vitiligo and clinical follow-up for segmental vitiligo
- For repigmentation of disease that has been stable for 12 months and resistant to topical treatment and/or phototherapy:
  - Optional: surgical techniques
- For depigmentation of disease that has been active/stable for 6 months:
  - Monobenzone
  - Pigment laser
  - Cryotherapy
- Corticosteroids
  - Topical corticosteroids are often used as first-line therapy and tend to have the highest response rates in newer lesions and lesions on the face and neck.
  - They are most useful for localized areas of involvement.
  - Side effects like dyspigmentation, striae, and atrophy can be minimized by not using them continuously.
  - More effective when combined with phototherapy.
- Topical calcineurin inhibitors
  - Efficacy similar to or slightly less than corticosteroids for lesions on the face and neck
  - More effective when combined with phototherapy
  - Can be alternated with topical corticosteroids on a rotating basis or used as maintenance therapy after repigmentation
- Topical JAK inhibitors
  - Topical JAK1/2 inhibitor (ruxolitinib) was FDA approved in 2022 for NSV affecting less than 10% of body surface area in patients ≥12 years old.
  - No randomized studies exist, but repigmentation rates and times with ruxolitinib appear similar to topical steroids and calcineurin inhibitors.
  - Generally used as second-line after corticosteroid or calcineurin inhibitor therapy.
  - Side effects include application site acne or erythema, pruritus, nasopharyngitis.[22]
- Phototherapy
  - Generally useful for more extensive cases. Administered two times to three times per week and may require 6 months to 2 years of treatment.
  - NBUVB[23]
    - Preferred first-line therapy for generalized or rapidly progressive vitiligo.
    - Starting dose and dose increments are based on patient's phototype and response.
    - Can be used in children, pregnant or lactating women, and individuals with hepatic or kidney dysfunction.
    - Home NBUVB units can increase patient compliance, though are expensive.
  - Excimer laser or lamp
    - Wavelength is close to NBUVB with equal to superior efficacy compared to NBUVB.[24,25]
    - Shorter duration of treatment than NBUVB and avoids darkening of unaffected skin.[23]
    - Primarily indicated for treating segmental vitiligo and other forms involving localized disease.[23]
  - Psoralen plus ultraviolet light therapy
    - No longer recommended for vitiligo considering the greater efficacy, ease of administration, and lack of systemic side effects of NBUVB but can be used for localized lesions

- Oral corticosteroid mini-pulse therapy
  - Indicated for rapidly progressive vitiligo, though investigation regarding efficacy and safety is needed.
  - Oral mini-pulses of betamethasone (5 mg) or dexamethasone (2.5-5 mg depending on body weight) twice weekly on 2 consecutive days per week for up to 3 to 6 months maximum. Alternatives to dexamethasone include methylprednisolone, prednisone, and prednisolone.[23]
- Investigational therapy: oral JAK inhibitors
  - Indicated for rapidly progressive vitiligo, but further investigation regarding efficacy and safety is needed.
  - Recently, a randomized phase 2b clinical trial in which patients with vitiligo received 200/50 mg oral ritlecitinib for 24 weeks with or without a 4-week loading dose demonstrated that oral ritlecitinib was effective and well-tolerated over 48 weeks in patients with active nonsegmental vitiligo.[26]
- Investigational therapy: afamelanotide (melanocyte-stimulating hormone analog)
  - When used in combination with NBUVB, afamelanotide has been shown to induce increased speed and extent of repigmentation in comparison to NBUVB therapy alone in patients with generalized vitiligo.[27]
  - However, afamelanotide-induced tanning in nonlesional skin can further accentuate the contrast with lesional, depigmented skin, particularly in patients with darker skin types.[28]
- Surgical therapies
  - Should be considered in patients with stable lesions that have been unresponsive to other treatments.
  - Techniques include blister grafting, punch grafting, autologous melanocyte suspension transplant, and grafting of individual hair to repigment vitiligo leukotrichia.
- Micropigmentation
  - Permanent dermal micropigmentation technique that utilizes a nonallergenic iron oxide to camouflage refractory areas of vitiligo
- Depigmentation
  - 20% monobenzyl ether of hydroquinone can be useful for patients with widespread involvement and few uninvolved sites.
  - Loss of pigmentation can occur at sites other than those that are treated.
  - Depigmentation is usually permanent, though repigmentation can sometimes occur with sun exposure.
- Camouflage
  - Options include makeup, self-tanning agents, and tattoos (see micropigmentation above). May help provide temporary or long-term relief.

## 2. Melasma

### 2.1. BACKGROUND

- Epidemiology
  - Most prevalent in young to middle-aged women with dark skin types including individuals who are Hispanic, Black, or of Asian or Middle Eastern descent
  - More common in women than in men
- Pathogenesis
  - It is hypothesized that UV irradiation or other triggering factors (pregnancy, oral contraceptive pills) cause hyperfunctional melanocytes to increase melanin production.

- Other proposed mechanisms of melasma include solar elastosis and increased mast cell presence with resultant hypervascularization and basement membrane damage.[29]
- Exacerbating factors include pregnancy, oral contraceptive pills, and sunlight.

## 2.2. CLINICAL PRESENTATION

- Characterized by light to dark brown or brown-gray macules and patches with irregular borders (Fig. 6-6).
- The face is most commonly affected and can display the following patterns:
  - Centrofacial (most common)—forehead, cheeks, nose, upper lip, chin
  - Malar—cheeks/nose
  - Mandibular—along jawline
- Less common sites of involvement include the extensor forearms and mid-upper chest.
- Often first appears or is first noticed with significant UV exposure or with pregnancy.
- Under the Wood lamp examination, melasma lesions with dermal melanin pigmentation are expected to appear blue or blend into unaffected skin, whereas melasma lesions with epidermal melanin pigmentation are expected to be further accentuated. However, further studies are needed to substantiate the clinical utility of the Wood lamp and its clinicopathologic correlations in assessing melasma lesions.

## 2.3. TREATMENT

- Sun protection, including sun-protective clothing, broad-spectrum sunscreen with physical blocker, and sun avoidance, can help prevent melasma. It is also essential for any other treatment to be effective.

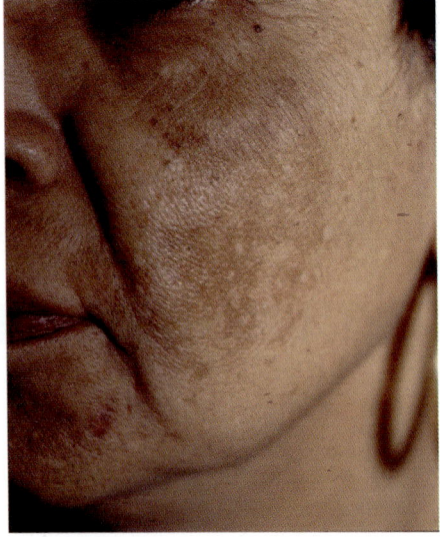

**Figure 6-6.** Melasma—brown macules and patches on the face.

- Combination products[30,31]
  - For moderate to severe melasma or mild melasma refractive to hydroquinone monotherapy, treat with triple combination therapy of hydroquinone, a retinoid, and a low-potency steroid.
  - Triple combination therapy is more effective in improving and clearing melasma than hydroquinone monotherapy (particularly in patients with darker skin tones) or any dual-combination of hydroquinone, retinoid, and/or topical steroid.[32-34]
  - May add a non–hydroquinone-based topical maintenance medication such as azelaic acid, kojic acid, niacinamide, and/or tranexamic acid (TXA) to reduce daily topical hydroquinone application.
  - Common side effects include erythema, scaling, dryness, burning sensation, and pruritus. Skin atrophy and telangiectasias may also result from prolonged steroid use.
- Hydroquinone[30,31]
  - Hydroquinone inhibits tyrosinase and is available in concentrations from 2% to 4%.
  - The most commonly reported short-term adverse effect associated with hydroquinone 4% or greater is an irritant contact dermatitis characterized by erythema, burning sensation, pruritus, and scaling.
  - Prolonged use can lead to hyperpigmentation (exogenous ochronosis).
- Topical retinoids[35]
  - Mechanisms of action thought to include tyrosinase inhibition, increased keratinocyte turnover, decreased melanosome transfer, melanin dispersion, and allowing other agents to more easily penetrate the stratum corneum.
  - Tretinoin is not as efficacious as hydroquinone monotherapy but can increase the effectiveness of and reduce the side effects of low concentration hydroquinone when used concomitantly.
  - Minimum treatment duration greater than 24 weeks to see improvement.
  - Adverse effects include erythema, dryness, flaking, photosensitivity, and sensations of burning and stinging but are generally well tolerated.
- Azelaic acid[31,35]
  - Inhibits tyrosinase.
  - Studies suggest that azelaic acid 20% cream is comparable or superior to hydroquinone 2% cream in reducing skin hyperpigmentation, but larger and randomized trials are needed to compare treatment efficacy.[36,37]
  - Due to its limited water solubility and poor skin permeability, azelaic acid is formulated at higher concentrations (10%-20%) to achieve desired clinical effects.
  - Generally well-tolerated. Most common side effects are mild, temporary, and include burning, itching, stinging, dryness, and erythema.
- Kojic acid[31,35]
  - Inhibits tyrosinase.
  - Studies suggest kojic acid as adjuvant therapy to enhance clinical efficacy of hydroquinone cream.
  - Kojic acid 1% or less is well-tolerated for up to 2 years, and the most common adverse reaction is irritant contact dermatitis characterized by localized pain, edema and pruritus.
- Glycolic acid[31,35]
  - An alpha-hydroxy acid that disrupts cell-adhesion, promoting skin desquamation, and inhibits tyrosinase activity.
  - May enhance the clinical effectiveness of hydroquinone, particularly in individuals with darker skin tones.
  - Adverse effects include mild to moderate erythema, pruritus, and inflammation.

- Salicylic acid[31]
  - A beta-hydroxy acid, lipid-soluble agent with keratolytic, antibacterial, and anti-inflammatory properties.
  - In a small prospective RCT, no difference in efficacy was seen between melasma lesions treated with salicylic acid peels and hydroquinone 4% cream versus hydroquinone 4% cream alone.[38]
  - Adverse reactions include erythema, burning sensation, irritation, peeling, blistering, and crusting. Contraindicated in pregnancy.
- Niacinamide (vitamin B3)[31]
  - Downregulates melanosome transfer from melanocytes to keratinocytes, thereby reducing accumulation of melanin in skin, and has anti-inflammatory and photoprotective properties.
  - Generally well-tolerated, and most common adverse reactions are mild burning, erythema, and pruritus.
- TXA (oral)[30,31,35]
  - An anti-fibrinolytic agent that inhibits plasminogen activator and interferes with the plasminogen/plasmin pathway, causing subsequent reduction in melanogenic factors.
  - For severe or refractory melasma, oral TXA 325 mg BID until maximum improvement achieved then taper to 325 mg QD for another 3 months to maintain results.
  - A randomized, placebo-controlled trial has shown benefit of 250 mg oral TXA twice daily for 1 month in reducing melasma severity in patients with moderate to severe melasma.[39]
  - Common adverse effects include heartburn, nausea, gastrointestinal discomfort, abdominal pain, and change in menstrual period.[30,39] Low risk of thrombotic events or relapse of hyperpigmentation with discontinuation.
  - Contraindicated in pregnant patients, patients trying to conceive, patients taking oral contraceptive pills, and patients with history of venous or arterial thromboembolism.[39]
- Chemical peels[31,35]
  - May be useful for patients who do not respond to skin-lightening agents or as treatment complementary to ongoing management of melasma.
  - Chemical peel options include glycolic acid, salicylic acid, or trichloroacetic acid.
  - Chemical peels can cause irritation, burning, and inflammation, leading to postinflammatory hyperpigmentation, especially in darker skin types. Often used concomitantly with skin-lightening agents to decrease this risk.
- Microneedling
  - Procedure that elicits physiological reaction by inducing wound repairment process and collagen and elastin synthesis
  - Suggested as a useful adjuvant to melasma topical therapies[40]

## 3. Oculocutaneous Albinism

### 3.1. BACKGROUND

- Approximately 1 in 17,000 to 20,000 people are affected worldwide with higher prevalence rates in African countries.[41,42]
- Due to defects in the melanin synthesis pathway leading to decreased melanin. Well-characterized forms are inherited in an autosomal recessive manner.

## 3.2. CLINICAL PRESENTATION

- Characterized by decreased or absent melanin with a normal number of melanocytes in the skin, hair, and eyes starting at birth.
- Ocular findings can include decreased visual acuity, photophobia, strabismus, and nystagmus.
- Patients are sensitive to sunlight and are at increased risk for skin cancers, particularly in those with minimal or no pigmentation.[42]

## 3.3. SUBTYPES

- Subtypes can be differentiated based on clinical features and genetic testing.
- Oculocutaneous albinism (OCA) types 1 and 2 are the most common forms worldwide.
- OCA type 1A (OCA1A) is the most severe form and is due to a complete loss of tyrosinase activity. Characterized by lack of pigment in skin and hair with blue-gray eyes at birth. Individuals with OCA1A may develop yellow-tinted hair with age due to hair keratin denaturation. Reduced visual acuity is most severe in individuals with OCA1A.[42]
- OCA type 1B (OCA1B) is due to decreased levels of tyrosinase. Usually with lack of pigment in skin and hair with blue eyes at birth. May eventually have increased pigment in skin, hair, and eyes during the first and second decades of life.[42]
- OCA type 2—due to mutations in the *OCA2* gene. Has a variable clinical phenotype—can vary from almost normal pigmentation to almost no pigmentation. Individuals with OCA type 2 may develop pigmented melanocytic nevi and lentigines in sun-exposed areas with time. Prader-Willi syndrome and Angelman syndrome, which present with hypopigmentation, have deletions involving the *OCA2* gene.[42]
- OCA type 3—due to mutations in tyrosinase-related protein 1 (TYRP1) gene. OCA type 3 is most common in Black individuals. Most common phenotype known as "rufous" and is characterized by red-bronze skin color, ginger-red hair, and blue or brown irides[42] (Fig. 6-7).
- OCA type 4—due to mutation in *SLC45A2* gene with a variable clinical phenotype. Hair color ranges from white to yellow brown, and patients may or may not increase pigmentation of skin and hair over time. Most common in individuals with albinism from Japan, China, or India.[42]
- OCA type 5—linked to chromosome 4q24, but exact gene has not yet been identified. OCA type 6—due to mutations in *SLC2A45*; OCA type 7—due to mutations in *LRMDA*; OCA type 8—due to mutations in *DCT (TYRP2)*.[43] Rare presentations.

## 3.4. TREATMENT

- Photoprotection should be strongly encouraged.
- All patients should undergo ophthalmologic evaluation early in life with continued, long-term care as needed.[42]
- Nitisinone is an FDA-approved inhibitor of tyrosine degradation and may prove to be a potential therapy for OCA1B patients. After 1 year of treatment with oral nitisinone, five patients with OCA1B had increased visual acuity, skin pigmentation, and hair pigmentation.[44]

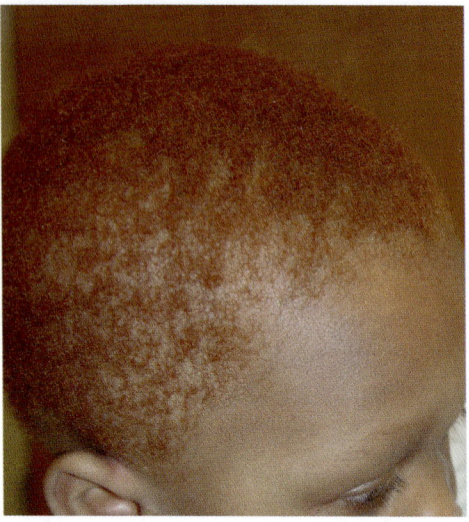

**Figure 6-7.** Red-bronze hair associated with OCA type 3.

# 4. Dermal Melanocytosis (Fig. 6-8)

## 4.1. CONGENITAL DERMAL MELANOCYTOSIS (MONGOLIAN SPOT)

- Most common in individuals with darker skin types including those of Asian and African descent.
- Due to presence of sparse dendritic melanocytes in the deep dermis.
- Characterized by blue to blue-gray patch or patches up to several centimeters in size. Most common locations include the lumbosacral area, buttocks, and back.
- Usually presents at birth or soon after and generally fades during childhood.[45]

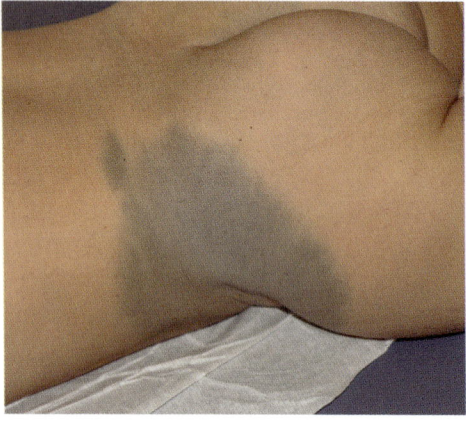

**Figure 6-8.** Dermal melanocytosis—blue-gray patch on the hip.

Chapter 6 • Disorders of Pigmentation | 137

## 4.2. NEVUS OF OTA

- Predominantly affects individuals with more pigmented skin, most commonly Asians. Majority of reported cases have occurred in women.
- Characterized histologically by scattered, pigmented, elongated dendritic melanocytes trapped between collagen bundles in the upper dermis. More dermal dendritic melanocytes are present than in dermal melanocytosis but less than in blue nevus.
- Characterized by blue to blue-black to blue-brown or slate-gray macules and patches in the V1 or V2 distribution of the face. Usually unilateral but can also be bilateral. Most patients also have involvement of the ipsilateral sclera. Some patients may develop glaucoma (Fig. 6-9).
- Most common ages of onset include infancy and puberty. Lesions tend to be persistent and may vary or darken in color with hormonal changes.[45]
- Melanoma develops rarely within these lesions, most often in the choroid, orbit, or meninges.[46]
  - The majority of melanomas associated are ocular melanomas, presenting either retro-orbitally (within the intraconal space) or within the choroid layer (uveal tract).
  - Melanoma in the skin often presents as a subcutaneous nodule.
  - Also associated with central nervous system melanomas.
- Acquired bilateral nevus of Ota-like macules (ABNOM; Hori nevus) are characterized by blue-gray to gray-brown macules acquired primarily in the bilateral malar areas and, less often, on the forehead, upper outer eyelids, and nose.[47]
- Q-switched lasers have been used to treat these lesions. In a case series, using picosecond laser to treat three Asian women with ABNOM was shown to improve the appearance of ABNOM.[48]

## 4.3. NEVUS OF ITO

- Has similar clinical appearance and histology as nevus of Ota but with a different distribution along lateral cutaneous brachial and posterior supraclavicular nerves and involves the supraclavicular, scapular, shoulder, and lateral neck regions[45] (Fig. 6-10)

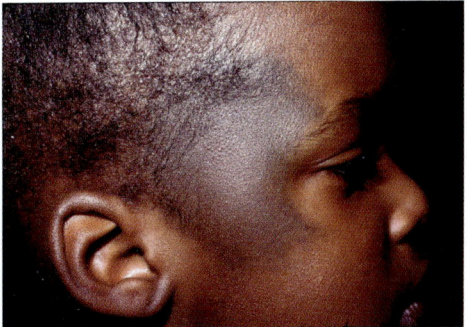

**Figure 6-9.** Blue-black nevus of Ota patch on V1-V2 distribution on the face.

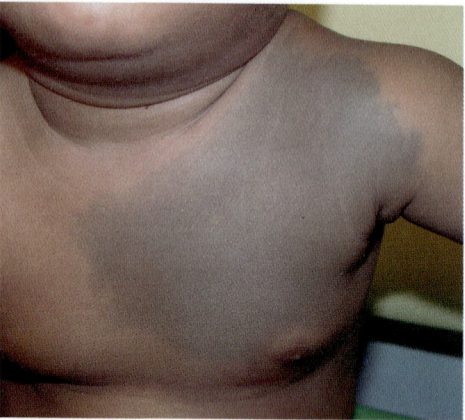

Figure 6-10. Blue-gray nevus of Ito patch on the unilateral shoulder and chest.

# 5. Drug-Induced Pigmentation

- Many medications and heavy metals can cause pigmentation changes.
- Pigmentation can be due to a combination of increased melanin, drug complex deposition, or heavy metal deposition.
- Involvement can be widespread or focal and can involve extracutaneous sites including the nails, mucosa, and sclera.
- In some cases, drug discontinuation leads to resolution.

## 5.1. COMMONLY IMPLICATED DRUGS/METALS

- Chemotherapeutic drugs: BCNU (carmustine), bleomycin, busulfan, cyclophosphamide, dactinomycin, daunorubicin, doxorubicin, 5-fluorouracil, hydroxyurea, imatinib (also dasatinib, gefitinib), mechlorethamine (nitrogen mustard), methotrexate
- Heavy metals: arsenic, bismuth, gold, iron, lead, mercury, silver
- Hormones: oral contraceptives, adrenocorticotropic hormone (ACTH)/melanocyte-stimulating hormone (MSH)
- Antimalarials: chloroquine, hydroxychloroquine, and quinacrine
- Tricyclic antidepressants/phenothiazines: amitriptyline, chlorpromazine, clomipramine, desipramine, imipramine, thioridazine
- Others: amiodarone, clofazimine, diltiazem, dioxins, eltrombopag, hydroquinone, interferon-alpha, imatinib, minocycline, nicotine, psoralens, prostaglandins, zidovudine

## 5.2. NOTABLE DRUGS/METALS AND THEIR PATTERN OF INVOLVEMENT

- Antimalarials—gray to blue-black pigmentation most commonly involving shins. Can also involve face, sclerae, oral mucosa, subungual areas, and extremities. Quinacrine is concentrated in the epidermis and can cause yellow to yellow-brown discoloration of skin and sclera (Fig. 6-11).

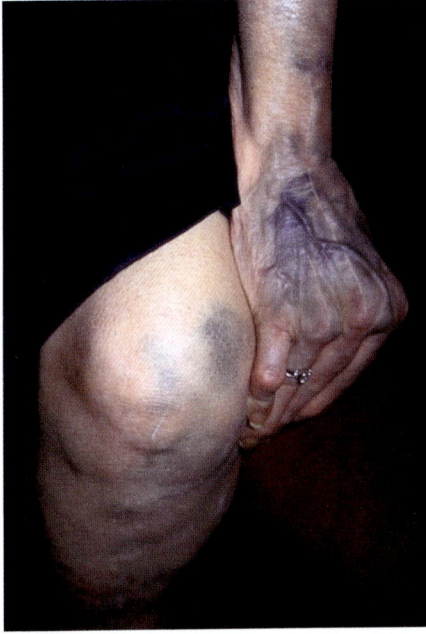

**Figure 6-11.** Gray-black quinacrine associated dyspigmentation on hands, forearms, and thighs.

- Amiodarone—photosensitivity leading to slate-gray to violaceous hyperpigmentation in sun-exposed areas.
- Hydroquinone—continuous topical application can lead to paradoxical hyperpigmentation (exogenous ochronosis).
- Minocycline—three patterns classically described. Type I with blue-black discoloration in areas of scarring and inflammation including acne scars, sarcoidal plaques, or surgical scars. Type II characterized by blue-gray pigmentation of the shins. Minocycline types I and II pigmentation can also affect the sclera, conjunctiva, bone, thyroid, ear cartilage, nail bed, oral mucosa, and permanent teeth. Type III described as a generalized "muddy brown" discoloration that is worse in sun-exposed areas (Fig. 6-12).
- Prostaglandin analogues—ophthalmic solutions used for glaucoma can lead to periocular hyperpigmentation and pigmentation of the iris.
- Silver (argyria)—diffuse slate-gray or blue-gray pigmentation that is accentuated in sun-exposed areas and is permanent. Occurs in two forms: local and systemic.
  - Local argyria is due to topical use of silver sulfadiazine or silver-containing dressings and clinically presents as blue-gray pigmentation at the site of application.
  - Systemic argyria can result from topical application (in patients with burn and epidermolysis bullosa), inhalation, mucosal application, or ingestion. Clinically presents as slate-gray or blue-gray skin, primarily in sun-exposed areas.
- Zidovudine (AZT)—blue or brown hyperpigmentation most commonly in nails. Diffuse hyperpigmentation, pigmentation of the lateral tongue, and increased tanning can occur as well. More commonly affects darker skin types. Hyperpigmentation is dose-dependent but will clear after discontinuing medication.[49]

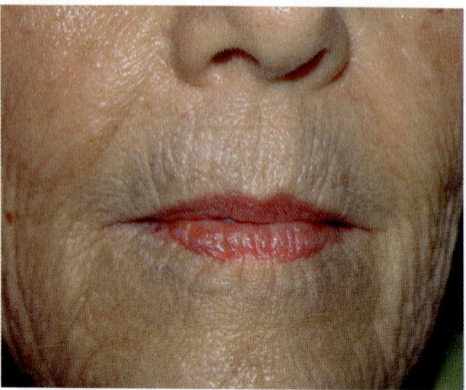

**Figure 6-12.** Blue-gray minocycline associated dyspigmentation around the mouth.

## 6. Erythema Dyschromicum Perstans

- Most prevalent in Latin American patients with type III and type IV skin.
- Clinical Presentation
  - Characterized by slowly progressive appearance of slate-gray to blue-brown oval, circular, or irregularly shaped macules and patches symmetrically distributed on the neck, trunk, and proximal extremities (Fig. 6-13).

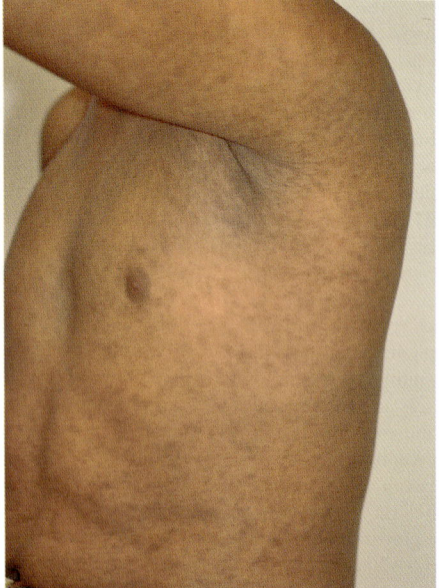

**Figure 6-13.** Erythema dyschromicum perstans—slate-gray patches on the trunk.

- Lesions typically measure up to several centimeters in size.
- During initial appearance of lesions, lesions may have a thin rim of raised erythema at the periphery.
- Most commonly presents during the second to third decade of life but may develop in younger children or older adults. Lesions may slowly progress and typically do not regress in adults.
- There is no consistent or generally effective treatment. Reported treatments include topical tacrolimus, NBUVB, oral dapsone, oral clofazimine, and oral isotretinoin.[49]

## 7. Idiopathic Guttate Hypomelanosis

- Most common in individuals over the age of 40 with increased prevalence with increasing age. Lesions occur in patients of all races and skin types and are most prominent on darker skin types due to chronic UV exposure and aging.
- Common disorder characterized by hypopigmented, sharply defined macules generally between 0.5 and 6 mm in size most commonly on shins and forearms. Hairs within lesions usually retain their pigment.
- Spontaneous repigmentation does not occur.[42]
- Photoprotection and use of physical barriers should be encouraged. As lesions are asymptomatic, treatments such as 5-fluorouracil tattooing are targeted to address cosmetic concerns.

## 8. Pityriasis Alba

- Occurs in children and adolescents, particularly those with an atopic diathesis.
- Thought to be due to postinflammatory hypopigmentation.
- Clinical presentation
  - Characterized by hypopigmented, slightly scaly, round to oval macules and patches that are ill-defined and variable in size (Fig. 6-14).
  - Most commonly presents on the cheeks but can also be present on the neck, trunk, and extremities.
  - Tends to be more pronounced in patients with darker skin types and during summer months.
- Generally clears spontaneously after puberty.
- Emollients and topical steroids often used for treatment.[42]

## 9. Postinflammatory Pigment Alteration

### 9.1. POSTINFLAMMATORY HYPERPIGMENTATION

- More common and more noticeable in patients with darker skin types, particularly types III to VI
- Can be caused by trauma to the skin and a variety of inflammatory skin conditions (eg, acne, insect bites, contact dermatitis, atopic dermatitis, psoriasis, lichen simplex chronicus, lichen planus, fixed drug eruption, discoid lupus)
- Clinical presentation
  - Characterized by hyperpigmented macules and patches due to acquired excess melanin pigment deposition in the epidermis and/or dermis (Fig. 6-15).

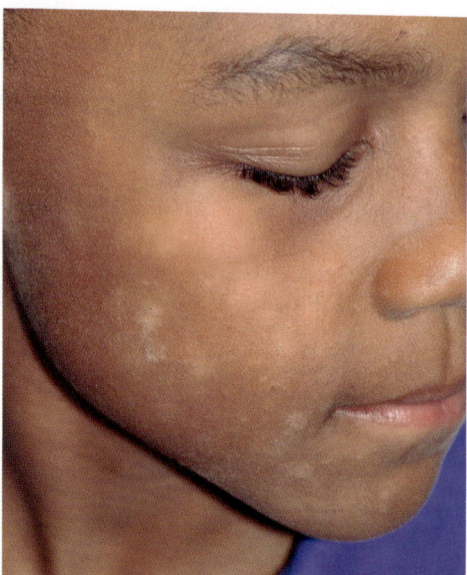

**Figure 6-14.** Hypopigmented ill-defined patches of pityriasis alba.

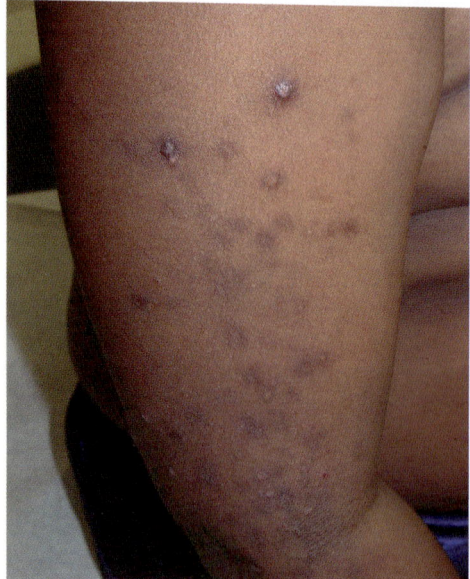

**Figure 6-15.** Postinflammatory hyperpigmented papules and patches secondary on the arm.

- Pigment in the epidermis is more likely to present as shades of brown. Dermal pigmentation often has a blue or gray appearance, though it can also have a brown appearance when melanin is in the superficial dermis.
- The primary condition leading to hyperpigmentation may or may not be evident. The size, shape, and distribution of the hyperpigmentation can often help determine the primary cause.[49]
- Increased epidermal melanin is more likely to resolve, while dermal melanin may last for years or may be permanent.
- Treatment
  - Treatment should first aim at managing the underlying cause.
  - Epidermal melanin may respond to hydroquinone along with other skin-lightening agents including azelaic acid and combinations of hydroquinone with corticosteroids and retinoids. Chemical peels and laser therapy may also provide some benefit for epidermal melanin but can also result in hyper- or hypopigmentation, especially in patients with darker skin types.[50]
  - Dermal pigmentation is not usually responsive to topical treatments.
  - Photoprotection can minimize further hyperpigmentation.[49]

### 9.2. POSTINFLAMMATORY HYPOPIGMENTATION

- Common causes include psoriasis, pityriasis alba, seborrheic dermatitis, atopic dermatitis, discoid lupus, and lichen sclerosus et atrophicus.
- Can occur after the underlying cause or present with it.
- Less common than postinflammatory hyperpigmentation.
- Presents with hypopigmented macules and patches with lesion size, shape, and distribution often reflecting the underlying etiology. More noticeable in patients with darker complexions.
- Treatment should aim at treating the underlying cause initially. UVB phototherapy or sun exposure can be helpful as well.[42]

## Acknowledgment

The authors would like to acknowledge Shaanan Shetty, MD, for their contributions to the previous edition.

## REFERENCES

1. Krüger C, Schallreuter KU. A review of the worldwide prevalence of vitiligo in children/adolescents and adults. *Int J Dermatol.* 2012;51(10):1206-1212.
2. Kyriakis KP, Palamaras I, Tsele E, Michailides C, Terzoudi S. Case detection rates of vitiligo by gender and age. *Int J Dermatol.* 2009;48(3):328-329.
3. Frisoli ML, Essien K, Harris JE. Vitiligo: mechanisms of pathogenesis and treatment. *Annu Rev Immunol.* 2020;38:621-648. doi:10.1146/annurev-immunol-100919-023531
4. Katz EL, Harris JE. Translational research in vitiligo. *Front Immunol.* 2021;12:624517. doi:10.3389/fimmu.2021.624517
5. Perez-Bootello J, Cova-Martin R, Naharro-Rodriguez J, Segurado-Miravalles G. Vitiligo: pathogenesis and new and emerging treatments. *Int J Mol Sci.* 2023;24(24):17306. doi:10.3390/ijms242417306
6. Spritz RA, Santorico SA. The genetic basis of vitiligo. *J Invest Dermatol.* 2021;141(2):265-273. doi:10.1016/j.jid.2020.06.004
7. Marchioro HZ, Silva de Castro CC, Fava VM, Sakiyama PH, Dellatorre G, Mito HA. Update on the pathogenesis of vitiligo. *An Bras Dermatol.* 2022;97(4):478-490. doi:10.1016/j.abd.2021.09.008

8. Ren Y, Yang S, Xu S, et al. Genetic variation of promoter sequence modulates XBP1 expression and genetic risk for vitiligo. *PLoS Genet.* 2009;5(6):e1000523. doi:10.1371/journal.pgen.1000523
9. Jin Y, Mailloux CM, Gowan K, et al. NALP1 in vitiligo-associated multiple autoimmune disease. *N Engl J Med.* 2007;356(12):1216-1225. doi:10.1056/NEJMoa061592
10. Alkhateeb A, Fain PR, Spritz RA. Candidate functional promoter variant in the FOXD3 melanoblast developmental regulator gene in autosomal dominant vitiligo. *J Invest Dermatol.* 2005;125(2):388-391. doi:10.1111/j.0022-202X.2005.23822.x
11. Riding RL, Harris JE. The role of memory $CD8^+$ T cells in vitiligo. *J Immunol.* 2019;203(1):11-19. doi:10.4049/jimmunol.1900027
12. Ezzedine K, Lim HW, Suzuki T, et al. Revised classification/nomenclature of vitiligo and related issues: the Vitiligo Global Issues Consensus Conference. *Pigment Cell Melanoma Res.* 2012;25(3):E1-E13. doi:10.1111/j.1755-148X.2012.00997.x
13. Manoj R, Singh S, Kothari R, Gupta A. Vitiligo. *J Am Acad Dermatol.* 2024;90(5):1106-1114. doi:10.1016/j.jaad.2023.12.040
14. Gan EY, Cario-André M, Pain C, et al. Follicular vitiligo: a report of 8 cases. *J Am Acad Dermatol.* 2016;74(6):1178-1184. doi:10.1016/j.jaad.2015.12.049
15. Ezzedine K, Mahé A, van Geel N, et al. Hypochromic vitiligo: delineation of a new entity. *Br J Dermatol.* 2015;172(3):716-721. doi:10.1111/bjd.13423
16. Böhm M, Schunter JA, Fritz K, et al. S1 Guideline: diagnosis and therapy of vitiligo. *J Dtsch Dermatol Ges.* 2022;20(3):365-378. doi:10.1111/ddg.14713
17. van Geel N, Speeckaert R. Segmental vitiligo. *Dermatol Clin.* 2017;35(2):145-150. doi:10.1016/j.det.2016.11.005
18. Lee JH, Ju HJ, Seo JM, et al. Comorbidities in patients with vitiligo: a systematic review and meta-analysis. *J Invest Dermatol.* 2023;143(5):777-789.e6. doi:10.1016/j.jid.2022.10.021
19. Dahir AM, Thomsen SF. Comorbidities in vitiligo: comprehensive review. *Int J Dermatol.* 2018;57(10):1157-1164. doi:10.1111/ijd.14055
20. Yuan J, Sun C, Jiang S, et al. The prevalence of thyroid disorders in patients with vitiligo: a systematic review and meta-analysis. *Front Endocrinol (Lausanne).* 2019;9:803. Published 2019 Jan 15. doi:10.3389/fendo.2018.00803
21. van Geel N, Speeckaert R, Taïeb A, et al. Worldwide expert recommendations for the diagnosis and management of vitiligo: position statement from the International Vitiligo Task Force Part 1: towards a new management algorithm. *J Eur Acad Dermatol Venereol.* 2023;37(11):2173-2184. doi:10.1111/jdv.19451
22. Rosmarin D, Passeron T, Pandya AG, et al. Two phase 3, randomized, controlled trials of ruxolitinib cream for vitiligo. *N Engl J Med.* 2022;387(16):1445-1455. doi:10.1056/NEJMoa2118828
23. Seneschal J, Speeckaert R, Taïeb A, et al. Worldwide expert recommendations for the diagnosis and management of vitiligo: position statement from the International Vitiligo Task Force-Part 2: Specific treatment recommendations. *J Eur Acad Dermatol Venereol.* 2023;37(11):2185-2195. doi:10.1111/jdv.19450
24. Lopes C, Trevisani VF, Melnik T. Efficacy and safety of 308-nm monochromatic excimer lamp versus other phototherapy devices for vitiligo: a systematic review with meta-analysis. *Am J Clin Dermatol.* 2016;17(1):23-32. doi:10.1007/s40257-015-0164-2
25. Poolsuwan P, Churee C, Pattamadilok B. Comparative efficacy between localized 308-nm excimer light and targeted 311-nm narrowband ultraviolet B phototherapy in vitiligo: a randomized, single-blind comparison study. *Photodermatol Photoimmunol Photomed.* 2021;37(2):123-130. doi:10.1111/phpp.12619
26. Ezzedine K, Peeva E, Yamaguchi Y, et al. Efficacy and safety of oral ritlecitinib for the treatment of active nonsegmental vitiligo: a randomized phase 2b clinical trial [published correction appears in J Am Acad Dermatol. 2023 Sep;89(3):639]. *J Am Acad Dermatol.* 2023;88(2):395-403. doi:10.1016/j.jaad.2022.11.005
27. Lim HW, Grimes PE, Agbai O, et al. Afamelanotide and narrowband UV-B phototherapy for the treatment of vitiligo: a randomized multicenter trial. *JAMA Dermatol.* 2015;151(1):42-50. doi:10.1001/jamadermatol.2014.1875
28. Passeron T. Indications and limitations of afamelanotide for treating vitiligo. *JAMA Dermatol.* 2015;151(3):349-350. doi:10.1001/jamadermatol.2014.4848
29. Artzi O, Horovitz T, Bar-Ilan E, et al. The pathogenesis of melasma and implications for treatment. *J Cosmet Dermatol.* 2021;20(11):3432-3445. doi:10.1111/jocd.14382
30. Kundu RV, Aderibigbe O, Riley JM. Managing facial hyperpigmentation. *JAMA Dermatol.* 2023;159(7):778-779. doi:10.1001/jamadermatol.2023.1414
31. González-Molina V, Martí-Pineda A, González N. Topical treatments for melasma and their mechanism of action. *J Clin Aesthet Dermatol.* 2022;15(5):19-28.
32. Chan R, Park KC, Lee MH, et al. A randomized controlled trial of the efficacy and safety of a fixed triple combination (fluocinolone acetonide 0.01%, hydroquinone 4%, tretinoin 0.05%) compared

with hydroquinone 4% cream in Asian patients with moderate to severe melasma. *Br J Dermatol.* 2008;159(3):697-703. doi:10.1111/j.1365-2133.2008.08717.x
33. Ferreira Cestari T, Hassun K, Sittart A, de Lourdes Viegas M. A comparison of triple combination cream and hydroquinone 4% cream for the treatment of moderate to severe facial melasma. *J Cosmet Dermatol.* 2007;6(1):36-39. doi:10.1111/j.1473-2165.2007.00288.x
34. Taylor SC, Torok H, Jones T, et al. Efficacy and safety of a new triple-combination agent for the treatment of facial melasma. *Cutis.* 2003;72(1):67-72.
35. Ghasmiyeh P, Fazlinejad R, Kiafar MR, Rasekh S, Mokhtarzadegan M, Mohammadi-Samani S. Different therapeutic approaches in melasma: advances and limitations. *Front Pharmacol.* 2024;15:1337282. doi:10.3389/fphar.2024.1337282
36. Farshi S. Comparative study of therapeutic effects of 20% azelaic acid and hydroquinone 4% cream in the treatment of melasma. *J Cosmet Dermatol.* 2011;10(4):282-287. doi:10.1111/j.1473-2165.2011.00580.x
37. Baliña LM, Graupe K. The treatment of melasma. 20% azelaic acid versus 4% hydroquinone cream. *Int J Dermatol.* 1991;30(12):893-895. doi:10.1111/j.1365-4362.1991.tb04362.x
38. Kodali S, Guevara IL, Carrigan CR, et al. A prospective, randomized, split-face, controlled trial of salicylic acid peels in the treatment of melasma in Latin American women. *J Am Acad Dermatol.* 2010;63(6):1030-1035. doi:10.1016/j.jaad.2009.12.027
39. Del Rosario E, Florez-Pollack S, Zapata L Jr, et al. Randomized, placebo-controlled, double-blind study of oral tranexamic acid in the treatment of moderate-to-severe melasma. *J Am Acad Dermatol.* 2018;78(2):363-369. doi:10.1016/j.jaad.2017.09.053
40. Bailey AJM, Li HO, Tan MG, Cheng W, Dover JS. Microneedling as an adjuvant to topical therapies for melasma: a systematic review and meta-analysis. *J Am Acad Dermatol.* 2022;86(4):797-810. doi:10.1016/j.jaad.2021.03.116
41. Kromberg JGR, Flynn KA, Kerr RA. Determining a worldwide prevalence of oculocutaneous albinism: a systematic review. *Invest Ophthalmol Vis Sci.* 2023;64(10):14. doi:10.1167/iovs.64.10.14
42. Seneschal J, Passeron T, Torrelo A, Ortonne JP. Vitiligo and other disorders of hypopigmentation. In: Bolognia JL, Cerroni L, eds. *Dermatology.* 5th ed. Elsevier; 2025:1098-1124. Accessed May 30, 2024.
43. James WD, Elston DM, Treat JR, Rosenbach MA, Neuhaus IM. Disturbances of Pigmentation. *Andrews' Diseases of the Skin.* 13th ed. Elsevier; 2020:862-880. Accessed May 30, 2024.
44. Onojafe IF, Adams DR, Simeonov DR, et al. Nitisinone improves eye and skin pigmentation defects in a mouse model of oculocutaneous albinism. *J Clin Invest.* 2011;121(10):3914-3923. doi:10.1172/JCI59372
45. Wiesner T, Barnhill RL. Benign melanocytic neoplasms and melanotic lesions. In: Bolognia JL, Cerroni L, eds. *Dermatology.* 5th ed. Elsevier; 2025:1973-2008. Accessed May 19, 2024.
46. Williams NM, Gurnani P, Labib A, Nuesi R, Nouri K. Melanoma in the setting of nevus of Ota: a review for dermatologists. *Int J Dermatol.* 2021;60(5):523-532. doi:10.1111/ijd.15135
47. Park JM, Tsao H, Tsao S. Acquired bilateral nevus of Ota-like macules (Hori nevus): etiologic and therapeutic considerations. *J Am Acad Dermatol.* 2009;61(1):88-93. doi:10.1016/j.jaad.2008.10.054
48. Wong THS. Picosecond laser treatment for acquired bilateral nevus of ota-like macules. *JAMA Dermatol.* 2018;154(10):1226-1228. doi:10.1001/jamadermatol.2018.2671
49. Weston GK, Chang MW. Disorders of hyperpigmentation. In: Bolognia JL, Cerroni L, eds. *Dermatology.* 5th ed. Elsevier; 2025:1125-1154. Accessed May 19, 2024.
50. Chaowattanapanit S, Silpa-Archa N, Kohli I, Lim HW, Hamvazi I. Postinflammatory hyperpigmentation: a comprehensive overview: treatment options and prevention. *J Am Acad Dermatol.* 2017;77(4):607-621. doi:10.1016/j.jaad.2017.01.036

# 7. Benign Skin Lesions

Aaron Russell, MD and M. Laurin Council, MD, MBA

Benign skin lesions are frequently encountered during the dermatologic examination. Although removal is often not necessary, it may be indicated for the treatment of symptomatic lesions. Additionally, when atypia or malignancy is suspected, a biopsy is indicated for definitive diagnosis.

## 1. Nevi

### 1.1. BACKGROUND

- Melanocytic nevi are congenital or acquired proliferations of pigmented cells (melanocytes). An acquired melanocytic nevus, often referred to as a mole, is a very common benign lesion with several subtypes, including junctional, compound, intradermal, blue, halo, and Spitz (Fig. 7-1).[1]

### 1.2. CLINICAL PRESENTATION

- **Junctional nevi**
  - Junctional nevi are tan or brown uniform macules with smooth regular borders. They are usually less than 6 mm in diameter. The term "junctional" refers to the histologic location of lesional melanocytes along the dermoepidermal junction (Fig. 7-1A).
- **Compound nevi**
  - Compound nevi are raised brown or tan papules. Histologically, melanocytes are found in both the dermis and the epidermis, hence the term "compound" (Fig. 7-1B).
- **Intradermal nevi**
  - Intradermal nevi are usually skin-colored, tan or light brown, well-demarcated, dome-shaped papules. The melanocytes of these nevi are located entirely within the dermis (Fig. 7-1C).
- **Blue nevi**
  - Blue nevi clinically appear as solitary, blue-black macules or papules (Fig. 7-1D). The two primary histologic variants are the common blue and the cellular blue nevus. Other less frequent histologic variants include sclerosing, amelanotic, and epithelioid blue nevus. Common blue nevi typically arise on the head and neck, whereas cellular blue nevi are more common on the lower trunk and buttocks. Atypical cellular blue nevi can be difficult to distinguish histologically from melanoma.
- **Halo nevi**
  - Halo nevi appear as brown macules or papules with a surrounding halo of depigmentation. The depigmentation is a result of an immune response to the melanocytes in the lesion. Histologically, a brisk lymphocytic infiltrate is typically seen within and around the nevus. Occasionally, the nevus will regress entirely.

---

*The authors would like to acknowledge the first edition author* Shayna Gordon.

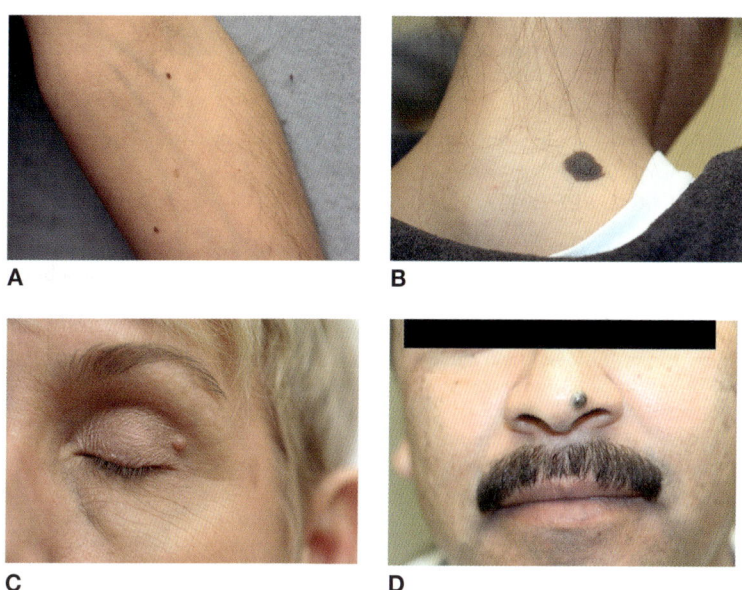

**Figure 7-1.** Spectrum of benign nevi. **A.** Junctional nevi. **B.** Compound nevus. **C.** Intradermal nevus. **D.** Blue nevus. (**C:** Courtesy of Eva Hurst, MD.)

- **Spitz nevi**
  - Spitz nevi are solitary pink papules usually on the face or scalp of a child or adolescent. Histologically, they are characterized by large nests of spindled and epithelioid melanocytes. Atypical Spitz nevi may be difficult to distinguish histologically from melanoma. Because Spitz nevi are rare in adulthood, some advocate for complete excision of these lesions.

## 1.3. EVALUATION

- Most nevi are benign and require only observation. Lesions with asymmetry, border irregularity, color variation, and diameter greater than 6 mm or lesions that are changing should be biopsied to rule out atypia or malignancy.
- A nevus that is different than the patient's other nevi is referred to as the "ugly duckling sign" and may necessitate a biopsy to rule out atypia or malignancy.

## 1.4. TREATMENT

- In general, any lesion deemed suspicious should be removed via deep shave or excisional biopsy and examined histologically to rule out malignancy.
- Surgical removal of benign lesions may be performed for cosmesis.

# 2. Seborrheic Keratosis

## 2.1. BACKGROUND

- Seborrheic keratoses are common acquired benign epidermal lesions.

## 2.2. CLINICAL PRESENTATION

- The classic lesion demonstrates a verrucous or waxy surface with a "stuck on" appearance (Fig. 7-2). Lesions may be skin-colored, tan, or brown and can appear anywhere on the body, sparing the palms and soles. Generally, these lesions appear after the third decade and increase in number with age.
- There are few histologic and clinically distinct variants of seborrheic keratoses.
  - Dermatosis papulosa nigra is a form of seborrheic keratosis that occurs in darker-pigmented individuals and presents as small dark brown or black papules on the face and neck. This condition tends to be familial.[2]
  - Stucco keratoses appear as rough, white papules that are easily scraped off and are frequently located on the lower extremities.
  - Rarely, the sudden appearance of multiple seborrheic keratoses may be a paraneoplastic manifestation of an internal malignancy, known as the sign of Leser-Trélat.[3]

## 2.3. EVALUATION

- Diagnosis can usually be made clinically, but a biopsy should be performed for confirmation of clinically suspicious lesions.

## 2.4. TREATMENT

- No treatment is necessary for seborrheic keratoses; however, removal may be requested for cosmesis, to decrease irritation or to rule out malignancy. Cryotherapy with liquid nitrogen is effective for most seborrheic keratoses, with the exception of extremely thick lesions. Repeat treatments may be necessary. Lesions can also be removed by curettage with or without electrocautery.

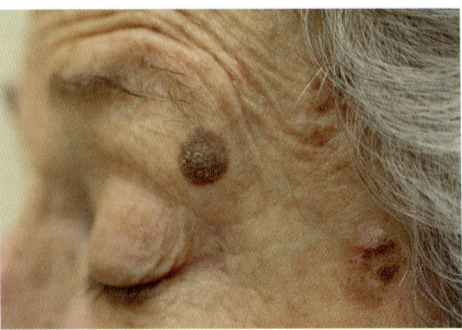

**Figure 7-2.** Seborrheic keratosis. (Courtesy of Eva Hurst, MD.)

# 3. Acrochordons

## 3.1. BACKGROUND

- Acrochordons, or skin tags, are pedunculated fibrous papules commonly occurring in skin folds (Fig. 7-3).

## 3.2. CLINICAL PRESENTATION

- Clinically, acrochordons appear as skin-colored or tan 1- to 5-mm pedunculated papules. They frequently appear in areas of friction. The axilla is the most common location, but these lesions can also appear along the neckline, eyelids, and inguinal and inframammary creases. Obesity is often a predisposing factor.[4] Lesions are usually asymptomatic but may become irritated and tender if traumatized by friction, jewelry, or clothing.[5]

## 3.3. EVALUATION

- Diagnosis can be made clinically, but a biopsy should be performed for confirmation of clinically suspicious lesions.

## 3.4. TREATMENT

- Asymptomatic lesions require no treatment. If lesions are irritated, or if removal is warranted for cosmesis, acrochordons can be removed via snip excision, using curved iris scissors. Electrosurgery or cryotherapy can also be used for removal.

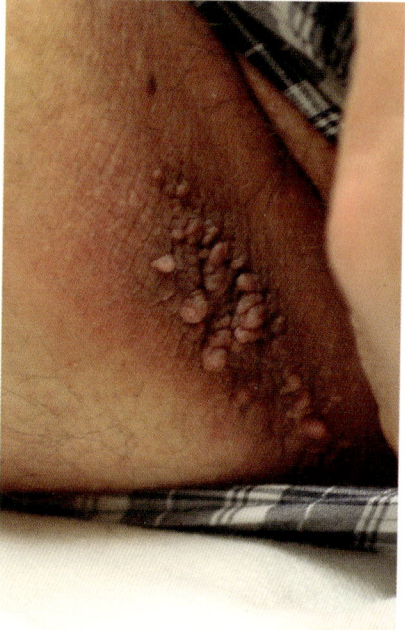

**Figure 7-3.** Plaque of acrochordons.

## 4. Angiomas

### 4.1. BACKGROUND

- Cherry angiomas are mature capillary proliferations.

### 4.2. CLINICAL PRESENTATION

- Cherry angiomas appear as 0.5- to 5-mm, bright red, maroon, or purple macules or papules and are most commonly located on the trunk or proximal extremities (Fig. 7-4). Lesions are usually asymptomatic but may bleed with trauma. Generally, cherry angiomas develop after the third decade, and the number of lesions increases with age.

### 4.3. EVALUATION

- Diagnosis can be made clinically, but a biopsy should be performed for confirmation of clinically suspicious lesions.

### 4.4. TREATMENT

- Patients may request removal of angiomas if they are cosmetically undesirable or chronically traumatized. Removal can be done by shave removal, electrodessication, or laser ablation with the pulsed dye laser.[6]

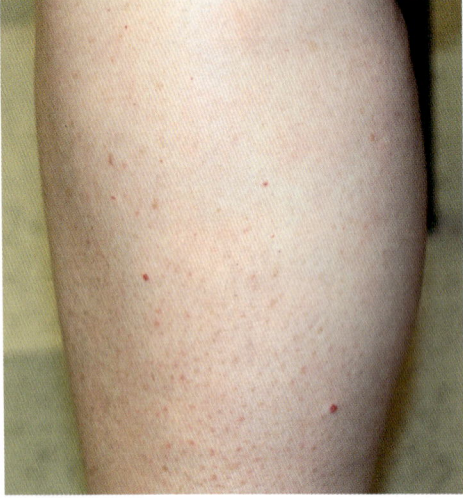

**Figure 7-4.** Angiomas.

## 5. Dermatofibroma

### 5.1. BACKGROUND

- A dermatofibroma is an area of focal dermal fibrosis. It is controversial whether the lesions are spontaneous benign neoplasms or rather a reactive fibrous hyperplasia due to injury or arthropod bite.[7]

### 5.2. CLINICAL PRESENTATION

- Dermatofibromas clinically appear as firm, discrete, asymptomatic nodules ranging in size from 3 to 10 mm in diameter (Fig. 7-5). Dermatofibromas can vary in color from pink to brown, often with a ring of hyperpigmentation. Most commonly, they appear on the lower legs and are usually asymptomatic, but occasionally tender.
- A helpful diagnostic test is the "dimple sign," in which the lesion dimples when lateral pressure is applied.

### 5.3. EVALUATION

- Diagnosis can be made clinically, but a biopsy should be performed of atypical or clinically suspicious lesions.

### 5.4. TREATMENT

- Treatment is not required unless the lesion is changing or symptomatic.

## 6. Lentigines

### 6.1. BACKGROUND

- Lentigines are hyperpigmented benign macules caused by a proliferation of melanocytes at the dermoepidermal junction (Fig. 7-6).

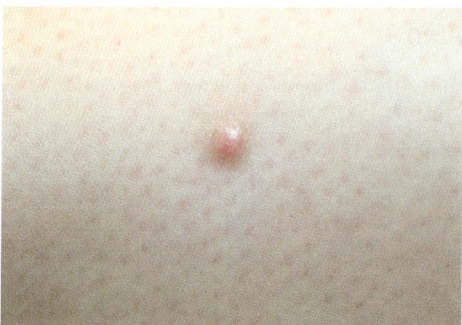

**Figure 7-5.** Dermatofibroma.

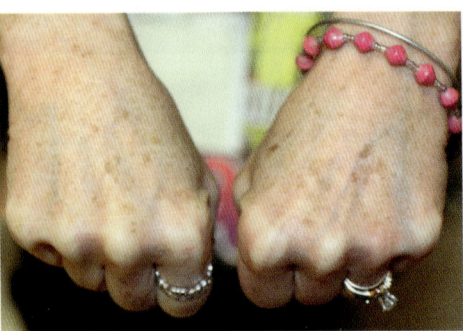

**Figure 7-6.** Lentigines.

## 6.2. CLINICAL PRESENTATION

- Lentigines are tan or brown macules located in sun-exposed areas such as the dorsal hands, forearms, upper chest, and shoulders.[8]

## 6.3. EVALUATION

- Diagnosis can be made clinically, but in cases of ambiguity, a biopsy should be performed to rule out lentigo maligna or melanoma in situ.

## 6.4. TREATMENT

- If there is no concern for malignancy, elective removal may be considered for cosmesis. Topical treatment with 2% to 4% hydroquinone, alone or in combination with a retinoid and steroid, may help lighten lesions. Laser destruction, chemical peels, and gentle freezing with liquid nitrogen are also effective. Strict photoprotection and the use of a high sun protection factor, and broad-spectrum sunscreen are necessary to prevent darkening of existing lentigines as well as the appearance of new lesions.

# 7. Sebaceous Hyperplasia

## 7.1. BACKGROUND

- Sebaceous hyperplasia is a common and benign proliferation of sebaceous glands.

## 7.2. CLINICAL PRESENTATION

- Sebaceous hyperplasia appears as a single lesion or as multiple soft white-yellow papules with a central umbilication (Fig. 7-7). Most lesions are 2 to 4 mm in diameter and appear on the forehead, cheeks, and nose of middle-aged and older adult patients.[9]

## 7.3. EVALUATION

- Diagnosis can be made clinically, but a biopsy should be performed for confirmation of clinically suspicious lesions. Sebaceous hyperplasia can sometimes be confused clinically with basal cell carcinoma.

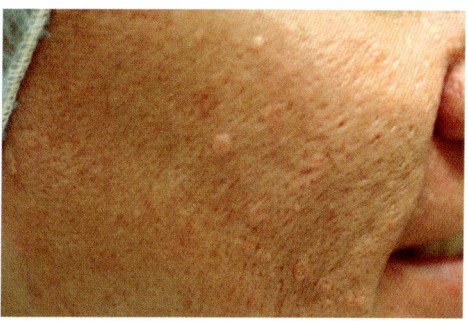

**Figure 7-7.** Sebaceous hyperplasia.

## 7.4. TREATMENT

- Treatment is not required but may be requested for cosmetic reasons. Elective removal may be accomplished with electrodessication, ablative laser surgery, cryosurgery, and shave excision with curettage.[10]

# 8. Keloids

## 8.1. BACKGROUND

- Keloids and hypertrophic scars represent an excessive wound healing response after injury to the skin (Fig. 7-8).
- The distinction between the two entities is clinical: hypertrophic scars remain confined to the boundaries of the original injury, while keloids extend beyond the margins of the initial insult.

## 8.2. CLINICAL PRESENTATION

- Keloids appear as firm, elevated, pink or dark brown nodules or plaques. The most common locations are the earlobes, upper chest, shoulders, and back. Keloids are more commonly found in individuals with darker skin types.[11] Lesions are usually asymptomatic but may be painful or pruritic.

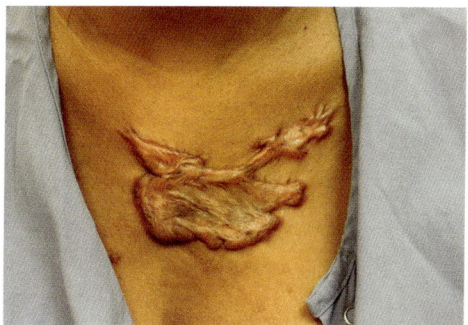

**Figure 7-8.** Keloid. (Courtesy of Eva Hurst, MD.)

## 8.3. EVALUATION

- Diagnosis can be made clinically, but a biopsy should be performed of clinically suspicious lesions.

## 8.4. TREATMENT

- Intralesional steroids may help flatten and soften hypertrophic scars and keloids and reduce any associated pruritus. Overtreatment with intralesional steroids can cause hypopigmentation and atrophy.[12] Keloids may be treated with excision, shave removal, or ablative laser, followed by serial injections with intralesional steroids to prevent recurrence.[13]

# 9. Cysts

## 9.1. BACKGROUND

- The most common types of cutaneous cysts are epidermal inclusion cysts (Fig. 7-9), pilar cysts, and milia cysts.

## 9.2. CLINICAL PRESENTATION

- **Epidermal inclusion cysts**
  - Epidermal inclusion cysts are common subcutaneous lesions that range in size from several millimeters to several centimeters in diameter. A helpful diagnostic clue is a central punctum that may drain a foul-smelling, cheesy substance. When inflamed, epidermal inclusion cysts can become quite painful, dramatically increase in size, and develop overlying erythema. At times, they may become secondarily infected.
- **Milia cysts**
  - Milia cysts are superficial epidermal inclusions cysts that are 1- to 2-mm white papules most commonly on the face of adults.
- **Pilar cysts**
  - Pilar (trichilemmal) cysts are firm mobile nodules commonly located on the scalp. They are typically seen in middle-aged women, and multiple lesions are frequent.

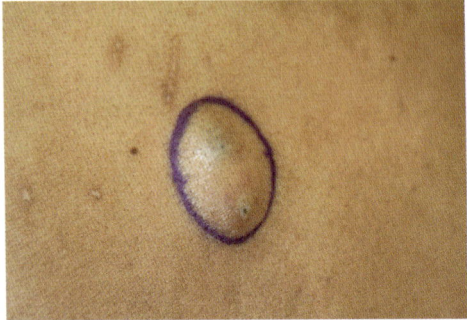

**Figure 7-9.** Epidermal inclusion cyst.

## 9.3. EVALUATION

- Diagnosis can be made clinically, but surgical removal is indicated for large, growing, symptomatic, or clinically atypical lesions.

## 9.4. TREATMENT

- **Epidermal inclusion cysts**
  - Inflamed epidermal inclusion cysts can be treated with intralesional steroids to decrease inflammation and tenderness. Severely inflamed lesions may also be treated with antibiotics.[14] Surgical excision is typically reserved for noninflamed lesions, due to increased risk of complications in acutely inflamed cysts. If active infection is suspected, an incision and drainage, with culture, can be performed.
- **Milia cysts**
  - Milia can be removed for cosmesis by puncturing the skin with a no. 11 blade or 19-gauge needle and then applying gentle pressure with a comedone extractor. Smaller lesions may respond to topical retinoid treatment.
- **Pilar cysts**
  - Pilar cysts can be easily removed by simple excision. Like epidermal inclusion cysts, surgery is reserved for noninflamed lesions.

# 10. Lipomas

## 10.1. BACKGROUND

- Lipomas are benign, subcutaneous tumors composed of mature adipose tissue (Fig. 7-10).

## 10.2. CLINICAL PRESENTATION

- A lipoma clinically appears as a painless, round, soft, mobile, subcutaneous nodule, often with doughy consistency. They are slow growing, and usually 1 to 3 cm in diameter, but can grow up to greater than 10 cm. They are most common in middle age and usually located on the shoulders, neck, trunk, and arms.
- Rarely, multiple lipomas can be associated with syndromes such as hereditary multiple lipomatosis, Banyan-Riley-Ruvalcaba, Gardner syndrome, adiposis dolorosa, and Madelung disease.[15]

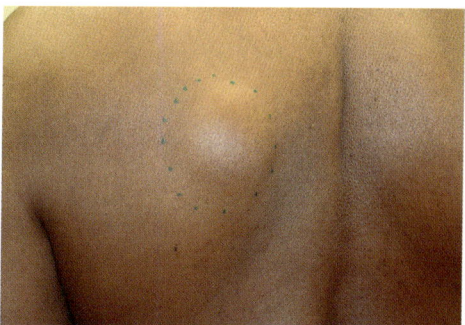

**Figure 7-10.** Lipoma.

## 10.3. EVALUATION

- Lipomas can usually be diagnosed clinically, but if a lesion is symptomatic or changing, a biopsy should be performed for histopathologic diagnosis.

## 10.4. TREATMENT

- Treatment for lipomas is not required but may be requested for cosmetic reasons. Most commonly, they are removed by simple surgical excision but can also be removed by liposuction.[16-18] Some histologic variants, such as the angiolipoma, may be painful. Surgical removal of these lesions can be performed.

# REFERENCES

1. Witt C, Krengel S. Clinical and epidemiological aspects of subtypes of melanocytic nevi (Flat nevi, Miescher nevi, Unna nevi). *Dermatol Online J.* 2010;16(1):1.
2. Lupo MP. Dermatosis papulosa nigra: treatment options. *J Drugs Dermatol.* 2007;6(1):29-30.
3. Husain Z, Ho JK, Hantash BM. Sign and pseudo-sign of Leser-Trélat: case reports and a review of the literature. *J Drugs Dermatol.* 2013;12(5):e79-e87.
4. Jindal A, Patel N, Shah R. Acrochordons as a cutaneous sign of metabolic syndrome: a case–control study. *Ann Med Health Sci Res.* 2014;4(2):202.
5. Luba MC, Bangs SA, Mohler AM, Stulberg DL. Common benign skin tumors. *Am Fam Physician.* 2003;67(4):729-738.
6. Pancar GS, Aydin F, Senturk N, Bek Y, Canturk MT, Turanli AY. Comparison of the 532-nm KTP and 1064-nm Nd:YAG lasers for the treatment of cherry angiomas. *J Cosmet Laser Ther.* 2011;20:1-4.
7. Zelger BG, Zelger B. Dermatofibroma (fibrous histiocytoma): an inflammatory or neoplastic disorder? *Histopathology.* 2001;38(4):379-381.
8. Praetorius C, Sturm RA, Steingrimsson E. Sun-induced freckling: ephelides and solar lentigines. *Pigment Cell Melanoma Res.* 2014;27(3):339-350.
9. Dent CD, Hunter WE, Svirsky JA. Sebaceous gland hyperplasia. *J Oral Maxillofac Surg.* 1995;53(8):936-938.
10. No D, McClaren M, Chotzen V, Kilmer SL. Sebaceous hyperplasia treated with a 1450-nm diode laser. *Dermatol Surg.* 2004;30(3):382-384.
11. KöSe O, Waseem A. Keloids and hypertrophic scars: are they two different sides of the same coin? *Dermatol Surg.* 2008;34(3):336-346.
12. Abdel-Meguid AM, Weshahy AH, Sayed DS, Refaiy EM, Awad SMI. Intralesional vs. contact cryosurgery in treatment of keloids: a clinical and immunohistochemical study. *Int J Dermatol.* 2015;54(4):468-475.
13. Shockman S, Paghdal KV, Cohen G. Medical and surgical management of keloids: a review. *J Drugs Dermatol.* 2010;9(10):1249-1257.
14. Poonawalla T, Uchida T, Diven DG. Survey of antibiotic prescription use for inflamed epidermal inclusion cysts. *J Cutan Med Surg.* 2006;10(2):79-84.
15. Nguyen T, Zuniga R. Skin conditions: benign nodular skin lesions. *FP Essent.* 2013;407:24-30.
16. Rao SS, Davison SP. Gone in 30 seconds: a quick and simple technique for subcutaneous lipoma removal. *Plast Reconstr Surg.* 2012;130(1):236e-238e.
17. Amber KT, Ovadia S, Camacho I. Injection therapy for the management of superficial subcutaneous lipomas. *J Clin Aesthet Dermatol.* 2014;7(6):46-48.
18. Ramakrishnan K. Techniques and tips for lipoma excision. *Am Fam Physician.* 2002;66(8):1405.

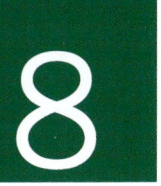

# Malignant Skin Lesions

Aubriana M. McEvoy, MD, MS, Ali Malik, MD, David Chen, MD, PhD, Amy Musiek, MD, and Lynn Cornelius, MD

Malignant skin lesions are divided generally into melanoma and nonmelanoma types. Nonmelanoma skin cancers (NMSCs), particularly keratinocyte carcinomas, basal cell and squamous cell carcinomas (SCCs), are the most common cancers in humans though this categorization includes a variety of rare cancers not discussed in this chapter. Correct identification of cancer type is of paramount importance to determining patient prognosis and appropriate management.

## 1. Basal Cell Carcinoma

- Basal cell carcinoma (BCC) is the most common cancer in the United States with over 3.6 million new cases estimated each year.[1] As there are no registries tracking BCC, estimates using claims data suggest that BCC is more common in men than in women and that its incidence is increasing in all age groups, particularly in women under 40 years of age.[2,3]

### 1.1. BACKGROUND

- **Risk factors**—a confluence of genetic factors and environmental exposures determines risk of developing BCC. Preventable environmental exposure to ultraviolet (UV) light from the sun or tanning beds confers significant risk for development of BCC. Approximately 98,000 additional cases of BCC in the United States each year are attributable to indoor tanning alone.[4] Additional risk factors include immunosuppression, advanced age, exposure to ionizing radiation or arsenic, and history of a prior NMSC. Genetic susceptibility to UV damage due to fair skin or hereditary disorders such as xeroderma pigmentosum (XP) confer independent risk for BCC. In another rare disorder, nevoid BCC syndrome (Gorlin syndrome), patients present with numerous, early-onset BCCs due to mutations in the patched 1 homolog (*PTCH1*) gene. Additional syndromes with early-onset BCC include Bazex-Dupre-Christol and Rombo syndromes. Therefore, patients with multiple or early BCC or extensive family history should be referred for dermatologic and genetic evaluation.
- **Pathogenesis**—the hedgehog pathway is aberrantly activated in nearly all instances of BCC. Approximately 90% of spontaneous BCCs have mutations in *PTCH1*, while an estimated 10% harbor mutations in the downstream smoothened gene (*SMO*). Additionally, tumor protein P53 gene (*TP53*) is frequently mutated, and in spontaneous BCC, *PTCH1* and *TP53* mutations appear to be induced by UV irradiation. Tumor maintenance depends on continued hedgehog pathway signaling.[5]

### 1.2. CLINICAL PRESENTATION

- **Clinical features**—BCC classically presents as a pink, translucent, or pearly papule or plaque with a rolled border and arborizing telangiectasias on sun-exposed skin

(Fig. 8-1A). Several common morphologic variants exist, including a pigmented variant, which can sometimes be mistaken for melanoma (Fig. 8-1B). Additionally, BCCs may have a scarlike appearance and can frequently be ulcerated. Superficial BCC may present as a scaly red plaque that may resemble inflammatory lesion as seen in psoriasis, though a rolled border would be suggestive of BCC (Fig. 8-1C). Finally, an uncommon and relatively indolent variant of BCC, known as the fibroepithelioma of Pinkus, can have a verrucous surface and is classically located on the lower back.

- **History**—patients may report a lesion that bleeds easily, does not heal, is slowly increasing in size, or is tender. Occasionally, patients present with a lesion growing for several years, given its relatively indolent nature.

## 1.3. EVALUATION

- **Biopsy is required for complete evaluation**—though in many instances the diagnosis of BCC is strongly suspected based on clinical appearance, biopsy confirms the diagnosis and provides valuable information to the treating physician(s). Metatypical, infiltrative, morpheaform, sclerosing, or micronodular features on histology represent an aggressive growth pattern and influence treatment decisions. Any one of several biopsy techniques is acceptable including shave, punch, incisional, and excisional biopsies.
- **BCCs tend to invade local tissue if untreated and very rarely metastasize.** Long-standing, large lesions, especially in high-risk patients, may merit further workup for local invasion into underlying structures. However, in the vast majority of BCC patients, imaging and further work up is not necessary.

## 1.4. TREATMENT

The National Comprehensive Cancer Network (NCCN) develops guidelines for the management of BCC.[6] Destructive and surgical techniques are the mainstay of therapy for BCC. Electrodesiccation and curettage provides an efficient and effective (>90% cure rate) method to treat BCCs with the following criteria: nonaggressive histology, low-risk location (trunk excluding genitals and extremities excluding hands and feet), size less than 2 cm. Surgical excision of such BCCs with a 4-mm margin provides a cure rate of more than 95%. For superficial BCC, topical 5-fluorouracil (5-FU) can eradicate approximately 90% of tumors, and clearance rates of superficial BCC with imiquimod are 43% to 100%.[7] Photodynamic therapy has demonstrated efficacy in clearing superficial BCC, though recurrence rates may be high. Cryotherapy, ablative laser therapy, and radiation therapy may be considered patients with low-risk BCCs and/or those who are poor surgical candidates.

- **Mohs micrographic surgery (MMS).** MMS allows for intraoperative evaluation of the entire peripheral and deep margin of the resected tumor specimen. BCCs with aggressive histologic characteristics, larger tumors (>2 cm) in any location, or any BCC in a high-risk location including the "mask areas" of the face or the genitals, tumors in an immunocompromised patient, and recurrent BCCs are appropriately treated with MMS. In a randomized, controlled trial of over 600 high-risk facial or recurrent facial BCCs, MMS was superior to surgical excision for primary (4.4% vs 12.2% 10-year recurrence risk) and recurrent (3.9% vs 13.5% 10-year recurrence risk) BCC.[8] Appropriate use of MMS for BCC (and other skin cancers) has been established and can be accessed via an American Academy of Dermatology mobile application.[9]

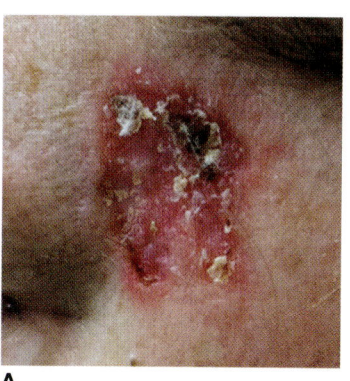

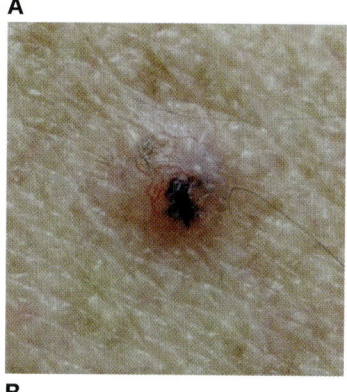

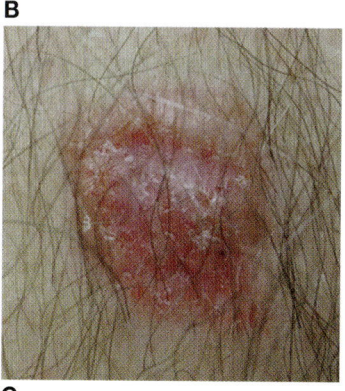

**Figure 8-1. A.** Basal cell carcinoma (BCC) with typical features. **B.** Pigmented BCC with arborizing telangiectasia and globular dark pigment. **C.** Superficial BCC with rolled borders at the periphery.

- **Locally advanced or metastatic BCC.** Rare cases of advanced BCC merit evaluation and management by a multidisciplinary team including dermatology, surgery, oncology, and radiation oncology as there are several treatment modalities available that may be tailored to each patient's case. Vismodegib is an inhibitor of smoothened (*SMO*) that results in decreased hedgehog pathway signaling and is an effective systemic treatment option for advanced BCC. In a multicenter, phase II clinical trial, vismodegib demonstrated objective response rates of 43% in locally advanced disease and 30% in metastatic disease.[10] Neoadjuvant use of vismodegib is currently under investigation. Unfortunately, patients taking vismodegib commonly experience alopecia, dysgeusia, ageusia, muscle spasms, fatigue, and other side effects that, in some instances, compel treatment cessation. The MIKIE trial demonstrated good response rates and reduction of side effects using an intermittent vismodegib dosing regimen.[11] Another hedgehog pathway inhibitor, sonidegib, demonstrated an overall response rate of 36% among patients with locally advanced or metastatic BCC, with a relatively favorable benefit-to-risk profile.[12] Immunotherapy with immune checkpoint blockade agents are approved for second-line therapy. Cemiplimab, an anti-Programmed Cell Death Protein (PD-1) antibody, demonstrates an overall response rate of 22% in patients that have progression or intolerance to hedgehog pathway inhibitors.[13,14]
- **Prognosis**—the prognosis for patients with BCC is excellent. Most patients with localized BCC are cured by the aforementioned modalities. If left untreated, BCCs continue to enlarge and are locally destructive. Metastases occur in less than 0.1% of patients and, although rare, are associated with a poor prognosis. Patients with metastatic BCC should be considered for systemic therapy with hedgehog pathway inhibitors like vismodegib or enrollment in a clinical trial, as there is no reliable cure.
- **Follow-up and prevention**—patients with a history of BCC have a 50% chance of developing a second BCC within 5 years.[15] Therefore, close follow-up is recommended with full skin examination every 6 to 12 months. Patients should be counseled to avoid sun exposure, tanning beds, and ionizing radiation.

## 2. Squamous Cell Carcinoma and Actinic Keratoses

- SCC is the second most common type of skin cancer in the United States after BCC, although recent studies suggest the ratio of BCC to SCC is decreasing and is close to 1 in the Medicare population.[16] The overwhelming majority of SCCs occur on chronically sun-exposed skin in older individuals. Men are twice as likely to develop SCC than women. Although SCC incidence is more than 20 times higher in individuals with lighter skin pigmentation, SCC is the most common skin cancer in black people. Incidence increases with latitudes closer to the equator, reflecting the importance of UV exposure in the pathogenesis of SCC.[17]

### 2.1. BACKGROUND

- **Risk factors.** Solar UV exposure is a major risk factor for the development of SCC. Therapeutic sources of UV radiation such as psoralen with UVA (PUVA) greatly increase the risk for SCC as do cosmetic sources of UV radiation. Indoor tanning accounts for approximately 72,000 excess cases of SCC each year.[4] UV-A exposure from nail salon lamps have even been studied as a risk factor for skin cancer development.[18] Other risk factors include immunosuppression especially in the context of solid organ transplantation, fair skin, exposure to ionizing radiation,

infection with certain human papillomavirus subtypes, burn scars, nonhealing ulcers, increased age, and hereditary disorders such as XP or recessive dystrophic epidermolysis bullosa.
- **Pathogenesis.** Cutaneous SCCs develop because of progressive genomic aberrations commonly induced by UV radiation and genomic instability. Mutations in tumor suppressor gene *TP53* are frequently observed (54%-95% of cases) as well as loss of function mutations in the Notch pathway (~80%). These mutations, resultant aberrant cellular networks, and interaction with stromal factors and the immune system are all contributing factors to development and maintenance of cutaneous SCC.[19] SCC on sun-exposed skin is generally thought to exist on a continuum from precursor actinic keratosis, to SCC in situ, to invasive SCC.

## 2.2. CLINICAL PRESENTATION

- **Clinical features.** SCC generally presents as a persistent, enlarging, erythematous, scaly papule or plaque on sun-exposed skin that may bleed and be tender (Fig. 8-2A). SCC may also present as a crusted, scaly nodule or a poorly healing ulcer. Specific presentations of SCC deserve mention. SCCs may develop within chronic ulcers of the lower leg, known as Marjolin ulcer, and are usually advanced at the time of diagnosis. On external genitalia, SCC may present as vegetative or verrucous nodules and plaques. Actinic keratoses (AKs) or SCC "precancers" are typically erythematous papules with adherent scale (Fig. 8-2B). In some instances, they may be less well-defined faint pink or tan patches with sandpaperlike scale that are more easily felt than seen. This may be difficult to distinguish from SCC in situ, which typically presents as an isolated, well-defined, red plaque with adherent scale (Fig. 8-2C).

## 2.3. EVALUATION

- **Biopsy is required for complete evaluation.** In most cases, AKs can be clinically diagnosed with confidence by an experienced clinician. However, any suspicion of SCC should prompt biopsy for definitive diagnosis. Persistent tenderness, rapid growth, size greater than 1 cm, and spontaneous bleeding are features of a lesion which should prompt biopsy. Several biopsy techniques are adequate including shave, punch, incisional, or excisional biopsies (without intent to cure). Histopathologic examination may differentiate in situ carcinoma from invasive carcinoma and provide further information to guide therapy by noting depth of invasion or aggressive histologic features such as perineural invasion. In addition to biopsy, a full dermatologic examination and palpation of the draining lymph nodes should be performed. Large tumors (>2 cm), tumors with aggressive histologic features (poor differentiation, perineural invasion), occurrence in a high-risk location, or clinical evidence of metastatic disease, especially in an immunosuppressed patient, are cases that merit consideration of further workup with imaging.[20]
- **Staging of cutaneous SCCs.** Two commonly utilized staging systems for SCC are based on the tumor, node, metastasis (TNM) system: the American Joint Committee on Cancer (AJCC) 8th edition and Brigham and Women's Hospital Tumor Staging System.[20,21] In 2010, AJCC guidelines were updated to stratify tumors based on tumor thickness, as it may have prognostic value.[22] One prospective study of SCC in 615 patients demonstrated no metastases in tumors less than 2.0 mm thick, while the rate increased to 4% in tumors 2.1 to 6.0 mm and 16% in tumors greater than 6.0 mm.[23] In the AJCC 8th edition staging system, primary tumors are staged using

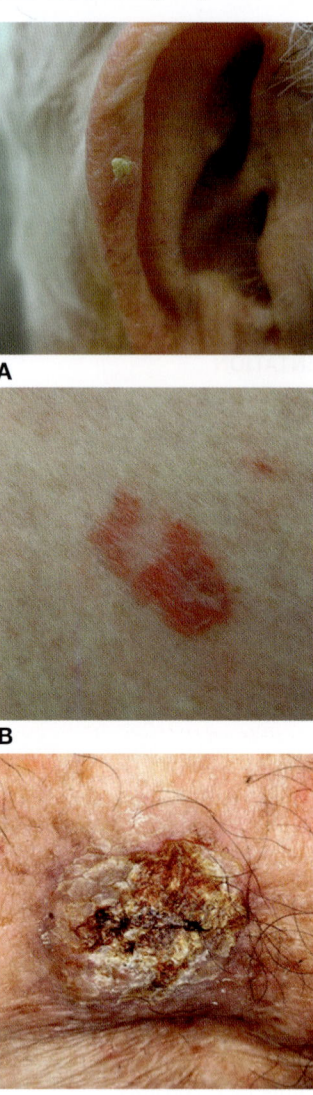

**Figure 8-2. A.** Squamous cell carcinoma. **B.** Hyperkeratotic papule, actinic keratosis. **C.** Red, minimally scaly plaque, squamous cell carcinoma in situ. (**A, C:** Courtesy of Arthur Z. Eisen, MD.)

the following criteria: T1 tumors are ≤2 cm; T2 tumors are greater than 2 cm; T3 tumors invade the orbit, maxilla, mandible, or temporal bone; and T4 tumors invade other bones or have direct perineural invasion of the skull base. High-risk SCC features in the AJCC 8th Edition Staging System include depth/invasion greater than 2 mm; Clark level ≥ IV (into reticular dermis or deeper); perineural invasion; anatomic location (primary site ear, primary site lip); and poor differentiation or undifferentiated.[21] High-risk SCC features in the Brigham and Women's Staging System include tumor diameter ≥2 cm, poorly differentiated histology, perineural invasion ≥0.1 mm, and tumor invasion beyond fat. In the Brigham and Women's System, primary tumors are staged based on the number of high-risk factors as follows: T1 tumors have 0 high-risk factors; T2a tumors have 1 high-risk factor; T2b tumors have 2 to 3 high-risk factors; and T3 tumors have ≥4 high-risk factors.[21]

## 2.4. TREATMENT

- **AKs.** Several methods exist for treatment of AKs. The most commonly used is destruction with liquid nitrogen cryotherapy, which is effective and has few adverse effects other than temporary pain and localized redness and blistering associated with the treatment. Electrodessication and curettage destruction may be employed and is useful for treatment of hyperkeratotic lesions. In individuals with significant UV exposure and/or immunosuppression, the phenomena of field cancerization can occur in which a broad area of skin (such as scalp, whole face, forearms) contains innumerable precancers with oncogenic mutations. The risk of any single actinic keratosis is relatively low for developing into SCC, approximately 0.025% to 16% per lesion, per year.[24,25] However, the cumulative risk of numerous lesions, especially in an immune suppressed individuals, merits discussion and consideration of treatment. Several effective field therapies may be applied, including the following:
  - 5-Fluorouracil. This antimetabolite topical therapy targets rapidly proliferating cells and is available as a cream to be supplied to the patient for self-application. It is effective in clearing clinically apparent AKs as well as subtle lesions that may not be clinically apparent within the treatment field. Side effects range from mild irritation to severe inflammation. Setting realistic patient expectations is critical prior to initiating treatment, as expected skin inflammation during treatment can be very uncomfortable for the patient. Testing small areas before wide application is one effective approach.

    Recently, the combination of topical 5-FU with topical calcipotriene demonstrated superior efficacy in treating areas of AKs (87.8% vs 26.3% mean reduction in the number of AKs), with shorter duration of treatment required (4 days vs 7-14 days of standard monotherapy), and fewer side effects.[26] Topical calcipotriene is thought to potentiate the action of 5-FU, though this combination is not yet available outside of compounding pharmacies. Therefore, patients mix the creams on application, and the combination may be more costly than 5-FU monotherapy.
  - Photodynamic therapy. Photosensitizers 5-aminolevulinic acid and methyl aminolevulinate cause preferential accumulation of protoporphyrin IX in neoplastic tissue, which is activated by blue or red visible light or pulsed dye laser to cause a reactive oxygen species–mediated phototoxic reaction. Clearance rates for AKs are similar to those from 5-FU application. Side effects include discomfort during treatment and ensuing mild irritation to severe inflammation.
  - Other topical therapies—have varying degrees of clearance. These include imiquimod (a Toll-like receptor 7 agonist that causes inflammatory destruction), diclofenac (an inhibitor of cyclooxygenase 2), ingenol mebutate (a natural extract

of the plant *Euphorbia peplus* that causes cytotoxic and inflammatory effects), and tirbanibulin (a microtubule inhibitor).
- **Localized SCC.** SCC in situ or low-risk SCC lesions in non–hair-bearing locations may be treated with electrodesiccation and curettage. Most lesions are removed surgically with 0.4-cm margins for lesions smaller than 2 cm in size and more than 0.6-cm margins for lesions larger than 2 cm or with ill-defined borders. Surgery with these margins is curative in greater than 90% of cases. MMS is recommended for lesions that are at high risk for recurrence and metastasis such as SCC on the central face, ears, eyelids, lips, or scalp; recurrent tumors; size larger than 2 cm; SCC with aggressive histology; SCC that develop in scars; or SCC in an immunocompromised patient. Additional therapies for SCC include cryosurgery, radiation, and, rarely, intralesional chemo- or immunotherapy. Radiation therapy is generally reserved for patients who are poor surgical candidates and can be used as adjuvant therapy in patients with metastatic disease or resected high-risk SCCs, including those with extensive perineural invasion. However, patients with XP, and other inherited disorders of nucleotide excision repair, should avoid radiation. The management of localized SCC (as well as metastatic SCC discussed in the subsequent section) is guided by NCCN guidelines.[20]
- **Metastatic cutaneous SCC.** In 2018, cemiplimab, a programmed death ligand-1 (PDL1) inhibitor, was the first immune checkpoint inhibitor approved for locally advanced or metastatic SCC. A phases I-II clinical trial demonstrated that cemiplimab induced a clinical response in about half of patients with advanced SCC.[27] Unfortunately, metastatic SCC is most often seen in patients with immunosuppression, such as patients with history of solid organ transplantation. Although immune-checkpoint inhibitor therapy trials had excluded such patients, there are promising studies of cemiplimab in immunosuppressed patients, and this is an ongoing area of research.[28,29] Platinum-based chemotherapy and epidermal growth factor receptor antagonist cetuximab have also demonstrated modest benefit for metastatic SCC.[30-32] Referral to a multidisciplinary management team or clinical trial is recommended.[20]
- **Prognosis.** Most cutaneous SCCs can be cured surgically. However, the incidence of local recurrence is 1% to 10% depending on the histologic variant and treatment modality and can be up to 20% in high-risk lesions. Overall, the incidence of metastasis in cutaneous SCC ranges from 2% to 4%,[33,34] typically affecting the first draining lymph node. SCCs with the following high-risk features may have a more aggressive course: location on the lip or ear, size greater than 2 cm, thick lesions, growth within scars, recurrent nature, perineural invasion, and any SCC in an immunosuppressed patient. The 5-year disease-specific survival rate of metastatic SCC is approximately 50% to 83%,[35,36] which underlines the critical importance of definitive management of early SCC, especially in immunosuppressed patients.
- **Follow-up and prevention**—patients with low-risk SCCs are followed up with full body skin examinations every 3 to 12 months for the first 2 years, every 6 to 12 months for the next 3 years, and annually thereafter. Patients with high-risk SCCs should be followed with complete skin and lymph node examination every 3 to 6 months for the first 2 years, every 6 to 12 months for the next 3 years, and then every 6 to 12 months thereafter according to the 2024 NCCN guidelines for cutaneous SCC.[20] Sun protection and sun avoidance need to be stressed in these patients. In high-risk patients, including solid organ transplant or otherwise immunosuppressed patients, precancerous AKs should be aggressively treated, and threshold for biopsy of suspicious lesions should be low.
  - **Chemoprevention**—Patients with high risk of developing cutaneous SCC, particularly solid organ transplant patients, may benefit from the use of oral

retinoids such as acitretin, oral nicotinamide (vitamin B3), and topical 5-FU.[37,38] Oral retinoid therapy may be associated with serum lipid abnormalities that may already be problematic in this patient population. In addition, the discontinuation of oral retinoid may be associated with a rebound development of SCCs.[38]

## 3. Melanoma

- Surveillance, Epidemiology and End Results Program data demonstrate a steady rise in the incidence of cutaneous melanoma since 1975 and a continued average of 1.1% year-over-year increase between 2012 and 2021.[39,40] The American Cancer Society estimates that in the year 2024, approximately 100,640 cases of melanoma will be diagnosed, and 8,290 individuals will die of melanoma. Melanoma is most common in individuals with light skin types, with an incidence of 34.7 per 100,000 for white men and 22.1 per 100,000 for white women.[39,40]

### 3.1. BACKGROUND

- **Risk factors**—there are clear genetic and environmental determinants of melanoma risk. Although familial melanoma is much less common than sporadic cases, mutations in the cyclin-dependent kinase inhibitor 2A (*CDKN2A*) tumor suppressor gene are present with some frequency in families with multiple affected family members or patients with multiple primary melanomas. Lower penetrance gene variants associated with increased melanoma risk include melanocortin 1 receptor (*MC1R*—the genetic determinant of skin/hair pigmentation type), tyrosinase (*TYR*), cyclin-dependent kinase 4 (*CDK4*), microphthalmia transcription factor (*MITF*), BRCA1-associated protein 1 (*BAP1*), and others.[41] Next-generation sequencing has led to the identification of new genetic risk determinants of melanoma. One study identified nongenic polymorphisms affecting the regulatory region in telomerase (*TERT*) in a family with multiple family members with melanoma.[42] Despite identification of such genetic risk factors, the utility of their detection has not been established. Therefore, without a significant personal history (multiple primary melanomas, pancreatic cancer) or significant family history of melanoma or other solid tumors, genetic testing is not a routine practice in the clinical setting, and clinical examination of patients and family members remains the standard of care.
- The most significant environmental exposure that drives melanoma is UV exposure. In fact, the World Health Organization has classified UV radiation between 100 nm and 400 nm as a known carcinogen. UV exposure, in collaboration with genetic risk factors, including fair skin, red hair (*MC1R* variants), and UV sensitivity syndromes like XP, increases melanoma risk. Individuals with light skin pigmentation living in lower latitudes such as New Zealand and Australia, or those who use tanning beds, are at increased risk. Personal history of melanoma confers a 10-fold risk of a subsequent melanoma (new primary) compared to the general population—an elevated risk state that likely reflecting a confluence of genetic factors and environmental exposure. Other risk factors include numerous nevi (>50), history of greater than five clinically atypical nevi, large congenital nevi (>20 cm), and immunosuppression.

### 3.2. CLINICAL PRESENTATION

- Cutaneous melanomas most commonly arise in the absence of a clinically apparent precursor, though in approximately 20% to 30% of cases, nevi are associated with melanoma on histologic examination. Patients may report the appearance of a new skin lesion or change in an existing lesion and will occasionally note associated symptoms such as itching and bleeding. Nonpigmented, or amelanotic, primary lesions constitute approximately 5% of cutaneous melanomas (Fig. 8-3A).

- **Clinical features.** While evaluating a pigmented skin lesion, the "ABCDE" morphologic criteria are helpful, but not absolute.
  ○ Asymmetry—one-half of the lesion does not match the other.
  ○ Border irregularity—the lesion has ragged or notched edges.
  ○ Color variation—pigmentation is a heterogeneous mixture of tan, brown, or black. Red, white, or blue discolorations are particularly of concern.
  ○ Diameter—larger than 6 mm.*
  ○ Evolution—change in characteristics of a lesion noted by the patient or physician.
- Particular attention should be given to lesions that by clinical documentation (ie, written or photographic records) or by patient report are evolving. Together, this set of criteria is sometimes known as the ABCDEs of melanoma. Lesions with one or more of these attributes should be brought to the attention of a physician, preferably a dermatologist, and evaluated for the possibility of melanoma (Fig. 8-3B). Other characteristics such as itching, bleeding, and the presence of ulceration should also prompt a careful evaluation for melanoma.

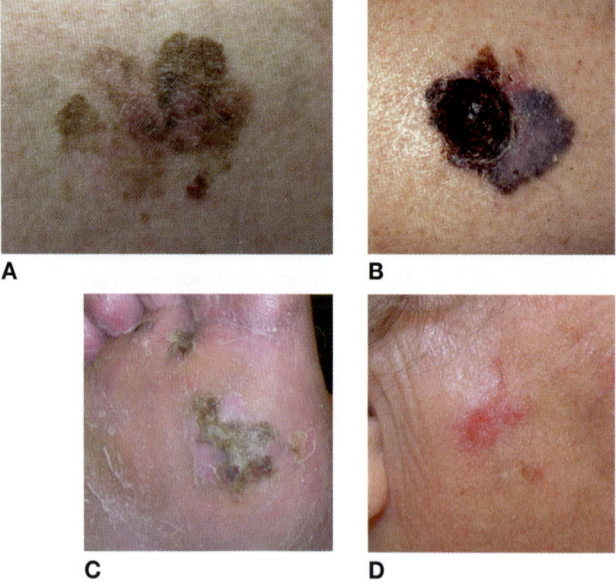

**Figure 8-3.** **A.** Multifocal, asymmetric, variably pigmented patch with border irregularity, representing typical in situ melanoma. **B.** Melanoma with variegated coloration, irregular borders with eccentric pigment, gray veil, and nodular component. **C.** Acral lentiginous melanoma. **D.** Amelanotic melanoma. (**B, D:** Courtesy of Arthur Z. Eisen, MD.)

---

*This parameter serves as a guideline only; melanomas may present clinically as smaller lesions.

## 3.3. EVALUATION

- A comprehensive skin examination—including scalp, hands and feet, genitalia, and oral cavity—performed by a dermatologist, is critical in evaluating and monitoring patients with multiple or atypical nevi, a history of excessive sun exposure, or a history of melanoma or NMSC.
- **Adequate biopsy is required for accurate diagnosis and staging.** The differential diagnosis of a pigmented skin lesion includes an atypical nevus as well as a benign growth such as melanocytic nevus, solar lentigo, seborrheic keratosis, angioma, and less commonly pigmented BCC or SCC. When a suspicious pigmented lesion is identified, the following biopsy techniques should be considered and pursued without delay.
    - **Excisional biopsy.** Full-thickness removal of the entire clinical lesion with 1- to 3-mm margins with consideration of patterns of lymphatic drainage is optimal for diagnosis and accurate staging by Breslow thickness and ultimately treatment. Elliptical excisions for diagnosis should avoid interruption of lymphatic channels to facilitate accurate sentinel lymph node mapping if later required.
    - **Incisional biopsy.** For large lesions or lesions on special sites like the palms and soles, face, ears, or digits, full-thickness incision or punch biopsy of the thickest/darkest clinical portion may be appropriate.
    - **Deep shave (saucerization).** Wide sampling is preferred in superficial lesions such as lentigo maligna, where atypical melanocytes may extend beyond the clinically observed lesion. In contrast, superficial shave biopsy is not recommended for any lesion suspected to be melanoma because if the lesion is transected, the Breslow thickness (a critically important determinant of prognosis and management) cannot be accurately determined.
- **Histologic reporting and classification.** Breslow thickness in millimeters, presence or absence of histologic ulceration, dermal mitotic rate (events per square millimeter), and presence or absence of tumor at the lateral or deep margins constitute the minimal elements that should be reported with the histologic evaluation of melanoma. Reports may include additional elements encouraged by the American Academy of Dermatology such as the presence or absence of regression, microsatellitosis, tumor infiltrating lymphocytes, lymphovascular invasion (LVI), neurotropism, and growth phase (radial vs vertical). The pathologist may also report the histologic subtypes, which include superficial spreading melanoma, nodular melanoma, lentigo maligna melanoma, and acral lentiginous melanoma. Superficial spreading melanoma is the most common subtype constituting 75% of all melanomas, while lentigo maligna constitutes 10% to 15% and is thought to have an extended radial growth phase. Nodular melanomas are, by definition, in vertical growth phase (Fig. 8-3B). Acral lentiginous melanoma (Fig. 8-3C) is the least common type in individuals with lighter skin types, but the most common subtype in persons of color and characteristically arises on specialized sites like palmar, plantar, and subungual locations. Aside from the four dominant subtypes, there are rare variants including nevoid melanoma and desmoplastic melanoma. Though histologically distinct, the subtype does not affect staging and does not influence management or prognosis with the exception of a purely desmoplastic melanoma, where sentinel lymph node biopsy (SLNB) may not be indicated due to the decreased propensity of this subtype to develop regional metastases.[43]
- **Staging.** The 8th edition of the AJCC staging system, updated in 2018, is used for the staging of melanoma.[44] The most important prognostic factors in staging are the thickness of the primary lesion measured in millimeters (Breslow thickness), the presence of histologic ulceration, and the presence of regional lymph node involvement

| TABLE 8-1 | Five-Year Disease-Specific Survival Statistics by AJCC 8th Edition Staging of Melanoma[44] |
|---|---|
| AJCC 8th Edition Stage | 5-Year Disease-Specific Survival |
| 0 | 100% |
| IA | 99% |
| IB | 97% |
| IIA | 94% |
| IIB | 87% |
| IIC | 82% |
| IIIA | 93% |
| IIIB | 83% |
| IIIC | 69% |
| IIID | 32% |
| IV | 16% |

and/or distant metastases. Prognosis varies significantly based on stage at diagnosis (Table 8-1). Patients with thin melanoma (<0.8 mm Breslow thickness, stage IA) have a 99% disease-specific survival rate, while only 16% of patients diagnosed with metastatic melanoma (stage IV) survive this cancer after 5 years.

- **SLNB.** Stages 0, I, and II melanomas are localized to the skin, while stage III melanoma denotes regional metastasis, which is detected by clinical examination or SLNB. Lymphoscintigraphy and SLNB are performed at the time of wide local excision and offer prognostic value to patients with primary melanoma greater than 1.0 mm (≥T2) or a thinner melanoma with ulceration (T1b). This is supported by multiple studies and reaffirmed in the final analysis of the Multicenter Selective Lymphadenectomy Trial-1. Generally, SLNB may be considered for primary for melanomas 0.8 to 1.0 mm based on the 2024 NCCN guidelines.[45]
- **Imaging.** Routine imaging is not recommended in stage I disease unless used to evaluate specific clinical signs and symptoms. The exception is ultrasonography of a nodal basin for an indeterminate lymph node clinical examination, which can help guide decisions for fine-needle aspiration (FNA) or lymph node biopsy. Positron emission tomography with computed tomography (PET-CT) offers no utility in detecting micrometastatic nodal disease. For stage III disease as determined by sentinel biopsy, clinically positive nodes, or in-transit metastases, baseline contrast-enhanced computer tomography (CT) examination is recommended, with or without PET-CT or magnetic resonance imaging (MRI), based on clinical context. For suspected stage IV disease, in addition to CT of the chest, abdomen, and pelvis, gadolinium-enhanced brain MRI is recommended in the initial staging because of its increased sensitivity for detecting small posterior fossa lesions (<1 cm) compared to head CT. PET-CT is also appropriate for initial staging in stages III and IV disease but has no utility in the determination of brain metastases.
- **FNA.** Suspected regional metastatic disease determined by clinical examination or imaging should be evaluated histologically by FNA or core biopsy. In the appropriate context, FNA or core needle biopsy can be performed for suspected stage IV disease except when archival tissue is not available for genetic testing (ie, for v-raf murine sarcoma viral oncogene homolog B, or BRAF, mutations). In this instance, open biopsy is preferred over FNA to facilitate genetic testing that may influence treatment decisions.

- **Lactate dehydrogenase (LDH).** Elevated serum levels of LDH are an independent predictor of poor outcome in stage IV disease. Monitoring LDH levels in patients with locoregional disease is not recommended to determine disease recurrence.
- **Gene expression profiling (GEP).** GEP tests have been developed in an effort to risk stratify stages I to II melanoma patients in terms of outcomes such as recurrence and death. However, as of 2024, the NCCN guidelines state "current GEP platforms do not provide clinically actionable prognostic information," and are not recommended.[45]

### 3.4. TREATMENT[45]

- **Wide local excision**. In stages 0, I, and II disease, wide local excision of the primary lesion with appropriate clinical margins provides the greatest chance of local control. As outlined in NCCN guidelines, excision margins are determined based upon tumor depth (Breslow thickness).[45,46] Margins of 0.5 to 1 cm are recommended for melanoma in situ (MIS). A margin of 1 cm is adequate for primary melanomas with a Breslow thickness of 1 mm or less, while melanomas between 1.01 and 2 mm thickness require a 1- to 2-cm margin. Any melanoma with a Breslow thickness of greater than 2 mm requires a 2-cm clinical margin. More aggressive margins than those recommended have not been demonstrated to improve survival. Conversely, margins may need to be compromised in sensitive areas to preserve function, for example, as in cases of periocular melanoma.
- **Staged excision ("Slow Mohs")** is a variation of the Mohs surgery technique that is used in some cases of lentigo maligna melanoma and MIS. Slow Mohs offers the tissue sparing benefit of MMS while also utilizing permanent sectioning of tissue (as opposed to frozen processing typically used in MMS). Permanent sectioning typically takes 1 to 2 days and allows for much better visualization of melanocytic tumors and therefore results in more accurate margin assessment. Current NCCN guidelines do not recommend MMS for invasive melanoma although studies have evaluated its potential.[47]
- **Nonsurgical therapy.** Although surgical excision is the standard of care for in situ melanoma, topical imiquimod may be considered for MIS or lentigo maligna (MIS on chronically UV-exposed skin such as the face) when surgical cure is not achievable.
- **Advanced melanoma.** Melanoma therapy is rapidly advancing owing to seminal discoveries in key signaling pathways and immunotherapy. Given the evolving landscape of advanced treatment in melanoma, it is important to consult up-to-date NCCN guidelines for current recommendations.[45] Patients with high-risk stage II disease (IIB/IIC) and those with metastatic melanoma (stages III and IV) may benefit from referral to a multidisciplinary management team for discussion of the use of targeted agents, immunotherapy, cellular therapy, or clinical trial. Early referral is preferred with rapidly developing evidence demonstrating the utility of neoadjuvant approaches for resectable, advanced melanoma, which require tight coordination between medical and surgical services. Around 50% of melanomas harbor activating mutations at $BRAF^{V600}$, which render these tumors exquisitely sensitive to inhibitors of the mutant kinase: vemurafenib and dabrafenib. BRAF inhibitors, when combined with MEK inhibitors (downstream kinase mitogen-activated protein kinase), demonstrated improved survival over monotherapy.[48] Immunomodulatory therapies like the CTLA-4 antagonist ipilimumab and PD-1 antagonists pembrolizumab and nivolumab have revolutionized the treatment of metastatic melanoma over the last decade.[49,50] Clinical trials evaluating both pembrolizumab and nivolumab plus ipilimumab in metastatic disease have demonstrated marked improvement in melanoma overall survival. These therapies are summarized in Figure 8-4.[51,52] In addition, adjuvant treatment of patients with surgically treated high-risk stage IIB/C

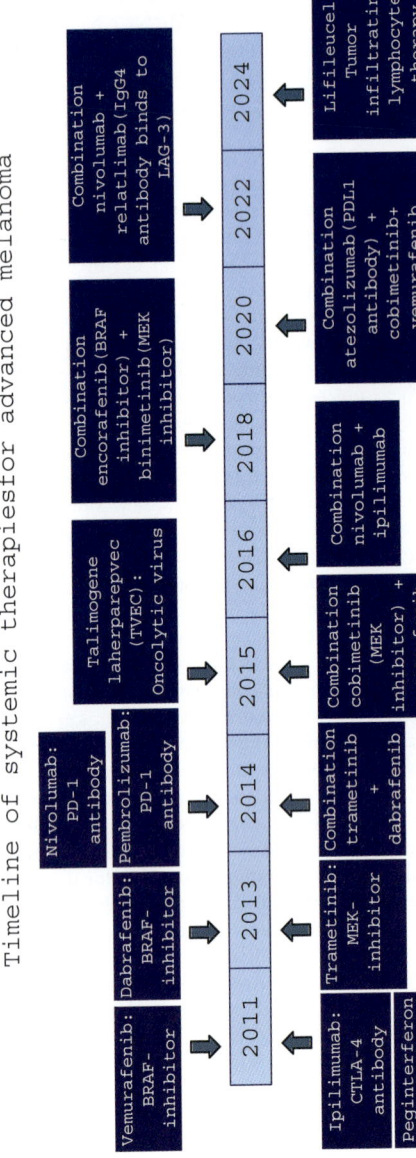

**Figure 8-4.** A recent timeline of FDA-approved systemic and adjuvant therapies for advanced melanoma.[51] Significant findings from clinical trials are highlighted here as well.

disease with checkpoint inhibitors has shown efficacy in improving recurrence-free survival (Keynote-716 and Checkmate 76k).[53,54] Furthermore, the combination of lymphocyte-activation gene 3 (LAG-3) antibody (relatlimab) has been combined with a PD-1 antagonist (nivolumab) and provided a greater benefit with regard to progression-free survival than PD-1 inhibition alone in patients with previously untreated metastatic or unresectable melanoma.[55] Recently, the FDA has approved cellular therapy (Lifileucel) for use in patients with unresectable melanoma or metastatic disease refractory to other treatments.[56]

These aforementioned therapies are typically managed by medical oncologists and administered via infusions. Intralesional (injected directly into tumor tissue) immunotherapy agents like talimogene laherparepvec (an oncolytic virus therapy made from a genetically modified herpes virus) represent an orthogonal class of therapies. It was approved in 2015 for the treatment of stages IIIB to IV unresectable melanoma.[57]

- **Follow-up and prevention.** Patients with a history of melanoma should be followed closely with comprehensive skin and lymph node examinations. They should be taught skin self-examination, as they are at increased risk for a second primary melanoma, as well as recurrence of disease. In addition, these patients need to be counseled regarding the daily use of a broad-spectrum sunscreen that blocks both UVA and UVB. Patients should also be taught sun avoidance strategies such as avoiding the midday sun (10 AM to 4 PM) and wearing protective clothing.
- Patients with stage 0 melanoma should be followed with periodic skin examinations for life. Current recommendations for stage IA to stage IIA with no evidence of disease are to have a history and physical examination every 6 to 12 months for the first 5 years, then annual skin examinations for life. Routine imaging is not recommended and should be considered only if new/concerning symptoms arise. Patients with stage IIB and greater melanoma with no evidence of disease warrant clinical examination every 3 to 6 months for the first 2 years after diagnosis, then every 3 to 12 months for 3 years, and then annually. According to NCCN guidelines, in patients with stage IIB-IV melanoma who are clinically disease-free, cross-sectional imaging (+/- brain MRI) with CT, or PET-CT every 3 to 12 months for 2 years, then every 6 to 12 months for another 3 years may be considered to assess for metastatic or recurrent disease.[45] Routine radiologic screening in stage IIB and higher is not recommended if rendered no evidence of disease after 5 years, unless symptoms warrant imaging. Circulating tumor DNA (ctDNA; the tumor derived fraction of circulating free DNA in the blood) is used most often for melanoma surveillance and may have future use as a prognostic marker.[58]

## 4. Merkel Cell Carcinoma

Merkel cell carcinoma (MCC) is a rare but aggressive skin cancer. The cell of origin is still unknown, but this tumor is referred to as a neuroendocrine cancer due to the appearance of the cells on electron microscopy and staining pattern on histopathology. In the past 20 years, the incidence of MCC has more than tripled to approximately 2,500 cases per year in the United States.[59-61] The risk of death from MCC is 2 to 3 times higher than that of invasive melanoma.

### 4.1. BACKGROUND

- **Risk factors.** Advanced age is a significant risk factor for MCC. The median age at diagnosis is 70 years, and there is a 5- to 10-fold increase in incidence after age 70.

Sun/UV exposure is also associated with increased risk of MCC (although not required), and 81% of MCC tumors are found on sun-exposed skin. Lastly, MCC is strongly associated with immunosuppression which includes HIV, lymphoma, organ transplant recipients, and immunosuppressive medications.[62]
- **Merkel Cell Polyomavirus (MCPyV).** Approximately 80% of MCC tumors have evidence of a key portion of the MCPyV (the oncoprotein or T-antigen).[63] Although a large proportion of the population has been exposed to MCPyV, this virus rarely causes signs or symptoms. MCPyV must integrate into host cell DNA to cause MCC. In the 20% of MCCs that do not demonstrate viral integration, UV-induced mutations are present at extremely high levels (on average, several times higher than in malignant melanoma).[64]

## 4.2. CLINICAL PRESENTATION

- **Primary tumor.** MCC typically appears as a red or purple, rapidly growing, nontender lesion (Fig. 8-5). One acronym, AEIOU, summarizes MCC significant features: Asymptomatic, Evolving rapidly, Immunosuppression, Older than 50 years, UV-exposed site.[62] Of note, in over one-half of MCC cases, the initial clinical impression was a benign diagnosis such as an inflamed cyst. There is no known precursor lesion.
- **Unknown primary.** In approximately 10% of MCC cases, patients present with bulky lymphadenopathy or other symptomatic noncutaneous manifestation of MCC. The unknown primary tumor phenomena is thought to be related to immune clearance of a previous cutaneous tumor, but persistence of lymph node or metastatic MCC. Patients with unknown primary tumors tend to have improved survival compared to patients with the same stage of disease and a known primary tumor likely related to a strong anti-MCC immune response.[65,66]

## 4.3. EVALUATION

- **Biopsy.** Tissue sampling is required for the diagnosis of MCC. For cutaneous lesions, various methods of skin biopsy are acceptable for obtaining the diagnosis:

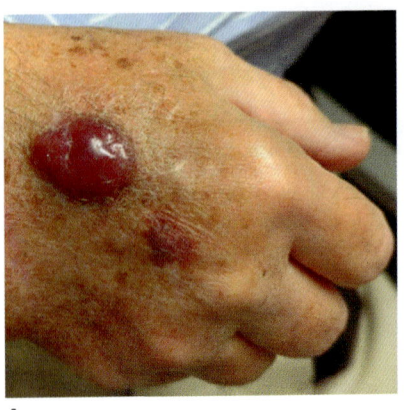
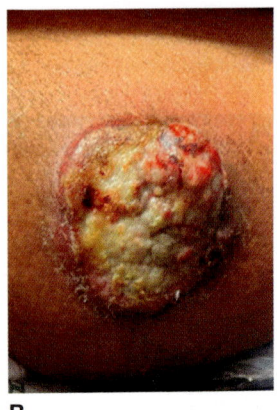

**A**  **B**

**Figure 8-5.** A representative image of Merkel cell carcinoma in an individual with (**A**) lighter skin type and (**B**) darker skin type.

shave, punch, incisional, or excisional biopsies. For patients who present with lymphadenopathy or other suspicious tumor/mass, various image-guided biopsy techniques can be employed. At the time of biopsy, lesion size should be noted as primary cutaneous lesions greater than 2 cm have a significantly poorer prognosis than smaller lesions.
- **Histopathologic evaluation.** MCC has a characteristic appearance on standard H&E staining but is confirmed by immunohistochemistry staining with cytokeratin-20, synaptophysin, and/or chromogranin. Unlike melanoma, Breslow depth is not integrated into MCC staging and is not commonly used for prognostication although there are data to suggest deeper Breslow depth is associated with worse outcomes. LVI is a very common feature in MCC (up to 90% of cases) even in small tumors.[67] LVI likely contributes to the high rates of recurrence (40%),[66] metastases and death from MCC.
- **Staging.** The AJCC 8th edition system for MCC uses TNM staging, with information from clinical examinations, imaging studies, and pathologic evaluation of the primary tumor, lymph nodes, and metastatic lesion(s). This most recent staging system reclassified patients with nodal MCC and unknown primary given their favorable prognosis.[68] Unlike other nonmelanoma skin cancers, there is a very strong rationale for baseline imaging in all cases of MCC for accurate staging. One study demonstrated that upstaging occurred in 13% of patients (and up to almost 30% in patients with large primary tumors).[69] CT scans are frequently used; however, PET-CT has shown higher sensitivity in detecting metastases.
- **Lymph node evaluation.** At diagnosis, the clinician should perform a thorough physical examination of lymph nodes—those draining the primary tumor as well as distant sites. If baseline imaging has not been performed, any clinically palpable nodes should prompt imaging studies. Even in the setting of clinically negative lymph nodes (based on physical examination and imaging), a SLNB should be performed on all MCC patients who are physically able. In fact, the current AJCC staging system for MCC separates patients into those who have been "pathologically" staged with SLNB and those who have only been "clinically" staged without SLNB. MCC is very likely to spread to lymph nodes without clinical signs/symptoms (~30% for the average 1.7 cm MCC).[70]

## 4.4. TREATMENT

- **Surgery.** Surgical excision with SLNB is the initial step in management of most cases of MCC. Optimal surgical margins for a wide local excision and the role of Mohs surgery for MCC are areas of ongoing research. NCCN guidelines suggest 1 to 2 cm margins when possible, and there are data to suggest that wider margins (2-3 cm) do not result in better disease control and are associated with higher morbidity.[71-73]
  As mentioned, SLNB should be performed at the time of surgery, if the patient is a surgical candidate. Completion lymphadenectomy is sometimes performed if there is clinically apparent involvement of the draining nodal bed. However, in one study, patient with nodal disease who underwent completion lymphadenectomy had comparable outcomes to those who received radiation therapy to the nodal bed without nodal surgery.[74]
- **Radiation therapy.** MCC is a very radiosensitive tumor, and there are several studies demonstrating acceptable treatment outcomes using radiation monotherapy.[74,75] In many of these cases, the tumor was deemed inoperable, and the radiation therapy

was given for palliation, but resulted in a durable response. Most commonly, radiation is used in the adjuvant setting after surgery. Several retrospective studies of adjuvant radiation demonstrate significant improvement in MCC locoregional recurrence rates; however, studies on the impact of radiation on survival show mixed results.[76-78]

- **Advanced therapies.** MCC patients diagnosed with locally advanced (stage II), nodal (stage III), or metastatic (stage IV) should be considered for systemic therapy. Immune checkpoint inhibitors were the first immunotherapy agents approved for MCC. In a multicenter clinical trial of stage IIIB to IV MCC, avelumab (an anti-PD1 antibody) resulted in a 73% objective response rate.[79] In another clinical trial in 2016, pembrolizumab (an anti-PD1 antibody) contributed to a partial or complete response in 56% of patients.[80] Chemotherapy is not recommended in MCC as it has not been shown to contribute any survival benefit and can result in significant morbidity. Although not approved for MCC, talimogene laherparepvec can be used for unresectable disease, and several promising cases have been reported.
- **Follow-up.** MCC has a very high rate of recurrence (approximately double that of melanoma), and greater than 90% of recurrences occur within the first 3 years after diagnosis.[66] Therefore, close surveillance of MCC patients during this timeframe is very important. NCCN guidelines recommend full body skin examinations (with lymph node examination) every 3 to 6 months for the first 3 years and then every 6 to 12 months thereafter.[71] Imaging with CT is generally performed every 6 months (although this varies by disease stage, treatment strategy, etc.) and/or based on clinical signs/symptoms. Antibodies to the MCPyV oncoprotein can be detected and measured using a clinically available serology test (AMERK). One management algorithm for the AMERK test suggests the following: baseline AMERK test at diagnosis to determine if a patient is an oncoprotein antibody producer (those who do not have a 40% higher risk of recurrence and should be followed more closely with scans, accordingly) and every 3 months thereafter for MCPyV oncoprotein antibody producers.[81] Recently, a blood test for ctDNA demonstrated high prognostic accuracy in detecting MCC recurrence and may be used to decrease frequency of surveillance imaging studies and to closely follow high-risk patients in between scans.[82] Lastly, a free, web-based recurrence risk calculator is available for providers to estimate an individual patient's risk of MCC recurrence at various time points after initial treatment.[83]

## 5. Cutaneous T-Cell Lymphoma

- Cutaneous T-cell lymphomas (CTCL) are a heterogeneous group of non-Hodgkin lymphomas that primarily involve the skin, though blood, lymph nodes, and viscera may also be affected. The two variants discussed in detail in this section are the most common clinical subtypes for the generalist to recognize—together, mycosis fungoides (MF) and Sézary syndrome (SS) constitute roughly 53% of cases of CTCL.[84]

### 5.1. BACKGROUND

- The median age for diagnosis of MF is between ages 55 and 60 years, and men are twice as likely to develop this condition than women. The exact cause is not known but may be due to chronic antigenic stimulation resulting in expansion of T helper cells.[84,85]

## 5.2. CLINICAL PRESENTATION

- MF and SS may mimic benign conditions such as eczema, psoriasis, vitiligo, folliculitis, and others. The mushroomlike tumors of late-stage MF were first described in 1806 by Alibert.[85] Despite the name, the most common clinical presentations of MF are patches and plaques of early-stage disease (see below and Fig. 8-6A). Progression to tumor stage often takes months to years, and in many cases, advanced disease never develops (Fig. 8-6B). Alternatively, MF may progress to erythroderma, or generalized redness of the skin, which signals advanced disease and is one of the diagnostic criteria for SS (Fig. 8-6C). MF and SS are thought to be separate entities with most cases of SS arising without preceding classical MF. The clinical staging of MF is assessed by the presence of the following:
  - **Patches**—nonindurated areas of erythema, hyperpigmentation, or hypopigmentation. These areas may develop scale and involve larger, though discrete, areas of the body.
  - **Plaques**—indurated areas of erythema, hyperpigmentation, or hypopigmentation. Plaque stage tends to have a more generalized distribution than does patch stage.
  - **Tumors**—nodular or exophytic growths greater than 1 cm.
  - **Erythroderma**—generalized redness of skin. This can exist concomitantly with plaques or tumors and is often associated with severe pruritus.
- **Secondary clinical characteristics**—while not specific to MF, features may suggest this diagnosis including alopecia, follicular-centered papules, and poikiloderma (hyper- and hypopigmentation with telangiectasias with associated atrophy). Generalized erythema with ectropion and/or palmoplantar hyperkeratosis is more frequently associated with SS.

## 5.3. EVALUATION

- The most common scenario for initial presentation of MF is a patient with long-standing, pruritic, nonspecific dermatitis in sun-protected areas that generally waxes and wanes but does not resolve despite repeated topical therapy. Clinical suspicion and careful clinicopathologic correlation is required to confirm the diagnosis of MF, often requiring the integration of longitudinal clinical examinations, skin biopsies (preferably off topical therapy), and laboratory evaluation. If there is clinical suspicion of CTCL, referral to a dermatologist with experience evaluating and treating this condition is strongly advised.
- **Physical examination**—full body skin and lymph node examination is required for accurate assessment and staging of disease. Complete staging requires determination of affected body surface area (BSA).
- **Biopsy and laboratory examination**—in early-stage or erythrodermic MF, nondiagnostic biopsies are common. It may be helpful to acquire biopsies of different concurrent morphologies of the eruption as well as from anatomically distinct sites. If a single biopsy is done, it should be of the most indurated area, as this likely represents the most advanced area of disease. Repeat biopsies are indicated if CTCL remains the favored diagnosis despite previously nondiagnostic biopsies. Histopathologic examination is the cornerstone for diagnosis, while immunophenotyping and assessment of T-cell clonality are supportive.
  - **Histopathology**—larger, atypical lymphocytes with cerebriform nuclei infiltrate the upper dermis and may line up along ("tag") the dermal-epidermal junction or even aggregate in the epidermis (Pautrier microabscess).

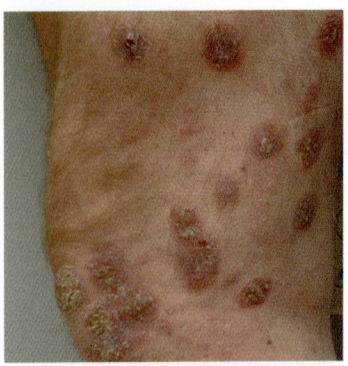

**A**

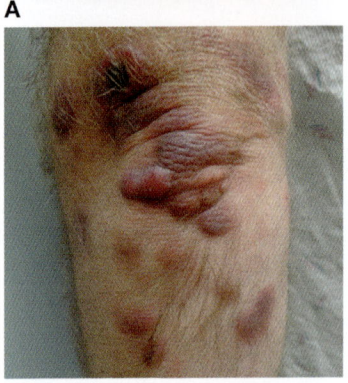

**B**

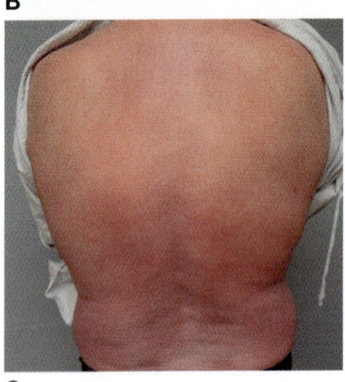

**C**

**Figure 8-6. A.** Scaly erythematous plaques of plaque stage mycosis fungoides (MF). **B.** Erythematous nodules, some ulcerated in tumor stage MF. **C.** Erythroderma in a patient with Sézary syndrome.

- **Immunophenotyping**—malignant cells typically express cluster of differentiation 3 (CD3) and CD4, while few cells will stain for CD8 and CD30. T-cell surface antigens CD2 and CD5 may be lost. Additionally, CD7, a marker for mature T cells, loss may be observed and may aid in distinguishing MF from a reactive lymphocytic infiltrate.
- **T-cell receptor gene rearrangement studies**—polymerase chain reaction analysis may be performed to assess clonality of the T-cell population in biopsy specimens. Caution is advised as nonmalignant conditions may demonstrate clonal T-cell populations, and conversely, not all CTCL has demonstrable clonality, particularly in early-stage MF.
- **Staging**—the International Society for Cutaneous Lymphomas and European Organization of Research and Treatment of Cancer created revised staging guidelines for MF- and SS-type CTCL in 2007 based on the tumor, node, visceral metastasis, and blood (TNMB) involvement.[86] T staging represents patches or plaques less than 10% BSA (T1) or greater than 10% BSA (T2), tumors (T3), or erythroderma (T4). Blood tumor burden with clonal population and Sézary cells at a concentration of 1,000 or greater cells per microliter (or its equivalent; see reference[86]) defines the B2 stage. Erythroderma and leukemic involvement of Sézary cells (T4B2) defines SS. Staging correlates to prognosis, with stage IA MF achieving life expectancy similar to matched control populations, while the 5-year survival for SS (stage IV) is 24%.[84]

## 5.4. TREATMENT

- CTCL is a treatable, but not curable, disease. Early-stage MF (stages I-IIA) typically responds well to skin-directed therapies, including topical medications, light therapy, nitrogen mustard or total skin electron beam radiation therapy for extensive or recalcitrant disease.
  - **Topical therapy**—mid-strength or super potent steroids, nitrogen mustards like mechlorethamine gel, and topical retinoids like bexarotene gel are effective as monotherapies for low-stage disease, or as adjuncts in higher-stage disease.
    - **Nitrogen mustard**—first described in 1959, nitrogen mustard or mechlorethamine gel functions as an alkylating agent and is a particularly effective treatment for plaque or patch-type disease and is also used in combination for more advanced disease. Nitrogen mustard is generally applied overnight and can be used as both a spot treatment or for total body application with minimal to no systemic absorption and no routine laboratory monitoring needed.
  - **Light therapy**—narrowband UVB or PUVA may provide long-term response in patch stage disease. PUVA may be effective in plaque stage disease. Both treatments are typically administered multiple times per week with a slow taper based on clinical response.
  - **Radiation therapy**—external beam radiation therapy is effective but is limited by systemic toxicity, including bone marrow suppression. It is most appropriate for localized tumor stage. Total skin electron beam therapy results in 56% to 96% complete response with IA to IIA disease, though relapse rates are high (reviewed in reference[85]). Total skin electron beam therapy may also be considered in generalized tumor stage.
- There is a wide array of treatment options for advanced stage MF and SS (stages IIB-IVB) with no sufficiently evidence-based treatment algorithms available.[87] Therapies range from oral retinoids to extracorporeal photopheresis, histone deacetylase inhibitors, interferons, single or multiagent chemotherapy, hematopoietic stem

cell transplant, and systemic therapies such as mogamulizumab and brentuximab. Benefits and risks of treatment approach are best addressed in the setting of a multidisciplinary specialty group including dermatology, medical oncology, and radiation oncology services. Importantly, immunomodulation is recommended prior to immunosuppression.

- **Retinoids**—oral bexarotene at a dose of 300 mg/m$^2$ can be given as a monotherapy for refractory or advanced-stage MF (stages IIB-IVB). Central hypothyroidism, hypercholesterolemia, and hypertriglyceridemia are common side effects requiring concomitant management.
- **Histone deacetylase inhibitors**—include oral vorinostat and intravenous romidepsin, which are given either as monotherapy or in combination for refractory CTCL. The most common side effects include gastrointestinal disturbances. Romidepsin is also known to cause QT prolongation.
- **Targeted systemic therapies**—include mogamulizumab and brentuximab vedotin, which are both FDA-approved agents for treating late-stage disease.
  - Mogamulizumab is a humanized antibody targeting CCR4 that is particularly effective for treating patients with SS. Rash and skin infections are the most common adverse events. Dose adjustments may be necessary to ameliorate such adverse events.
  - Brentuximab vedotin is an anti-CD30 monoclonal antibody that is an effective treatment for MF and lymphoproliferative disorders such as Hodgkin lymphoma and anaplastic large cell lymphoma. Use of this therapy requires a thorough discussion of risk and benefits. For example, its use should be minimized in lymphomatoid papulosis, which manifests with recurrent but often self-healing lesions. Peripheral neuropathy is a common side effect and can be prevented by increasing the dosing interval or decreasing the dose administered.

# REFERENCES

1. The Skin Cancer Foundation. *Our New Approach to a Challenging Skin Cancer Statistic*. Accessed July 1, 2024. https://www.skincancer.org/blog/our-new-approach-to-a-challenging-skin-cancer-statistic/
2. Christenson LJ, Borrowman TA, Vachon CM, et al. Incidence of basal cell and squamous cell carcinomas in a population younger than 40 years. *JAMA*. 2005;294(6):681-690. doi:10.1001/jama.294.6.681
3. Lukowiak TM, Aizman L, Perz A, et al. Association of age, sex, race, and geographic region with variation of the ratio of basal cell to cutaneous squamous cell carcinomas in the United States. *JAMA Dermatol*. 2020;156(11):1192-1198. doi:10.1001/jamadermatol.2020.2571
4. Wehner MR, Shive ML, Chren MM, Han J, Qureshi AA, Linos E. Indoor tanning and non-melanoma skin cancer: systematic review and meta-analysis. *BMJ*. 2012;345:e5909. doi:10.1136/bmj.e5909
5. Epstein EH. Basal cell carcinomas: attack of the hedgehog. *Nat Rev Cancer*. 2008;8(10):743-754. doi:10.1038/nrc2503
6. National Comprehensive Cancer Network. *Basal Cell Skin Cancer (Version 3.2024)*. Accessed July 1, 2024. https://www.nccn.org/professionals/physician_gls/pdf/nmsc.pdf
7. Love WE, Bernhard JD, Bordeaux JS. Topical imiquimod or fluorouracil therapy for basal and squamous cell carcinoma: a systematic review. *Arch Dermatol*. 2009;145(12):1431-1438. doi:10.1001/archdermatol.2009.291
8. van Loo E, Mosterd K, Krekels GA, et al. Surgical excision versus Mohs' micrographic surgery for basal cell carcinoma of the face: a randomised clinical trial with 10 year follow-up. *Eur J Cancer*. 2014;50(17):3011-3020. doi:10.1016/j.ejca.2014.08.018
9. American Academy of Dermatology Association. *Mohs Surgery Appropriate Use Criteria (AUC) App*. Accessed July 1, 2024. https://www.aad.org/member/publications/apps/mohs
10. Sekulic A, Migden MR, Oro AE, et al. Efficacy and safety of vismodegib in advanced basal-cell carcinoma. *N Engl J Med*. 2012;366(23):2171-2179. doi:10.1056/NEJMoa1113713
11. Dreno B, Kunstfeld R, Hauschild A, et al. Two intermittent vismodegib dosing regimens in patients with multiple basal-cell carcinomas (MIKIE): a randomised, regimen-controlled, double-blind, phase 2 trial. *Lancet Oncol*. 2017;18(3):404-412. doi:10.1016/S1470-2045(17)30072-4

12. Migden MR, Guminski A, Gutzmer R, et al. Treatment with two different doses of sonidegib in patients with locally advanced or metastatic basal cell carcinoma (BOLT): a multicentre, randomised, double-blind phase 2 trial. *Lancet Oncol.* 2015;16(6):716-728. doi:10.1016/S1470-2045(15)70100-2
13. Stratigos AJ, Sekulic A, Peris K, et al. Cemiplimab in locally advanced basal cell carcinoma after hedgehog inhibitor therapy: an open-label, multi-centre, single-arm, phase 2 trial. *Lancet Oncol.* 2021;22(6):848-857. doi:10.1016/S1470-2045(21)00126-1
14. Lewis KD, Peris K, Sekulic A, et al. Final analysis of phase II results with cemiplimab in metastatic basal cell carcinoma after hedgehog pathway inhibitors. *Ann Oncol.* 2024;35(2):221-228. doi:10.1016/j.annonc.2023.10.123
15. Lewis KG, Weinstock MA. Trends in nonmelanoma skin cancer mortality rates in the United States, 1969 through 2000. *J Invest Dermatol.* 2007;127(10):2323-2327. doi:10.1038/sj.jid.5700897
16. Rogers HW, Weinstock MA, Feldman SR, Coldiron BM. Incidence estimate of nonmelanoma skin cancer (keratinocyte carcinomas) in the U.S. population, 2012. *JAMA Dermatol.* 2015;151(10):1081-1086. doi:10.1001/jamadermatol.2015.1187
17. Qureshi AA, Laden F, Colditz GA, Hunter DJ. Geographic variation and risk of skin cancer in US women. Differences between melanoma, squamous cell carcinoma, and basal cell carcinoma. *Arch Intern Med.* 2008;168(5):501-507. doi:10.1001/archinte.168.5.501
18. Curtis J, Tanner P, Judd C, Childs B, Hull C, Leachman S. Acrylic nail curing UV lamps: high-intensity exposure warrants further research of skin cancer risk. *J Am Acad Dermatol.* 2013;69(6):1069-1070. doi:10.1016/j.jaad.2013.08.032
19. Ratushny V, Gober MD, Hick R, Ridky TW, Seykora JT. From keratinocyte to cancer: the pathogenesis and modeling of cutaneous squamous cell carcinoma. *J Clin Invest.* 2012;122(2):464-472. doi:10.1172/JCI57415
20. National Comprehensive Cancer Network. *Squamous Cell Skin Cancer (Version 1.2024).* July 1, 2024.
21. Karia PS, Jambusaria-Pahlajani A, Harrington DP, Murphy GF, Qureshi AA, Schmults CD. Evaluation of American Joint Committee on Cancer, International Union Against Cancer, and Brigham and Women's Hospital tumor staging for cutaneous squamous cell carcinoma. *J Clin Oncol.* 2014;32(4):327-334. doi:10.1200/JCO.2012.48.5326
22. Karia PS, Morgan FC, Califano JA, Schmults CD. Comparison of tumor classifications for cutaneous squamous cell carcinoma of the head and neck in the 7th vs 8th edition of the AJCC Cancer Staging Manual. *JAMA Dermatol.* 2018;154(2):175-181. doi:10.1001/jamadermatol.2017.3960
23. Brantsch KD, Meisner C, Schonfisch B, et al. Analysis of risk factors determining prognosis of cutaneous squamous-cell carcinoma: a prospective study. *Lancet Oncol.* 2008;9(8):713-720. doi:10.1016/S1470-2045(08)70178-5
24. Glogau RG. The risk of progression to invasive disease. *J Am Acad Dermatol.* 2000;42(1 Pt 2):23-24. doi:10.1067/mjd.2000.103339
25. Marks R, Rennie G, Selwood TS. Malignant transformation of solar keratoses to squamous cell carcinoma. *Lancet.* 1988;1(8589):795-797. doi:10.1016/s0140-6736(88)91658-3
26. Cunningham TJ, Tabacchi M, Eliane JP, et al. Randomized trial of calcipotriol combined with 5-fluorouracil for skin cancer precursor immunotherapy. *J Clin Invest.* 2017;127(1):106-116. doi:10.1172/JCI89820
27. Migden MR, Rischin D, Schmults CD, et al. PD-1 blockade with cemiplimab in advanced cutaneous squamous-cell carcinoma. *N Engl J Med.* 2018;379(4):341-351. doi:10.1056/NEJMoa1805131
28. Verkerk K, Geurts BS, Zeverijn LJ, et al. Cemiplimab in locally advanced or metastatic cutaneous squamous cell carcinoma: prospective real-world data from the DRUG Access Protocol. *Lancet Reg Health Eur.* 2024;39:100875. doi:10.1016/j.lanepe.2024.100875
29. Kuzmanovszki D, Kiss N, Toth B, et al. Real-world experience with cemiplimab treatment for advanced cutaneous squamous cell carcinoma—a retrospective single-center study. *J Clin Med.* 2023;12(18). doi:10.3390/jcm12185966
30. Bauman JE, Eaton KD, Martins RG. Treatment of recurrent squamous cell carcinoma of the skin with cetuximab. *Arch Dermatol.* 2007;143(7):889-892. doi:10.1001/archderm.143.7.889
31. Maubec E, Petrow P, Scheer-Senyarich I, et al. Phase II study of cetuximab as first-line single-drug therapy in patients with unresectable squamous cell carcinoma of the skin. *J Clin Oncol.* 2011;29(25):3419-3426. doi:10.1200/JCO.2010.34.1735
32. Cranmer LD, Engelhardt C, Morgan SS. Treatment of unresectable and metastatic cutaneous squamous cell carcinoma. *Oncologist.* 2010;15(12):1320-1328. doi:10.1634/theoncologist.2009-0210
33. Chuang TY, Popescu NA, Su WP, Chute CG. Squamous cell carcinoma. A population-based incidence study in Rochester, Minn. *Arch Dermatol.* 1990;126(2):185-188. doi:10.1001/archderm.126.2.185
34. Schmults CD, Karia PS, Carter JB, Han J, Qureshi AA. Factors predictive of recurrence and death from cutaneous squamous cell carcinoma: a 10-year, single-institution cohort study. *JAMA Dermatol.* 2013;149(5):541-547. doi:10.1001/jamadermatol.2013.2139
35. Tokez S, Wakkee M, Kan W, et al. Cumulative incidence and disease-specific survival of metastatic cutaneous squamous cell carcinoma: a nationwide cancer registry study. *J Am Acad Dermatol.* 2022;86(2):331-338. doi:10.1016/j.jaad.2021.09.067

36. Brunner M, Veness MJ, Ch'ng S, Elliott M, Clark JR. Distant metastases from cutaneous squamous cell carcinoma—analysis of AJCC stage IV. *Head Neck*. 2013;35(1):72-75. doi:10.1002/hed.22913
37. Chen AC, Martin AJ, Choy B, et al. A phase 3 randomized trial of nicotinamide for skin-cancer chemoprevention. *N Engl J Med*. 2015;373(17):1618-1626. doi:10.1056/NEJMoa1506197
38. Harwood CA, Leedham-Green M, Leigh IM, Proby CM. Low-dose retinoids in the prevention of cutaneous squamous cell carcinomas in organ transplant recipients: a 16-year retrospective study. *Arch Dermatol*. 2005;141(4):456-464. doi:10.1001/archderm.141.4.456
39. National Cancer Institute Surveillance, Epidemiology, and End Results Program. *Cancer Stat Facts: Melanoma of the Skin*. Accessed July 1, 2024. https://seer.cancer.gov/statfacts/html/melan.html
40. SEER Program (National Cancer Institute (U.S.)), National Cancer Institute (U.S.), National Cancer Institute (U.S.). Surveillance Program. *SEER Cancer Statistics Review 1975-2017*. NIH publication. U.S. Dept. of Health and Human Services, Public Health Service, National Institutes of Health, National Cancer Institute U.S. National Cancer Institute; 2020.
41. Bishop DT, Demenais F, Iles MM, et al. Genome-wide association study identifies three loci associated with melanoma risk. *Nat Genet*. 2009;41(8):920-925. doi:10.1038/ng.411
42. Horn S, Figl A, Rachakonda PS, et al. TERT promoter mutations in familial and sporadic melanoma. *Science*. 2013;339(6122):959-961. doi:10.1126/science.1230062
43. Hawkins WG, Busam KJ, Ben-Porat L, et al. Desmoplastic melanoma: a pathologically and clinically distinct form of cutaneous melanoma. *Ann Surg Oncol*. 2005;12(3):207-213. doi:10.1245/ASO.2005.03.022
44. Gershenwald JE, Scolyer RA, Hess KR, et al. Melanoma staging: evidence-based changes in the American Joint Committee on Cancer eighth edition cancer staging manual. *CA Cancer J Clin*. 2017;67(6):472-492. doi:10.3322/caac.21409
45. National Comprehensive Cancer Network. *Melanoma: Cutaneous (Version 2.2024)*. Accessed July 1, 2024. https://www.nccn.org/professionals/physician_gls/pdf/cutaneous_melanoma.pdf
46. Eggermont AM. Randomized trials in melanoma: an update. *Surg Oncol Clin N Am*. 2006;15(2):439-451. doi:10.1016/j.soc.2005.12.001
47. Theunissen CCW, Lee MH, Murad FG, Waldman AH. Systematic review of the role of Mohs micrographic surgery in the management of early-stage melanoma of the head and neck. *Dermatol Surg*. 2021;47(9):1185-1189. doi:10.1097/DSS.0000000000003126
48. Robert C, Karaszewska B, Schachter J, et al. Improved overall survival in melanoma with combined dabrafenib and trametinib. *N Engl J Med*. 2015;372(1):30-39. doi:10.1056/NEJMoa1412690
49. Hodi FS, Sileni VC, Lewis KD, et al. Long-term survival in advanced melanoma for patients treated with nivolumab plus ipilimumab in CheckMate 067. *J Clin Oncol*. 2022;40(16_suppl):9522. doi:10.1200/JCO.2022.40.16_suppl.9522
50. Robert C, Carlino MS, McNeil C, et al. Seven-year follow-up of the phase III KEYNOTE-006 study: pembrolizumab versus ipilimumab in advanced melanoma. *J Clin Oncol*. 2023;41(24):3998-4003. doi:10.1200/jco.22.01599
51. Knight A, Karapetyan L, Kirkwood JM. Immunotherapy in melanoma: recent advances and future directions. *Cancers (Basel)*. 2023;15(4). doi:10.3390/cancers15041106
52. Wolchok JD, Kluger H, Callahan MK, et al. Nivolumab plus ipilimumab in advanced melanoma. *N Engl J Med*. 2013;369(2):122-133. doi:10.1056/NEJMoa1302369
53. Luke JJ, Rutkowski P, Queirolo P, et al. Pembrolizumab versus placebo as adjuvant therapy in completely resected stage IIB or IIC melanoma (KEYNOTE-716): a randomised, double-blind, phase 3 trial. *Lancet*. 2022;399(10336):1718-1729. doi:10.1016/S0140-6736(22)00562-1
54. Kirkwood JM, Del Vecchio M, Weber J, et al. Adjuvant nivolumab in resected stage IIB/C melanoma: primary results from the randomized, phase 3 CheckMate 76K trial. *Nat Med*. 2023;29(11):2835-2843. doi:10.1038/s41591-023-02583-2
55. Tawbi HA, Schadendorf D, Lipson EJ, et al. Relatlimab and nivolumab versus nivolumab in untreated advanced melanoma. *N Engl J Med*. 2022;386(1):24-34. doi:10.1056/NEJMoa2109970
56. Sarnaik AA, Hamid O, Khushalani NI, et al. Lifileucel, a tumor-infiltrating lymphocyte therapy, in metastatic melanoma. *J Clin Oncol*. 2021;39(24):2656-2666. doi:10.1200/JCO.21.00612
57. Andtbacka RH, Kaufman HL, Collichio F, et al. Talimogene laherparepvec improves durable response rate in patients with advanced melanoma. *J Clin Oncol*. 2015;33(25):2780-2788. doi:10.1200/JCO.2014.58.3377
58. Lee RJ, Gremel G, Marshall A, et al. Circulating tumor DNA predicts survival in patients with resected high-risk stage II/III melanoma. *Ann Oncol*. 2018;29(2):490-496. doi:10.1093/annonc/mdx717
59. Hodgson NC. Merkel cell carcinoma: changing incidence trends. *J Surg Oncol*. 2005;89(1):1-4. doi:10.1002/jso.20167
60. Lemos B, Nghiem P. Merkel cell carcinoma: more deaths but still no pathway to blame. *J Invest Dermatol*. 2007;127(9):2100-2103. doi:10.1038/sj.jid.5700925
61. Paulson KG, Park SY, Vandeven NA, et al. Merkel cell carcinoma: current US incidence and projected increases based on changing demographics. *J Am Acad Dermatol*. 2018;78(3):457-463 e2. doi:10.1016/j.jaad.2017.10.028

62. Heath M, Jaimes N, Lemos B, et al. Clinical characteristics of Merkel cell carcinoma at diagnosis in 195 patients: the AEIOU features. *J Am Acad Dermatol.* 2008;58(3):375-381. doi:10.1016/j.jaad.2007.11.020
63. Rodig SJ, Cheng J, Wardzala J, et al. Improved detection suggests all Merkel cell carcinomas harbor Merkel polyomavirus. *J Clin Invest.* 2012;122(12):4645-4653. doi:10.1172/JCI64116
64. Goh G, Walradt T, Markarov V, et al. Mutational landscape of MCPyV-positive and MCPyV-negative Merkel cell carcinomas with implications for immunotherapy. *Oncotarget.* 2016;7(3):3403-3415. doi:10.18632/oncotarget.6494
65. Kotteas EA, Pavlidis N. Neuroendocrine Merkel cell nodal carcinoma of unknown primary site: management and outcomes of a rare entity. *Crit Rev Oncol Hematol.* 2015;94(1):116-121. doi:10.1016/j.critrevonc.2014.12.005
66. McEvoy AM, Lachance K, Hippe DS, et al. Recurrence and mortality risk of merkel cell carcinoma by cancer stage and time from diagnosis. *JAMA Dermatol.* 2022;158(4):382-389. doi:10.1001/jamadermatol.2021.6096
67. Kukko HM, Koljonen VS, Tukiainen EJ, Haglund CH, Bohling TO. Vascular invasion is an early event in pathogenesis of Merkel cell carcinoma. *Mod Pathol.* 2010;23(8):1151-1156. doi:10.1038/modpathol.2010.100
68. Harms KL, Healy MA, Nghiem P, et al. Analysis of prognostic factors from 9387 merkel cell carcinoma cases forms the basis for the new 8th Edition AJCC Staging System. *Ann Surg Oncol.* 2016;23(11):3564-3571. doi:10.1245/s10434-016-5266-4
69. Singh N, Alexander NA, Lachance K, et al. Clinical benefit of baseline imaging in Merkel cell carcinoma: analysis of 584 patients. *J Am Acad Dermatol.* 2021;84(2):330-339. doi:10.1016/j.jaad.2020.07.065
70. Gupta SG, Wang LC, Penas PF, Gellenthin M, Lee SJ, Nghiem P. Sentinel lymph node biopsy for evaluation and treatment of patients with Merkel cell carcinoma: the Dana-Farber experience and meta-analysis of the literature. *Arch Dermatol.* 2006;142(6):685-690. doi:10.1001/archderm.142.6.685
71. National Comprehensive Cancer Network. *Merkel Cell Carcinoma (Version 1.2023).* Accessed July 1, 2024. https://merkelcell.org/wp-content/uploads/2022/04/NCCN-Guidelines-for-Merkel-Cell-Carcinoma-v1.2023.pdf
72. Schmults CD, Blitzblau R, Aasi SZ, et al. NCCN guidelines(R) insights: merkel cell carcinoma, Version 1.2024. *J Natl Compr Canc Netw.* 2024;22(1D):e240002. doi:10.6004/jnccn.2024.0002
73. Tarabadkar ES, Fu T, Lachance K, et al. Narrow excision margins are appropriate for Merkel cell carcinoma when combined with adjuvant radiation: analysis of 188 cases of localized disease and proposed management algorithm. *J Am Acad Dermatol.* 2021;84(2):340-347. doi:10.1016/j.jaad.2020.07.079
74. Fang LC, Lemos B, Douglas J, Iyer J, Nghiem P. Radiation monotherapy as regional treatment for lymph node-positive Merkel cell carcinoma. *Cancer.* 2010;116(7):1783-1790. doi:10.1002/cncr.24919
75. Mortier L, Mirabel X, Fournier C, Piette F, Lartigau E. Radiotherapy alone for primary Merkel cell carcinoma. *Arch Dermatol.* 2003;139(12):1587-1590. doi:10.1001/archderm.139.12.1587
76. Longo MI, Nghiem P. Merkel cell carcinoma treatment with radiation: a good case despite no prospective studies. *Arch Dermatol.* 2003;139(12):1641-1643. doi:10.1001/archderm.139.12.1641
77. Mojica P, Smith D, Ellenhorn JD. Adjuvant radiation therapy is associated with improved survival in Merkel cell carcinoma of the skin. *J Clin Oncol.* 2007;25(9):1043-1047. doi:10.1200/JCO.2006.07.9319
78. Allen PJ, Bowne WB, Jaques DP, Brennan MF, Busam K, Coit DG. Merkel cell carcinoma: prognosis and treatment of patients from a single institution. *J Clin Oncol.* 2005;23(10):2300-2309. doi:10.1200/JCO.2005.02.329
79. Bhatia S, Nghiem P, Veeranki SP, et al. Real-world clinical outcomes with avelumab in patients with Merkel cell carcinoma treated in the USA: a multicenter chart review study. *J Immunother Cancer.* 2022;10(8):e004904. doi:10.1136/jitc-2022-004904
80. Nghiem PT, Bhatia S, Lipson EJ, et al. PD-1 Blockade with pembrolizumab in advanced Merkel-cell carcinoma. *N Engl J Med.* 2016;374(26):2542-2552. doi:10.1056/NEJMoa1603702
81. Paulson KG, Lewis CW, Redman MW, et al. Viral oncoprotein antibodies as a marker for recurrence of Merkel cell carcinoma: a prospective validation study. *Cancer.* 2017;123(8):1464-1474. doi:10.1002/cncr.30475
82. Akaike T, Thakuria M, Silk AW, et al. Circulating tumor DNA assay detects merkel cell carcinoma recurrence, disease progression, and minimal residual disease: surveillance and prognostic implications. *J Clin Oncol.* 2024;42(26):3151-3161. doi:10.1200/JCO.23.02054
83. McEvoy AM, Hippe DS, Lachance K, et al. Merkel cell carcinoma recurrence risk estimation is improved by integrating factors beyond cancer stage: a multivariable model and web-based calculator. *J Am Acad Dermatol.* 2024;90(3):569-576. doi:10.1016/j.jaad.2023.11.020
84. Jawed SI, Myskowski PL, Horwitz S, Moskowitz A, Querfeld C. Primary cutaneous T-cell lymphoma (mycosis fungoides and Sezary syndrome): part I. Diagnosis: clinical and histopathologic features and new molecular and biologic markers. *J Am Acad Dermatol.* 2014;70(2):205.e1-205.e16; quiz 221-222. doi:10.1016/j.jaad.2013.07.049

85. Siegel RS, Pandolfino T, Guitart J, Rosen S, Kuzel TM. Primary cutaneous T-cell lymphoma: review and current concepts. *J Clin Oncol*. 2000;18(15):2908-2925. doi:10.1200/JCO.2000.18.15.2908
86. Olsen E, Vonderheid E, Pimpinelli N, et al. Revisions to the staging and classification of mycosis fungoides and Sezary syndrome: a proposal of the International Society for Cutaneous Lymphomas (ISCL) and the cutaneous lymphoma task force of the European Organization of Research and Treatment of Cancer (EORTC). *Blood*. 2007;110(6):1713-1722. doi:10.1182/blood-2007-03-055749
87. Jawed SI, Myskowski PL, Horwitz S, Moskowitz A, Querfeld C. Primary cutaneous T-cell lymphoma (mycosis fungoides and Sezary syndrome): part II. Prognosis, management, and future directions. *J Am Acad Dermatol*. 2014;70(2):223.e1-223.e17; quiz 240-242. doi:10.1016/j.jaad.2013.08.033

# Disorders of the Hair and Nails

Caroline Mann, MD and Aaron Russell, MD

Disorders of the hair and nails are common dermatologic concerns, particularly of the female patient. While some of these conditions are idiopathic, others may signify an underlying systemic condition.

## 1. Androgenetic Alopecia

- Progressive, androgen-dependent form of hair loss with distinctive patterns in males and females (Fig. 9-1)

### 1.1. BACKGROUND

- Pathogenesis involves the conversion of terminal hairs into "miniaturized" or vellus hairs.
- 5-Alpha reductase is an enzyme in hair follicles that converts testosterone into dihydrotestosterone and is implicated in the pathophysiology of androgenetic alopecia (AGA).
- Levels of 5-alpha reductase and dihydrotestosterone are increased in scalp hairs of men with AGA.[1]

### 1.2. CLINICAL PRESENTATION

- "Male-type" pattern usually involves thinning at the frontotemporal and vertex scalp.
- "Female-type" pattern typically preserves the anterior hairline and involves diffuse thinning at the crown, often in a "Christmas tree" pattern.
- No inflammation is seen.

### 1.3. EVALUATION

- Diagnosis is made by clinical history and examination.
  - Histopathology is not usually necessary except in women who present with an atypical pattern.
- Clinical history often includes a positive family history; however, a negative family history does not exclude the diagnosis.
- Associated comorbidities include metabolic disorders and benign prostatic hypertrophy; an association with cardiovascular disease remains controversial.[2]

### 1.4. TREATMENT

- Treatment of AGA is aimed at maintaining current hair density and does not return scalp to normal hair density or reverse areas of alopecia.

---

*The authors would like to acknowledge the first edition authors Katherine Moritz and Ann Martin.*

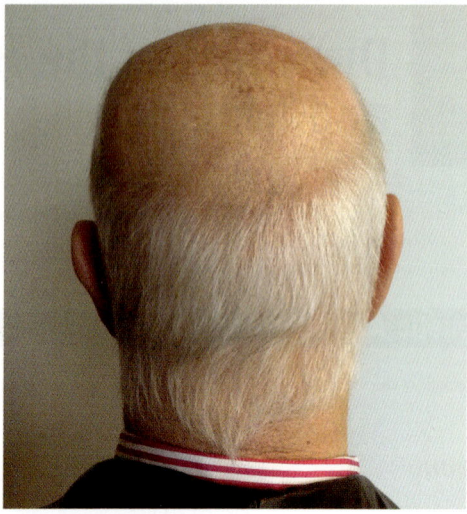

**Figure 9-1.** Androgenetic alopecia. (Courtesy of M. Laurin Council, MD.)

- Discontinuing effective treatment will cause progression of alopecia to the level it would have been without treatment.
- The two Food and Drug Administration–approved drugs for the treatment of AGA in men are topical 5% minoxidil applied 1 to 2 times daily and oral finasteride 1 mg daily.
- For female pattern hair loss, Food and Drug Administration–approved therapy includes both 2% and 5% topical minoxidil solution applied 1 to 2 times daily. The 5% concentration however demonstrated significantly superior efficacy over the 2% in a double-blind, placebo-controlled trial of 381 female patients with AGA.[3] Facial hypertrichosis is a more common side effect in women.
- Low-dose oral minoxidil (0.625-5 mg daily) may be used off-label for treatment of AGA in both males and females. The most common adverse effect is hypertrichosis, which may be undesirable in females.[4]
- Platelet-rich plasma injections may be used off-label for treatment of AGA on both men and women. This is an office-based procedure that involves drawing blood from the patient and separating out the plasma via centrifugation. The platelet-rich plasma is then injected into the scalp. Treatments are typically repeated every 4 to 6 weeks.[5] Cost may be prohibitive.
- Photobiomodulation (low-level light therapy) includes several commercially available LED devices that emit red or near-infrared light. The absorption of light energy within this spectrum is thought to cause a number of beneficial biochemical events that may inhibit androgen-mediated hair loss, although its exact influence on the pilosebaceous unit remains uncertain.[6]
- See Table 9-1 for a list of most commonly used treatments.

## TABLE 9-1. Treatments for Male and Female Pattern Hair Loss

| Males | Females |
|---|---|
| Topical minoxidil 5%[a] | Topical minoxidil 2%[a] or 5%[a] |
| Finasteride 1 mg daily[a] | Finasteride 2.5-5 mg daily (in postmenopausal women) |
| Dutasteride | Dutasteride 0.5-2.5 mg daily |
| Low-dose oral minoxidil | Spironolactone 200 mg daily |
| Surgical treatment | Low-dose oral minoxidil |
| Topical ketoconazole | Topical ketoconazole |
| Wigs, camouflages | Surgical treatment |
| Platelet-rich plasma injections | Wigs, camouflages |
| | Platelet-rich plasma injections |

[a]Food and Drug Administration approval for androgenetic alopecia.

# 2. Alopecia Areata

- Nonscarring form of autoimmune alopecia mediated by T cells (Fig. 9-2).
- Alopecia areata has a lifetime prevalence of approximately 1.7%.[7]

## 2.1. CLINICAL PRESENTATION

- Most commonly presents as round to oval, nonscarring patches of alopecia, most commonly on the scalp > beard > eyebrows > extremities.
  - Variable disease course, approximately 50% recover in 1 year without treatment; however, relapses are common.
  - Asymptomatic.
- Alopecia totalis is loss of all hair on the scalp. Alopecia universalis is loss of all scalp and body hair.
  - Ophiasis pattern involves bandlike alopecia in the parietooccipital scalp and is particularly refractory to treatment.
- May be associated with diffuse nail pitting as well as atopic disease and other autoimmune diseases.

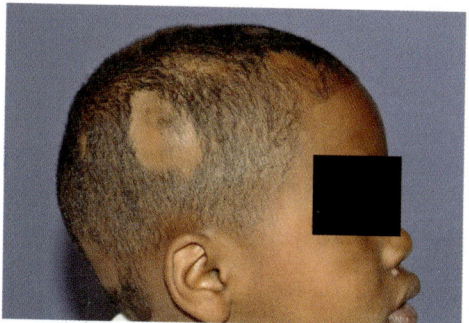

**Figure 9-2.** Alopecia areata. (Courtesy of Susan J. Bayliss, MD.)

### TABLE 9-2  Treatments for Alopecia Areata

Topical and intralesional corticosteroids
Topical irritants (anthralin 1%)
Topical immunotherapy (squaric acid dibutyl ester and diphencyprone)
Topical minoxidil (2% and 5%)
Topical Janus kinase (JAK) inhibitors
Psoralen plus ultraviolet A (topical or oral)
Photodynamic therapy
Pulsed corticosteroids
Oral JAK inhibitors
Systemic cyclosporine
Targeted immunomodulators ("biologics")

## 2.2. EVALUATION

- Diagnosis is usually based on clinical examination.
- Punch biopsy of acutely affected areas shows peribulbar lymphocytic infiltrate.

## 2.3. TREATMENT

- Topical and intralesional corticosteroids are appropriate for patchy disease.
  - Intralesional triamcinolone acetonide 3 to 5 mg/mL can be injected every 4 to 8 weeks.
- Topical irritants such as anthralin 1% cream and topical immunotherapy such as squaric acid dibutyl ester may be first-line choices in treating widespread scalp involvement.
- Oral Janus kinase inhibitors may be considered for severe or widespread disease.
- Please refer to Table 9-2 for a more extensive list of treatments.

# 3. Telogen Effluvium

- Excessive shedding of scalp hairs due to a precipitating event

## 3.1. BACKGROUND

- Hair loss normally occurs in an asynchronous manner to maintain a stable density of scalp hair.
- In telogen effluvium (TE), an inciting event drives an abnormally large amount of anagen (growing) phase hairs into telogen (resting) phase causing synchronous shedding.
  - Common causes include stress, surgery, fever, childbirth, infections, medications, and dietary changes.
  - See Table 9-3 for list of common causes of TE.

## 3.2. CLINICAL PRESENTATION

- Diffuse hair loss usually begins approximately 3 months after a particular stressor occurs and usually lasts for 3 to 6 months.

| TABLE 9-3 | Common Causes and Basic Laboratory Evaluation of Telogen Effluvium |
|---|---|
| **Common Causes** | **Lab Workup** |
| Stress | CBC, ferritin |
| Iron deficiency | ESR |
| Febrile illness | TSH |
| Postpartum | |
| Major surgery | |
| Hypothyroidism | |
| Malnutrition or crash diets | |
| Medications (includes initiation, cessation, or change in dose): | |
| • Oral contraceptives | |
| • Anticoagulants | |
| • Systemic retinoids | |
| • Anticonvulsants | |
| • Lithium | |

- A chronic form of TE can affect women, usually age 30s to 60s, in which hair shedding may occur for years.
  - May be due to multifactorial causes; however, these patients generally have a good prognosis, and progression to baldness does not occur.

### 3.3. EVALUATION

- If there is no clear cause, basic workup involves ruling out iron deficiency and hypothyroidism.

### 3.4. TREATMENT

- Treatment involves reassurance and eliminating any underlying cause if possible.
- Eventual hair regrowth can be expected.

## 4. Anagen Effluvium

- Diffuse loss of anagen (growth phase) hairs due to abrupt cessation of mitotic activity, most commonly from direct toxic effect from antineoplastic agents, radiation, or environmental toxins, particularly ingestion of heavy metals.[8]
- Given that 90% of human scalp hairs are in anagen phase at any time, a high volume of hair is rapidly lost, usually within a few weeks of insult.
- Treatment consists of reassurance and removal of toxin if possible.

## 5. Trichotillomania

- Impulse control disorder with repetitive self-induced manipulation of hair from scalp, eyebrows, eyelashes, beard, or other areas of the body (Fig. 9-3).
- Patients pull out or twist off hairs.
- Can be an isolated disorder or part of an obsessive-compulsive disorder.
- More common in females.

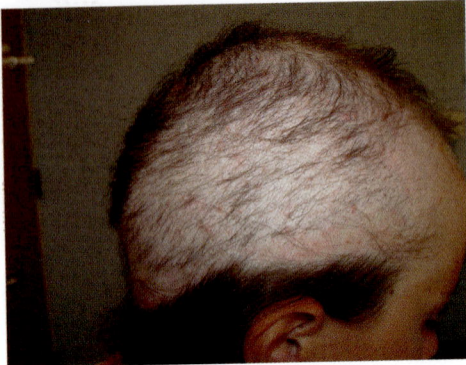

**Figure 9-3.** Trichotillomania. (Courtesy of Susan J. Bayliss, MD.)

## 5.1. CLINICAL FINDINGS

- Single or multiple well-defined patches of alopecia, often with a geometric pattern
- Contain broken hairs of various lengths

## 5.2. EVALUATION

- Diagnosis is by clinical history and examination.
- Punch biopsy may reveal distorted hair follicles, pigmented hair casts, perifollicular hemorrhage, and a predominance of catagen hairs.

## 5.3. TREATMENT

- Treatment is difficult and involves specialized behavioral modification therapy.
- Selective serotonin reuptake inhibitors and clomipramine have been used with partial success.[9]

# 6. Central Centrifugal Cicatricial Alopecia

- Most common form of scarring alopecia among Black women (Fig. 9-4)

## 6.1. BACKGROUND

- Pathogenesis involves predisposition toward premature desquamation of the follicular internal root sheath.[10] Loss-of-function mutations in *PADI3*, a protein involved in hair shaft formation, have been discovered in women with central centrifugal cicatricial alopecia, suggesting a possible genetic basis of this disease.[11]
- Damage to the already abnormal hair follicle may be exacerbated by use of chemical or thermal relaxers, straighteners, and high-tension hair styles.

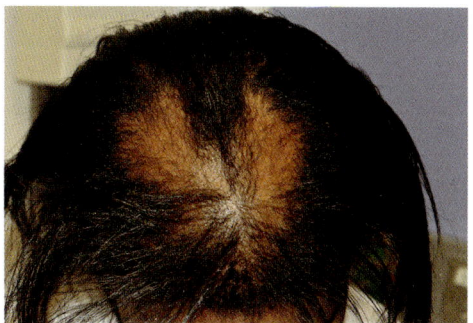

**Figure 9-4.** Central centrifugal cicatricial alopecia. (Courtesy of Susan J. Bayliss, MD.)

## 6.2. CLINICAL PRESENTATION

- Scarring alopecia of the crown and vertex scalp that progresses centrifugally from the center of the scalp.
  - Active inflammation in a roughly circular perimeter surrounding central patch of alopecia
- Often asymptomatic, however, may be associated with burning and itching.
- Loss of follicular ostia is a marker of the cicatricial (scarring) nature of the disease, and scattered tufted hairs are often seen within the alopecic area.
- Disease usually slowly progresses despite cessation of harsh hair care practices.

## 6.3. EVALUATION

- Diagnosis is made by clinical history and examination.
- A punch biopsy should be done at the periphery of the spreading alopecic plaque where the active inflammation is occurring.

## 6.4. TREATMENT

- High-potency topical steroids may be first-line treatment, such as clobetasol propionate 0.05% solution or fluocinonide 0.05% solution applied twice daily to active areas.
- Monthly injections of triamcinolone acetonide 3 to 5 mg/mL to the hair-bearing areas surrounding the central alopecic patch help halt active inflammation.
- Topical or intralesional corticosteroids are usually given in conjunction with a tetracycline antibiotic such as doxycycline hyclate 50 to 100 mg BID for several months.
- Highly inflammatory or purulent cases may be due to bacterial superinfection and require antistaphylococcal therapy.
- Topical or oral metformin (500 mg daily) has been shown to be beneficial as an adjunctive treatment for central centrifugal cicatricial alopecia.

## 7. Discoid Lupus Erythematosus (See Chapter 10)

- Form of chronic cutaneous lupus erythematosus that may cause scarring alopecia
  - Majority of patients do not have systemic involvement; however, approximately 10% of patients will progress to develop systemic disease.

### 7.1. BACKGROUND

- Pathogenesis of discoid lupus erythematosus is unknown but involves perivascular and periadnexal lymphocytic inflammation and may be an immunologic reaction to an unknown antigenic trigger.

### 7.2. CLINICAL PRESENTATION

- Patients present with erythematous alopecic plaques with follicular plugging and occasional scale on scalp, face, ears, neck, and other sun-exposed areas.
  - Progresses to depigmented, scarred atrophic plaques
- Pruritus and tenderness of lesions are common.

### 7.3. EVALUATION

- Diagnosis requires histologic confirmation and cannot be made by clinical examination alone.
  - Punch biopsy should be done in area of active erythema, avoiding scarred or depigmented areas.
- A complete blood count, creatinine, urinalysis, antinuclear antibodies, and extractable nuclear antigens should be checked upon initial evaluation.

### 7.4. TREATMENT

- High-potency topical steroids and intralesional corticosteroids may be used as first-line treatment.
- Antimalarials such as hydroxychloroquine and chloroquine are often used in conjunction with topical corticosteroids.
- Strict avoidance of sun exposure as well as smoking cessation are imperative for treatment success.
  - See Table 9-4 for list of therapies.

## 8. Lichen Planopilaris

- Follicular variant of lichen planus that results in a scarring alopecia (Fig. 9-5)

### 8.1. BACKGROUND

- More common in females than males
- More common in Caucasians

### 8.2. CLINICAL PRESENTATION

- In the early stages of classic lichen planopilaris, patients complain of increased hair loss, scalp pruritus, and tenderness.

### TABLE 9-4 Treatments for Discoid Lupus Erythematosus

High-potency topical corticosteroids
- Clobetasol propionate 0.05% solution or ointment BID
- Fluocinonide 0.05% solution BID

Triamcinolone acetonide 3-5 mg/mL injections q4-6wk
- Antimalarials
- Hydroxychloroquine 200 mg BID (6.5 mg/kg/d)
- Chloroquine (4.5 mg/kg/d)
- Quinacrine 100 mg qd

Other:
Retinoids such as acitretin
Dapsone
Thalidomide
Methotrexate
Mycophenolate mofetil

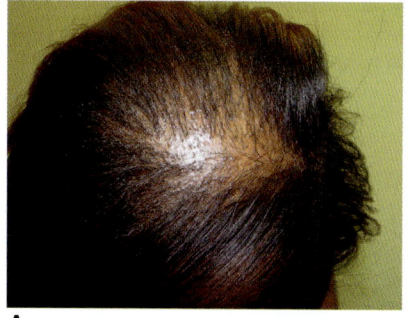

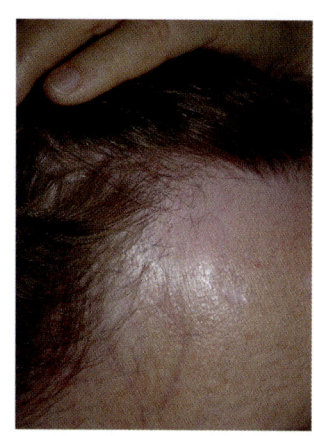

**Figure 9-5. A.** Lichen planopilaris, classic. **B.** Lichen planopilaris, frontal fibrosing variant. (**A, B:** Courtesy of Susan J. Bayliss, MD.)

| TABLE 9-5 | Treatment of Lichen Planopilaris and Frontal Fibrosing Alopecia |
|---|---|

High-potency topical corticosteroids
- Clobetasol propionate 0.05% solution or ointment BID
- Fluocinonide 0.05% solution BID

Triamcinolone acetonide 3-5 mg/mL injections q4-6wk
Hydroxychloroquine 200 mg BID (6.5 mg/kg/d)
Minocycline 100 mg BID
Topical minoxidil 2%-5% BID
Pioglitazone hydrochloride
Acitretin

- Patchy alopecia of the frontal and vertex scalp with perifollicular erythema and follicular hyperkeratosis is most common, progressing eventually into scarred plaques with surrounding active inflammation.
- Up to 50% of patients will exhibit lichen planus-type lesions elsewhere on the skin at some point in the disease process.
- The frontal fibrosing variant demonstrates the above clinical features but stays limited to the anterior and temporal hairlines and is most common in postmenopausal Caucasian women.
  - Loss of eyebrows is common.

### 8.3. EVALUATION

- Diagnosis requires histologic confirmation.
  - A punch biopsy should be taken at the edge of the alopecic plaque where the inflammation is most prominent.

### 8.4. TREATMENT

- Treatment of lichen planopilaris can be difficult, and subtle disease progression may occur in the absence of clinical signs of inflammation.[12]
  - See Table 9-5 for treatment options.

## 9. Dissecting Cellulitis

- Chronic and relapsing suppurative disease of the scalp (Fig. 9-6)
  - Evolves to scarring alopecia
- Commonly presents in young Black males in 20s to 30s

### 9.1. BACKGROUND

- Pathogenesis involves follicular hyperkeratosis with retention of keratin, predisposing to bacterial superinfection and follicular rupture. Keratin debris in the dermis leads to a foreign body–type reaction and eventual scarring.
- Dissecting cellulitis is considered part of the "follicular occlusion tetrad" along with hidradenitis suppurativa, acne conglobata, and pilonidal cysts.[7]

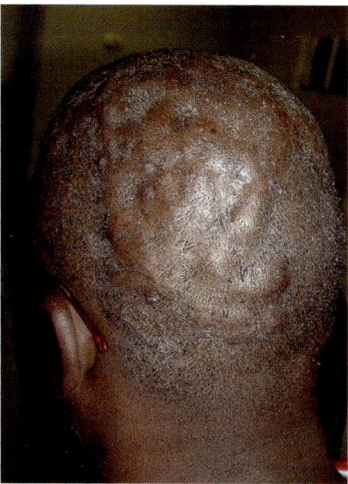

**Figure 9-6.** Dissecting cellulitis. (Courtesy of Susan J. Bayliss, MD.)

## 9.2. CLINICAL PRESENTATION

- Fluctuant nodules and plaques with draining sinus tracts that eventually progress to scarring and hair loss
- Can be painful or asymptomatic

## 9.3. EVALUATION

- Diagnosis is based on clinical history and examination.

## 9.4. TREATMENT

- First-line treatment is oral isotretinoin 1 mg/kg daily for 6 to 12 months.[12]
  - Can be used in conjunction with intralesional injections of triamcinolone acetonide (10-40 mg/mL)
- Other treatments include oral antibiotics such as doxycycline hyclate 100 mg BID.

# 10. Folliculitis Decalvans

- Highly inflammatory form of scarring alopecia most commonly seen in young to middle-aged adults

## 10.1. BACKGROUND

- *Staphylococcus aureus* and an abnormal host immune response are thought to be driving factors in the pathogenesis of this disorder.[13]

## 10.2. CLINICAL PRESENTATION

- Begins as a painful and purulent folliculitis most prominent on vertex and occipital scalp that progresses to boggy scarred plaques of alopecia
  - Tufting of hairs within scars as well as hemorrhagic crusts and erosions may be seen.

## 10.3. EVALUATION

- Bacterial culture swab of the scalp or an intact pustule is recommended to rule out staph infection.
- Punch biopsy at the hair-bearing periphery of an active area shows a neutrophilic inflammatory infiltrate.

## 10.4. TREATMENT

- Treatment is directed at eradicating *S aureus* infection and controlling inflammation.
  - Rifampicin 300 mg BID along with clindamycin 300 mg BID × 10 to 12 weeks has been reported to be successful.
  - Long-term doxycycline (100 mg BID) may be needed to suppress disease activity.
  - PO antibiotics can be used in conjunction with class I or II topical corticosteroids such as clobetasol 0.05% solution BID or intralesional triamcinolone acetonide 10 mg/mL injections q 4 to 6 weeks.

# 11. Secondary Scarring Alopecias

- Deep burns
- Radiation dermatitis
- Cutaneous sarcoidosis
- Cutaneous malignancies, both primary and metastatic
- Infections, including bacterial and fungal

# 12. Hypertrichosis

- Excessive hair growth that may be generalized or local. It may also be inherited or acquired. The excess hair may be lanugo, vellus, or terminal. Lanugo hair is the fine, nonpigmented downy hair that is normally shed in utero or in neonatal period.
  - Congenital forms of hypertrichosis are very rare. More commonly seen are acquired variants, often as side effects of medications (Table 9-6).

# 13. Hirsutism

- Excess growth of terminal hair in a male pattern in female patients
- Indicative of androgen excess and affects approximately 5% of women of reproductive age[14]

### TABLE 9-6. Common Causes of Hypertrichosis

**Congenital forms:**

**Porphyrias (can be acquired as in pseudoporphyria)**
- Sun-exposed areas

**Universal hypertrichosis**
- Rare, autosomal dominant

**Congenital hypertrichosis lanuginosa**
- Rare, autosomal dominant

**Becker nevus**
- Congenital hamartoma of upper trunk, usually in males
- Hyperpigmented patch that develops hypertrichosis after puberty

**Acquired forms:**

**Acquired hypertrichosis lanuginosa**
- Paraneoplastic disorder associated with lung, colon, and breast cancer
- May be accompanied by fissured tongue

**Drug induced:**
- Phenytoin
- Cyclosporine
- Minoxidil
- Diazoxide
- Streptomycin
- Glucocorticosteroids
- Psoralens
- Interferon alpha
- Epidermal growth factor receptor inhibitors

**Malnutrition (anorexia nervosa)**
**Repeated friction, trauma, or inflammation (eg, under a cast)**
**Posttraumatic brain injury**

## 13.1. BACKGROUND

- The source of the excess androgens is most often ovarian or adrenal; however, female patients may have features of hirsutism in the absence of significant hormonal imbalance, that is, constitutional hirsutism.
  - SAHA syndrome (seborrhea, acne, hirsutism, alopecia) may be an isolated clinical finding.
- See Table 9-7 for a list of causes of hirsutism.

### TABLE 9-7. Causes of Hirsutism

**Ovarian causes:**
- Polycystic ovarian syndrome
- Ovarian tumors
- Ovarian hyperthecosis

**Adrenal causes:**
- Congenital adrenal hyperplasia
- Adrenal tumors
- Hypercortisolism (Cushing syndrome)

**Iatrogenic:**
- Anabolic steroids (danazol)
- Glucocorticoids
- Oral contraceptives with progesterone

**Hyperprolactinemia**
**Acromegaly**
**Severe insulin resistance**

## 13.2. CLINICAL PRESENTATION

- Hirsutism may be accompanied by other signs of virilization such as acne, male pattern AGA, oligo- or amenorrhea, and increased muscle mass.
- An adrenal cause of hirsutism should be considered in any female patient presenting with terminal hair growth in a central distribution—anterior neck to upper pubic area.
- An ovarian cause of hirsutism usually presents with lateral distribution of hair growth (sides of face, neck, and on breasts) and may be accompanied by menstrual abnormalities and obesity.

## 13.3. EVALUATION

- A thorough clinical history should be taken, taking into account the patient's age, ethnicity, medications, family history of hirsutism, and menstrual cycles.
- Physical examination should look for signs of virilization, peripheral hyperandrogenism, and insulin resistance.
- Basic laboratory evaluation should include total and free testosterone as well as DHEA-S, prolactin, and Δ-4-androstenedione.
  - DHEA-S is a marker of adrenal gland androgens.
  - Δ-4-androstenedione is indicative of an ovarian source of androgens.
- If significant abnormalities are found, referral to an endocrinologist or gynecologic endocrinologist should be considered.

# 14. Nail Disorders

- The nails often give many diagnostic clues about a patient's underlying health status, including inflammatory, traumatic, environmental, neoplastic, drug-induced, and psychiatric disease[15,16] (Table 9-8).

### TABLE 9-8 Common Nail Signs

| Nail Disorder | Physical Finding | Causes and Associated Diseases | Image |
|---|---|---|---|
| **Beau lines** | Transverse depression of nail plate due to temporary decrease in mitosis in nail matrix | *Multiple nails:* may be due to severe systemic illness, drug, high fever, viral infection<br>*Single nail:* trauma to matrix or paronychia | |
| **Onychomadesis** | Proximal shedding of nail | *Multiple nails:* usually due to systemic illness, high fever<br>*Single nail:* most often traumatic or paronychia | |

## TABLE 9-8  Common Nail Signs (continued)

| Nail Disorder | Physical Finding | Causes and Associated Diseases | Image |
|---|---|---|---|
| **Pitting** | Multiple punctate depressions of nail plate | *Psoriasis:* irregular pitting often in association with oil spots and onycholysis. Pitting also can be seen in alopecia areata (AA) | |
| **Onychorrhexis** | Nail brittleness and fragility in longitudinal direction | May be due to severe nail dryness and often is normal finding in older patients. Can be seen with lichen planus | |
| **Leukonychia** | White discoloration of nail due to either nail bed abnormalities (*apparent leukonychia*) or nail plate abnormalities (*true leukonychia*) | *Terry nails:* apparent leukonychia of proximal two-thirds of nail associated with liver cirrhosis. *Half and half nails:* proximal half of nail is white, common in hemodialysis patients. *Muehrcke lines:* transverse white bands often seen with cirrhosis or due to chemotherapy | |
| **Trachyonychia** (20-nail dystrophy) | Rough, sandpapered appearance of all 20 nails | Most commonly associated with AA, also seen with lichen planus, psoriasis, or eczema | |

*(continued)*

## TABLE 9-8  Common Nail Signs (*continued*)

| Nail Disorder | Physical Finding | Causes and Associated Diseases | Image |
|---|---|---|---|
| **Onycholysis** | Detachment of distal nail plate | Trauma, psoriasis, onychomycosis, tumors (solitary affected nail), or drug induced Tetracyclines (often after exposure to ultraviolet light) Fluoroquinolones Psoralens Nonsteroidal anti-inflammatory drugs | |
| **Subungual hyperkeratosis** | Accumulation of keratin debris under nail causing detachment and thickening of nail | Onychomycosis, psoriasis, trauma | |
| **Paronychia** | Erythema, swelling, and pain of nail folds, usually absent cuticle | *Acute paronychia:* often one nail affected, due to bacterial infection  *Chronic paronychia:* often one or more nails due to chronic irritation from manicures, exposure to water, often with yeast colonization  *Other causes:* epidermal growth factor receptor inhibitors, retinoids, indinavir | |

## TABLE 9-8    Common Nail Signs (*continued*)

| Nail Disorder | Physical Finding | Causes and Associated Diseases | Image |
|---|---|---|---|
| **Green nail syndrome** | Green-brown discoloration of nail due to pyocyanin pigment produced by *Pseudomonas aeruginosa* infection Often with onycholysis and paronychia | Predisposing factors include prolonged exposure to water, trauma, health care work. Treatment includes 4% thymol iodide in absolute alcohol applied to nail BID and dilute acetic acid soaks | |
| **Longitudinal melanonychia** | Brown-black pigmented streak on nail, common in dark-skinned patients | *Multiple streaks:* may be due to medications or systemic disease *Single streak:* may be due to subungual nevus or melanocyte hyperplasia, need to rule out subungual melanoma | |
| **Subungual malignant melanoma** | May present as brown-black longitudinal streak, often irregular, or subungual pigmented ulcer, or amelanotic lesion resembling a pyogenic granuloma | *Hutchinson sign:* extension of pigmentation onto periungual skin, suggestive of melanoma when seen with longitudinal melanonychia | |

Onychorrhexis image from Mohr WK. *Psychiatric-Mental Health Nursing*. 8th ed. Wolters Kluwer Health; 2013:532. Figure 26.6C; Green Nail Syndrome image from Goodheart HP, Gonzalez ME. *Goodheart's Photoguide to Common Pediatric and Adult Skin Disorders*. 4th ed. Wolters Kluwer Health; 2016. Figure 22-4.
Images courtesy of David Sheinbein, MD, Susan Bayliss, MD, and M. Laurin Council, MD.

- Involvement of all or most of the fingernails and/or toenails indicates a systemic cause of dystrophy, while involvement of one or two nails usually suggests exogenous source of injury, neoplasm, or local infection.

## Acknowledgment

The authors would like to acknowledge Katherine Moritz and Ann Martin for their contributions to the previous edition.

## REFERENCES

1. Sawaya ME, Price VH. Different levels of 5alpha-reductase type I and II, aromatase, and androgen receptor in hair follicles of women and men with androgenetic alopecia. *J Invest Dermatol*. 1997;109:296-300.
2. Arias-Santiago S, Buendía-Eisman A, Gutiérrez-Salmerón MT, Serrano-Ortega S. Male androgenetic alopecia. In: Preedy VR, ed. *Handbook of Hair in Health and Disease*. Wageningen Academic Publishers; 2012:98-116.
3. Lucky AW, Piacquadio DJ, Ditre CM, et al. A randomized, placebo-controlled trial of 5% and 2% topical minoxidil solutions in the treatment of female pattern hair loss. *J Am Acad Dermatol*. 2004;50(4):541-553.
4. Devjani S, Ezemma O, Kelley KJ, Stratton E, Senna M. Androgenetic alopecia: therapy update. *Drugs*. 2023;83(8):701-715.
5. Avram MR, Finney R. Platelet-rich plasma therapy for male and female pattern hair loss. *Dermatol Surg*. 2019;45(1):80-82.
6. Glass GE. Photobiomodulation: the clinical applications of low-level light therapy. *Aesthet Surg J*. 2021;41(6):723-738.
7. Sperling LC, Sinclair RD, El Shabrawi-Caelen L. Alopecias. In: Bolognia JL, Jorizzo JL, Schaffer JV, eds. *Dermatology*. 3rd ed. Elsevier Saunders; 2012:1093-1109.
8. Trueb RM. Diffuse hair loss. In: Blume-Peytavi U, Tosti A, Whitting DA, Trüeb RM, eds. *Hair Growth and Disorders*. Springer; 2008:259-272.
9. Ravindran AV, da Silva TL, Ravindran LN, Richter MA, Rector NA. Obsessive-compulsive spectrum disorders: a reviewed of the evidence-based treatments. *Can J Psychiatry*. 2009;54:331-343.
10. Gathers RC, Lim HW. Central centrifugal cicatricial alopecia: past, present, and future. *J Am Acad Dermatol*. 2009;60(4):660-668.
11. Malki L, Sarig O, Romano MT, et al. Variant PADI3 in central centrifugal cicatricial alopecia. *N Engl J Med*. 2019;380(9):833-841.
12. Harries MJ, Sinclair RD, Whiting DA, Griffiths CEM, Paus R. Management of primary cicatricial alopecias: options for treatment. *Br J Dermatol*. 2008;159(1):1-22.
13. Otberg N, Kang H, Alzolibani AA, Shapiro J. Folliculitis decalvans. *Dermatol Ther*. 2008;21:238-244.
14. Camacho-Martinez FM. Hypertrichosis and hirsutism. In: Bolognia JL, Jorizzo JL, Schaffer JV, eds. *Dermatology*. 3rd ed. Elsevier Saunders; 2012:1115-1127.
15. Piraccini BM. *Nail Disorders: A Practical Guide to Diagnosis and Management*. Springer; 2014.
16. Tosti A, Piraccini BM. Nail disorders. In: Bolognia JL, Jorizzo JL, Schaffer JV, eds. *Dermatology*. 3rd ed. Elsevier Saunders; 2012:1129-1144.

# 10 Cutaneous Manifestations of Systemic Disease

Amy Musiek, MD

It is important to not think of the skin as an isolated organ. Many systemic disorders have an associated skin involvement including autoimmune connective tissue disease and sarcoidosis, where cutaneous signs can aid in diagnosis. There are also primary skin conditions with secondary systemic involvement such as autoimmune blistering disease. Examples of these and further evaluation and management are reviewed here.

## 1. Lupus

### 1.1. BACKGROUND[1,2]

- Multisystem autoimmune disorder, characterized by presence of multiple antibodies.
- Skin involvement can be seen in up to 85% of patients with lupus; with four cutaneous signs included in the classification criteria for systemic lupus erythematosus (SLE).[3]
- Cutaneous lupus can be subdivided into three categories: acute, subacute, and chronic. Chronic cutaneous lupus contains multiple subtypes, including discoid lupus, that have different clinical manifestations.

### 1.2. CLINICAL PRESENTATION

- Acute cutaneous lupus erythematosus
  - Bilateral malar erythema, classically sparing the nasolabial folds following sun exposure
  - May also occur as a generalized photosensitive eruption, often involving the extensor forearms and dorsal hands
  - Is a manifestation of SLE
- Subacute cutaneous lupus erythematosus (SCLE) (Fig. 10-1)
  - Annular pink, scaly plaques, typically photodistributed on the upper chest and back.
  - Drug-induced variant: known drug triggers include proton pump inhibitors, hydrochlorothiazide, terbinafine, calcium channel blockers, antiepileptics, anti–tumor necrosis factor alpha agents.[4]
  - Neonatal lupus is a form of SCLE in neonates that can occur in mothers with anti-SSA antibodies. The eruption is like that of SCLE, with a predilection for the scalp and periorbital areas. Internal organ involvement can be seen with congenital heart block (with a mortality of 20% if untreated), hepatobiliary disease, and thrombocytopenia.
- Chronic lupus erythematous
  - Discoid lupus erythematosus (Fig. 10-2): indurated, erythematous thin papules and plaques with adherent scale on the face, scalp, and/or ears. Lesions heal with

*The authors would like to acknowledge the first edition author* Urvi Patel.

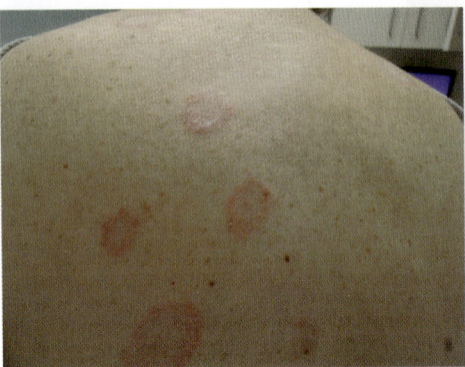

**Figure 10-1.** Subacute cutaneous lupus erythematosus. Nonscarring, erythematous, scaly, annular plaques on the back.

scarring, and 25% of patients can have oral involvement. There is increased risk of developing squamous cell carcinoma in scars or chronically inflamed lesions.

### 1.3. EVALUATION

- Skin biopsy can help differentiate cutaneous lupus from other skin disorders.
- Each subtype of lupus has a varying risk of developing systemic lupus.
- Blood tests
  - Acute lupus erythematosus
    - Antinuclear antibody (ANA), double-stranded DNA, Sjögren syndrome–related antigen A and B (SS-A and SS-B), Smith antibody, U1 small nuclear ribonucleoprotein, histone antibodies, complete blood count, complete metabolic panel, urinalysis, and complement levels
  - Subacute cutaneous lupus erythematosus
    - ANA, SS-A, and SS-B.
    - 18% to 50% of patient will possess the criteria for SLE.[5]

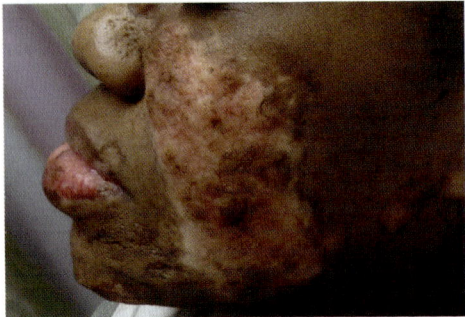

**Figure 10-2.** Discoid lupus erythematosus. Erythematous to hyperpigmented plaques with central scarring and atrophy.

- Discoid lupus erythematosus
  - ANA often negative
  - 5% to 15% risk of developing SLE

## 1.4. TREATMENT[6]

- Lifestyle: strict photoprotection and smoking cessation.
- First-line agents: topical or intralesional steroids, class 1 steroid often required.
- Antimalarial agents are standard of care when systemic therapy is needed.
  - First line: hydroxychloroquine at 200 mg twice a day for most patients.
  - Alternative: chloroquine.
  - Quinacrine may be added to either of the above agents.
- Antimalarial-resistant lupus
  - Methotrexate
  - Thalidomide
  - Mycophenolate mofetil
  - Dapsone
  - Anifrolumab

# 2. Dermatomyositis

## 2.1. BACKGROUND[7]

- Autoimmune inflammatory myopathy with cutaneous findings and systemic involvement, currently with unknown pathogenesis.
- Skin manifestations and pathogenic autoantibodies can help differentiate dermatomyositis (DM) from other autoimmune disorders as well as different subtypes of DM.

## 2.2. CLINICAL PRESENTATION

- Classic dermatomyositis (Fig. 10-3)
  - Gottron papules: violaceous papules overlying the dorsal interphalangeal or metacarpophalangeal, elbow, or knee joints
  - Linear extensor erythema: erythema running along the extensor tendons on the hands
  - Heliotrope rash: violaceous erythema and edema involving the periorbital region and eyelids
  - Shawl sign: pink poikiloderma across the upper back
  - V-distributed erythema: photo-distributed pink and erythematous patches on the mid- to upper chest
  - Holster sign: erythematous patches on the hips
  - Mechanic's hands: erythematous, scaly, hyperkeratotic papules and plaques on the palms and lateral surfaces with fissuring
  - Periungual telangiectasias and "ragged" cuticles
  - Calcinosis cutis
- Antisynthetase syndrome[8]
  - Mechanic's hands: most characteristic finding of antisynthetase syndrome
  - Other cutaneous features: Gottron papules and Raynaud phenomenon
  - Extracutaneous findings: interstitial lung disease (ILD), arthritis, myositis, and fever

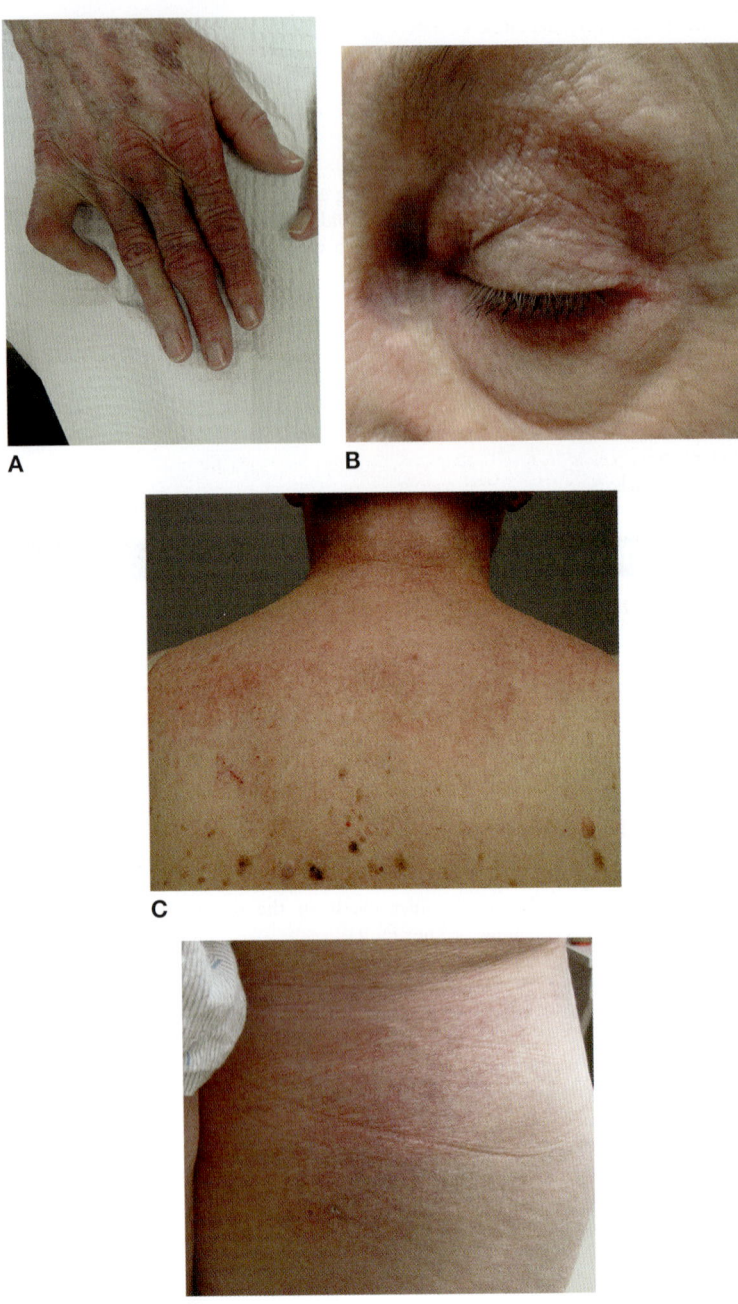

**Figure 10-3.** Dermatomyositis. **A.** Linear extensor erythema. **B.** Heliotrope rash. **C.** Shawl sign. **D.** Holster sign.

- Associated antibodies: to aminoacyl transfer ribonucleic acid synthetases, including Jo-1, OJ, KJ, PL-7, and PL-12
- Amyopathic dermatomyositis
  - Typical skin findings noted above, without the findings of muscle involvement within 6 months after onset of skin findings.
  - Associated antibodies: transcriptional intermediary factor 1-γ antibody (TIF1-γ; 80% of patients) and clinically amyopathic dermatomyositis-140 (CADM-140) antibodies (10%-15% of patients). Those with CADM-140 antibodies have a risk of severe, progressive ILD that can lead to death from respiratory failure.
- Immune-mediated necrotizing myopathy
  - Patients with anti-HMGCR antibodies may have atypical skin findings.[9]
  - Manifestations include ashlike scales, nonscaly red patches, and lumps, predominantly on the neck and back.
  - Histopathological examination of these skin lesions often reveals Bcl-2–positive lymphocytic infiltrations.
- Dermatomyositis and malignancy[10,11]
  - In adults, there is an increased risk (5%-7%) of developing a malignancy.
  - Most common malignancies: ovarian, lung, pancreatic, stomach, and colorectal carcinomas.
  - Can present anywhere from 2 years preceding to 3 years after presentation of DM.
  - Poorer prognostic factors include older age, male, cutaneous ulceration, and dysphagia.
  - Associated antibodies: TIF1-γ (formerly known as p-155).
- Extracutaneous involvement
  - Musculoskeletal: symmetric, proximal muscle weakness initially but can progress to all muscle groups
  - Pulmonary: ILD, pulmonary hypertension, and pneumothorax
  - Gastrointestinal: dysphagia secondary to pharyngeal muscle involvement, esophageal reflux, and dysmotility
  - Cardiac: arrhythmias and conduction defects
- Drug induced[12]
  - Hydroxyurea and statins (per above) are the most common culprits.

## 2.3. EVALUATION[7]

- Skin biopsy can help point toward a diagnosis of DM.
- Muscle involvement: serum creatinine kinase and aldolase, electromyography, magnetic resonance imaging, and muscle biopsy.
- Serology testing
  - ANA positive less than 10% of the time.
  - Other myositis antibodies (as above) may be helpful, but they are not always widely available.
- Refer for pulmonary function testing to evaluate for ILD.
- Physical examination and history, age-appropriate malignancy screening, computed tomography (CT) scan of the chest, abdomen, and pelvis in patient at risk for malignancy, and a pelvic ultrasound.

## 2.4. TREATMENT[7]

- Muscle disease is more responsive to treatment than is cutaneous disease.
- Initial (acute) therapy: corticosteroids.

- Steroid-sparing agents
  - First line: hydroxychloroquine—helpful for cutaneous disease, questionable efficacy for muscle disease
  - Second line: methotrexate, azathioprine, mycophenolate mofetil, intravenous immunoglobulin, rituximab, anifrolumab

# 3. Sarcoidosis

## 3.1. BACKGROUND[13]

- A chronic, granulomatous multisystem disorder with unclear etiology.
- Cutaneous disease is present in at least 20% of patients and can be the initial sign in one-third of these patients.
- Ninety to ninety-five percent of patient with skin disease will have pulmonary involvement.
- Cutaneous manifestations can vary greatly.

## 3.2. CLINICAL PRESENTATION

- Classically red-brown to violaceous indurated papules and plaques (Fig. 10-4).
- Lupus pernio
  - Violaceous papules and plaques favoring the nose, ears, and cheeks. The classic presentation is a beaded appearance around the nasal rim.
  - Association with chronic sarcoidosis of the lungs (~75% of patients) and of the upper respiratory tract (~50% of patients).
  - Can heal with scarring.
- Papular sarcoidosis
  - Skin-colored papules typically on the face, specifically on the eyelid and nasolabial folds, that heals without scarring
  - Favorable disease prognosis
- Darier-Roussy
  - Skin-colored, subcutaneous, firm, mobile nodules on the extremities; usually painless (differentiating it from erythema nodosum)

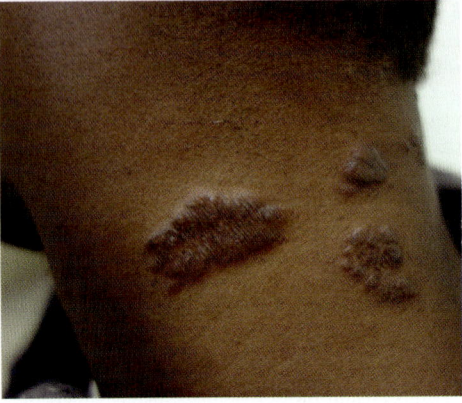

**Figure 10-4.** Sarcoid. Hyperpigmented, dermal plaques.

- Löfgren syndrome
  - Acute form of sarcoidosis that includes erythema nodosum, polyarthralgias, and bilateral hilar lymphadenopathy
- Scar sarcoidosis
  - Infiltration of sarcoidal granulomas in previous surgical sites, tattoos, piercings, and other sites of trauma
- Higher incidence in African Americans and women.
- African Americans have more severe disease.
- Japanese patients are more likely to have cardiac and ocular involvement.

### 3.3. EVALUATION

- Skin biopsy should show noncaseating granulomas with no or sparse surrounding inflammation.
- Labs: complete metabolic panel, serum calcium, 1,25 dihydroxyvitamin D, and angiotensin-converting enzyme level (may decline with therapy, but does not have prognostic value).
- Chest radiograph or high-resolution CT scan of the chest to determine nodal and parenchymal involvement.
- Pulmonary function testing and carbon monoxide diffusion capacity.
- Electrocardiogram to evaluate cardiac involvement.

### 3.4. TREATMENT

- Topical and intralesional steroids for limited cutaneous involvement
- Systemic steroids for widespread or disfiguring involvement
- Hydroxychloroquine, methotrexate, tetracyclines, and tumor necrosis factor-alpha inhibitors for maintenance

## 4. Scleroderma and Related Disorders

### 4.1. BACKGROUND

- Scleroderma describes fibrosis of the dermis and subcutaneous tissue. Scleroderma can be classified as either localized cutaneous disease or cutaneous with systemic disease.
- Morphea is also known as localized scleroderma. It is generally self-limiting and typically appears as solitary and linear plaques.[14]
- Systemic sclerosis includes both limited scleroderma (CREST) and progressive systemic sclerosis.[15]
- Lichen sclerosus et atrophicus (LSA) is another inflammatory skin disorder that affects superficial dermis and mucosa leading to atrophic scarring.[16]

### 4.2. CLINICAL PRESENTATION

- Morphea[14]
  - Begins as erythematous to violaceous plaques that evolve into white, sclerotic plaques and will resolve as hyperpigmented atrophic plaques
- Scleroderma[15]
  - Limited scleroderma (CREST)
    - Calcinosis cutis, Raynaud phenomenon, esophageal dysmotility, sclerodactyly, telangiectasia

- Progressive systemic sclerosis
  - Hallmarks are sclerodactyly and digital pitting scars.
  - Other features include taut and waxy skin, calcinosis cutis, nail fold capillary changes, matlike telangiectasias, Raynaud phenomenon, and salt and pepper dyspigmentation.
  - Morbidity and mortality are from pulmonary, renal, cardiac, and gastrointestinal involvement.
- The physician should differentiate between morphea and systemic sclerosis. Systemic involvement, sclerodactyly, nail fold changes, and Raynaud phenomenon are not seen in morphea but are seen in systemic sclerosis.
- Lichen sclerosus et atrophicus[16] (LSA)
  - Erythematous patches that evolve into atrophic white plaques. Lesions are more commonly located in the anogenital area and can have significant pruritus.
  - This can be complicated by fissuring, fusion of labia minora to majora, introital narrowing, phimosis, dyspareunia, and dysuria.
  - Increased risk of developing squamous cell carcinoma in anogenital lesions.
  - Women with genital LSA should have alternate evaluations with dermatology and gynecology.

## 4.3. EVALUATION

- These are clinical diagnoses, where skin biopsies can be supportive but not diagnostic among this group of disorders.
- No further evaluation for LSA and morphea.
- Systemic sclerosis[15]
  - ANA, anticentromere antibody (CREST), and antitopoisomerase I (aka Scl-70) antibodies
  - Pulmonary involvement: chest radiograph, pulmonary function testing, and high-resolution CT
  - Gastrointestinal involvement: esophagogram, esophagoduodenoscopy, and small bowel series

## 4.4. TREATMENT

- Morphea[17]
  - First line: topical steroids and topical calcineurin inhibitors
  - Refractory disease: phototherapy and methotrexate
  - Physical therapy in the case of contractures
- Scleroderma[15]
  - No agent reverses the process. Disease-modifying agents that have been used with mixed success include methotrexate and cyclophosphamide. In the most severe cases, stem cell transplantation has also been used in clinical trials, but currently is not the standard of care.
  - Proton pump inhibitors and/or $H_2$ blocker for gastroesophageal reflux disease symptoms. Esophageal strictures may need esophageal dilation. Metoclopramide and erythromycin can promote upper gastrointestinal motility. Octreotide is useful to lower gastrointestinal motility.
  - Angiotensin-converting enzyme inhibitors to prevent scleroderma renal crisis.
  - Prostacyclin analogs, bosentan, and sildenafil have been used for pulmonary hypertension.
  - Treatment of digital ulceration includes proper wound care and treatment of bacterial superinfections.

- Lichen sclerosus at atrophicus[16]
  - First line: topical steroids and topical calcineurin inhibitors
  - Second line: phototherapy

# 5. Bullous Disorders

## 5.1. BACKGROUND

- A heterogeneous group of acquired disorders consisting of bullous cutaneous findings secondary to autoantibodies to antigens in the epidermis and basement membrane
- Pemphigus vulgaris (PV) and pemphigus foliaceus (PF)[18]
  - Due to IgG autoantibodies to proteins important in cell-to-cell adhesion
    PF: desmoglein 1
    PV: desmoglein 3
- Bullous pemphigoid[19]
  - Most common immunobullous disorder, typically affecting the older adults (Fig. 10-5)
  - Antibodies to bullous pemphigus (BP) antigen 230 (aka BPAg1) and BP antigen 180 (BPAg2) located in the basement membrane
- Dermatitis herpetiformis (DH)[20]
  - Autoimmune disorder due to IgA antibodies to epidermal transglutaminase (also known as tissue transglutaminase 3)

## 5.2. CLINICAL PRESENTATION

- PV and foliaceus[18]
  - Skin findings consist of flaccid blisters and erosions in both types.
  - Mucosal involvement is only seen in PV and presents as painful erosions.
- Bullous pemphigoid[19]
  - Tense vesicles and bullae on erythematous, urticarial, or eczematous plaques
  - Association with neurologic disorders, specifically Parkinson disease, dementia, psychiatric disorders, stroke, and multiple sclerosis
- Dermatitis herpetiformis[20]
  - Grouped erythematous papules and vesicles commonly on bilateral extensor surfaces, scalp, and buttocks. Lesions are very pruritic and are replaced with erosions and excoriations. These erosions can be the initial presentation.
  - All patients with DH have celiac disease, which can be clinically silent.
  - Associated disorders include type 1 diabetes mellitus and Hashimoto thyroiditis.
  - Patients have a higher risk of non-Hodgkin lymphoma, particularly enteropathy-associated T-cell lymphoma.

## 5.3. EVALUATION

- Skin biopsy for H&E and for direct immunofluorescence
  - A biopsy for direct immunofluorescence should be perilesional (contain normal skin).
- PV and PF[18]
  - ELISA for desmogleins 1 and 3
- BP[16]
  - Indirect immunofluorescence
  - ELISA for BP180 and BP230

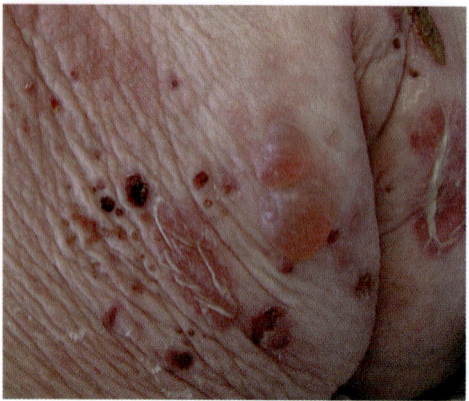

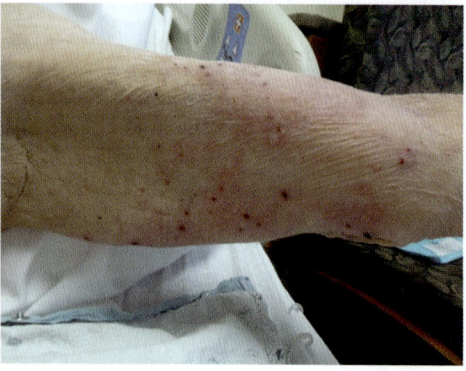

Figure 10-5. Bullous pemphigoid. **A.** Erythematous, urticarial plaque with tense vesicles. **B.** Tense bullae on erythematous background.

- DH[17]
  - Total IgA level.
  - Antitissue transglutaminase (tTG2), IgA, and IgG.
  - Antiepidermal transglutaminase (tTG3), IgA, and IgG.
  - Antiendomysial IgA and IgG.
  - Check for associated disorders, that is, thyroid function testing, blood glucose tolerance, and complete blood count.

## 5.4. TREATMENT

- PV and foliaceus[21]
  - First line: rituximab and oral corticosteroids
  - Second line: intravenous immunoglobulin, azathioprine, and mycophenolate mofetil

- Bullous pemphigoid[19]
  - First line: topical and oral steroids
  - Second line: mycophenolate mofetil, azathioprine, **omalizumab, dupilumab,** and methotrexate
- Dermatitis herpetiformis[22]
  - First line: adherence to gluten-free diet and dapsone

## 6. Nutritional Deficiencies[23]

- Most nutritional deficiencies have cutaneous manifestations, and some are pathognomonic for specific deficiencies (Table 10-1).

| TABLE 10-1 | Nutritional Deficiencies | | |
|---|---|---|---|
| Deficiency | Clinical Manifestation | Treatment | Misc. |
| Vitamin A | Aka phrynoderma; keratotic, follicular papules typically extremities and buttocks | Vitamin A 50,000-200,000 IU/d depending on age and clinical severity | Can have night blindness, keratomalacia, and stunted growth |
| Vitamin K | Purpura and ecchymoses | Phytonadione: Newborn: 0.5-1.0 mg Children: 2 mg Adults: 5-10 mg Fresh frozen plasma in cases of acute hemorrhage | Will have elevated prothrombin time and INR |
| Vitamin $B_1$ (thiamine) | Aka beriberi; glossitis and skin breakdown | Thiamine 100 mg TID IV × several days, then switch to 100 mg/d | |
| Vitamin $B_2$ (riboflavin) | Aka oral-ocular-genital syndrome; angular stomatitis (macerated papules and fissuring at corners of the mouth), cheilitis (erythema and fissuring of lips), glossitis, crusted and erythematous patches and plaques in the inguinal folds extending to vulva/scrotum and inner thighs, photophobia, and conjunctivitis | Riboflavin: Infants and children: 1.0-2.0 mg/d Adults: 10-20 mg/d | |

*(continued)*

| TABLE 10-1 | Nutritional Deficiencies (*continued*) | | |
|---|---|---|---|
| Deficiency | Clinical Manifestation | Treatment | Misc. |
| Vitamin $B_3$ (niacin or nicotinic acid) | Aka pellagra; photodistributed erythematous and hyperpigmented plaques on face, chest, neck, and dorsal hands | Nicotinamide (aka nicotinic acid) 500 mg daily for several weeks | Classic tetrad: dermatitis, dementia, diarrhea, death |
| Vitamin $B_6$ (pyridoxine) | Seborrheic dermatitis including face and perineum, angular cheilitis, glossitis with ulceration | Pyridoxine 100 mg daily | |
| Vitamin $B_{12}$ (cobalamin) | Glossitis with fissuring, hyperpigmentation | Cyanocobalamin 1 mg weekly × 1 month, then monthly if persistent | |
| Vitamin C | Aka scurvy; ecchymoses and follicular petechiae and hyperkeratosis; corkscrew hairs (Fig. 10-6) | Ascorbic acid 100-300 mg/d | |
| Folic acid (vitamin $B_9$) | Cheilitis, glossitis with mucosal erosions, and hyperpigmentation | Folic acid 1-5 mg daily | |
| Biotin (vitamin $B_7$) | Erythema and crusting in seborrheic and periorificial distribution, alopecia | Biotin 150 μg daily | |
| Iron | Pallor, koilonychia, glossitis, angular cheilitis, alopecia | Elemental iron: 100-200 mg of elemental iron daily | |
| Zinc | Periorificial eczematous plaques that become eroded and macerated, alopecia, diarrhea | Elemental zinc: Inherited: 3 mg/kg daily Acquired in children: 0.5-1 mg/kg/d Acquired in adults: 15-30 mg/d | Can be an acquired or inherited deficiency, latter of which is known as acrodermatitis enteropathica |
| Marasmus | Dry, wrinkled, and loose skin; aged facial appearance due to loss of buccal fat pads, alopecia | Slow replacement of protein and calories | Total nutrient deficiency |
| Kwashiorkor | Desquamation and erosions | Aggressive nutritional replacement | Hypoproteinemia |

Of note, Vitamin D and E deficiencies do not have cutaneous manifestations.
Reprinted with permission from Schaefer SM, Hivnor CM. Nutritional diseases. In: Bolognia JL, Jorizzo JL, Schaffer JV, eds. *Dermatology*. 3rd ed. Elsevier Saunders; 2012:737-751. Table 51-2.

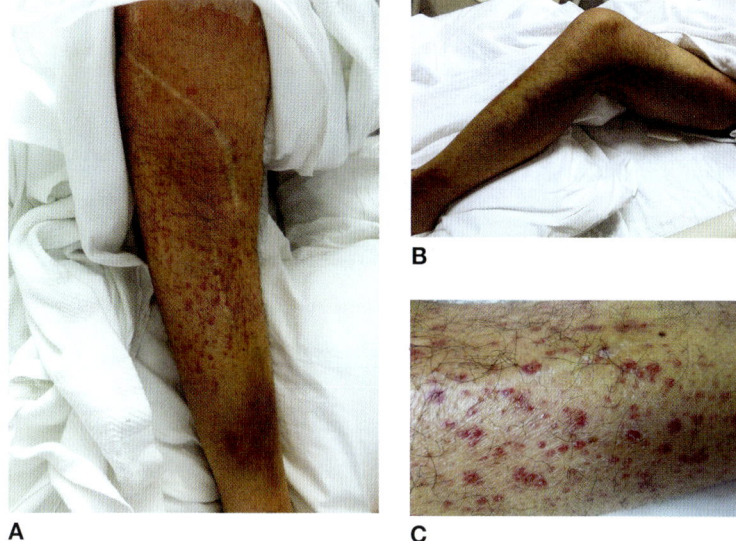

**Figure 10-6.** Scurvy. **A.** Petechiae. **B.** Extensive ecchymoses. **C.** Perifollicular petechiae with corkscrew hairs.

# REFERENCES

1. Rothfield N, Sontheimer RD, Bernstein M. Lupus erythematosus: systemic and cutaneous manifestations. *Clin Dermatol.* 2006;24(5):348-362.
2. Lee LA, Werth BP. Lupus erythematosus. In: Bolognia JL, Jorizzo JL, Schaffer JV, eds. *Dermatology.* 3rd ed. Elsevier Saunders; 2012:615-629.
3. Aringer M, Costenbader K, Daikh D, et al. 2019 European League against rheumatism/American College of Rheumatology Classification Criteria for systemic lupus erythematosus. *Ann Rheum Dis.* 2019;78(9):1151-1159.
4. Poh YJ, Alrashid A, Sangle SR, et al. Proton pump inhibitor induced subacute cutaneous lupus erythematosus: clinical characteristics and outcomes. *Lupus.* 2022;31(9):1078-1083. doi:10.1177/09612033221104237
5. Grönhagen CM, Fored CM, Granath F, Nyberg F. Cutaneous lupus erythematosus and the association with systemic lupus erythematosus: a population-based cohort of 1088 patients in Sweden. *Br J Dermatol.* 2011;164(6):1335-1341.
6. Kuhn A, Ruland V, Bonsmann G. Cutaneous lupus erythematosus: update of therapeutic options part I. *J Am Acad Dermatol.* 2011;65(6):e179-e193.
7. Kovacs SO, Kovacs SC. Dermatomyositis. *J Am Acad Dermatol.* 1998;39:899-920.
8. Katzap E, Barilla-LaBarca ML, Marder G. Antisynthetase syndrome. *Curr Rheumatol Rep.* 2011;13(3):175-181.
9. Kurashige T, Nakamura R, Murao T, et al. Atypical skin conditions of the neck and back as a dermal manifestation of anti-HMGCR antibody-positive myopathy. *BMC Immunol.* 2024;25(1):30. doi:10.1186/s12865-024-00622-2
10. Hill CL, Zhang Y, Sigurgeirsson B, et al. Frequency of specific cancer types in dermatomyositis and polymyositis: a population-based study. *Lancet.* 2001;357(9250):96-100.
11. Wang J, Guo G, Chen G, Wu B, Lu L, Bao L. Meta-analysis of the association of dermatomyositis and polymyositis with cancer. *Br J Dermatol.* 2013;169(4):838-847.
12. Seidler AM, Gottlieb AB. Dermatomyositis induced by drug therapy: a review of case reports. *J Am Acad Dermatol.* 2008;59(5):872-880.
13. Haimovic A, Sanchez M, Judson MA, Prystowsky S. Sarcoidosis: a comprehensive review and update for the dermatologist: part I. Cutaneous disease. *J Am Acad Dermatol.* 2012;66(5):699.e1-699.e18.
14. Fett N, Werth VP. Update on morphea: part I. Epidemiology, clinical presentation, and pathogenesis. *J Am Acad Dermatol.* 2011;64(2):217-228.

15. Chung L, Lin J, Furst DE, Fiorentino D. Systemic and localized scleroderma. *Clin Dermatol.* 2006;24(5):374-392.
16. Meffert JJ, Davis BM, Grimwood RE. Lichen sclerosus. *J Am Acad Dermatol.* 1995;32(3):393-416.
17. Fett N, Werth VP. Update on morphea: part II. Outcome measures and treatment. *J Am Acad Dermatol.* 2011;64(2):231-242.
18. Ruocco V, Ruocco E, Lo Schiavo A, Brunetti G, Guerrera LP, Wolf R. Pemphigus: etiology, pathogenesis, and inducing or triggering factors: facts and controversies. *Clin Dermatol.* 2013;31(4):374-381.
19. Di Zenzo G, Della Torre R, Zambruno G, Borradori L. Bullous pemphigoid: from the clinic to the bench. *Clin Dermatol.* 2012;30(1):3-16.
20. Bolotin D, Petronic-Rosic V. Dermatitis herpetiformis. Part I. Epidemiology, pathogenesis, and clinical presentation. *J Am Acad Dermatol.* 2011;64(6):1017-1024.
21. Cianchini G, Lupi F, Masini C, Corona R, Puddu P, De Pità O. Therapy with rituximab for autoimmune pemphigus: results from a single-center observational study on 42 cases with long-term follow-up. *J Am Acad Dermatol.* 2012;67(4):617-622.
22. Bolotin D, Petronic-Rosic V. Dermatitis herpetiformis. Part II. Diagnosis, management, and prognosis. *J Am Acad Dermatol.* 2011;64(6):1027-1033.
23. Jen M, Yan AC. Syndromes associated with nutritional deficiency and excess. *Clin Dermatol.* 2010;28(6):669-685.

# 11 Dermatologic Surgery

Ali Malik, MD, Aubriana M. McEvoy, MD, MS, and M. Slade Stratton, MD

Cutaneous surgery is an important part of dermatology and is the mainstay of treatment for many benign and malignant neoplasms. Understanding key principles of dermatologic surgery is important for both primary care physicians and dermatologists.

## 1. Preoperative Assessment

- A careful preoperative patient evaluation is the first step to ensuring optimal surgical outcomes.
- In addition to a comprehensive review of past medical and surgical history, special attention should be paid to several areas outlined below.

### 1.1. CARDIOVASCULAR RISK AND ANTICOAGULANT USE

- The surgeon must understand a patient's history in regard to cardiovascular disease, hypercoagulability, anticoagulant medications and supplements, and the presence of implantable cardiac devices (pacemakers and defibrillators).
- Pertinent cardiovascular disease history includes myocardial infarction, stroke, transient ischemic attack, atrial fibrillation, and cardiac or vascular stents. This information is crucial to determine the appropriateness of preoperative continuation of anticoagulants and medications that increase the risk of bleeding. Additionally, this history can guide whether medications such as tranexamic acid are used to control bleeding intra- and postoperatively.
  - In patients without cardiovascular disease or the conditions listed above, it is acceptable to hold preventative aspirin as well as vitamin E, multivitamins, fish oil, and omega-3 fatty acid supplements for 14 days leading up to surgical excision.[1,2] Given the minimal risk, surgeons may also choose to allow patients to continue supplements in the perioperative period.
  - Reversible platelet inhibitors such as nonaspirin nonsteroidal anti-inflammatory drugs are typically held only 2 days prior to a procedure, by surgeons and patients choosing to do so.[3]
  - Anticoagulation is typically not discontinued for small procedures such as biopsies, regardless of their indication.
  - Patients may be on medications other than anticoagulants which increase the risk of bleeding (ie, ibrutinib). The risks and benefits of continuing or discontinuing the medication in the perioperative period should be discussed with the patient and/or prescribing physician.
  - In patients who have a history of cardiovascular disease or hypercoagulability of any type, it is important to continue regimens such as aspirin, warfarin, direct oral anticoagulants, and clopidogrel because the risk of serious life-threatening events outweighs the benefit of minimizing minor bleeding complications.[4]

---

*The authors would like to acknowledge the first edition authors* Chris Urban and Eva Hurst.

- The surgeon must also assess a patient's history of bleeding disorders or thrombocytopenia.
  - Guidelines set forth by the American Society of Clinical Oncology state that major invasive procedures may safely be performed with platelet counts of 40,000 to 50,000.[5]
  - Platelet transfusion should be considered for patients with platelets under 30,000 for excisions, although small biopsies can likely be performed with care in patients with even lower levels when utilizing meticulous hemostasis.

## 1.2. IMPLANTABLE CARDIAC DEVICES

- In patients without implanted electrical devices, electrocoagulation is used to stop normal bleeding.
- The concern with using electrosurgery in patients with implanted electrical devices is that the newly introduced current may be detected and interpreted as cardiac electrical activity. Although this is unlikely, it could theoretically alter pacemaker function or stimulate the activation of a defibrillator and result in harm to the patient.
- In patients with a pacemaker but no defibrillator, it is safe to use unipolar electrocoagulation or electrodessication in short bursts of less than a few seconds at the lowest effective settings as long as the treatment area is not directly over the cardiac device.
- In patients who have a defibrillator, the safest option is to use heat cautery only, although a recent study suggests bipolar electrocautery devices are safe.[6]

## 1.3. INFECTION PRECAUTIONS

- Several variables should be considered in the preoperative and intraoperative setting to determine a patient's risk of postoperative infection including site of surgery, depth of surgery, patient comorbidities, etc.
- Most wounds in dermatologic surgery are created on normal skin using clean or sterile technique and are considered clean wounds. The infection rate is very low, and prophylactic antibiotics are typically not necessary.
- Wounds on the oral cavity, axilla, and perineum are considered clean-contaminated, and the infection rate approaches 10%.[7]
- Risk factors for postoperative wound infection include diabetes, immunocompromised states secondary to immune deficiency or medications, smoking, malnutrition, and concurrent malignancies.
- Patients who have had joint replacement surgery with insertion of artificial joints within the past 6 months should be given prophylactic oral antibiotics preoperatively.
  - An appropriate preoperative, prophylactic regimen is cephalexin 2 g at least 60 minutes before surgery. Clindamycin 600 mg can be used in patients with a penicillin or cephalosporin allergy.[8]
- If there is concern or risk for methicillin-resistant *Staphylococcus aureus* or MRSA infection, doxycycline can be used as an empiric treatment.
- Bacterial endocarditis prophylaxis may be considered for high-risk patients who have prosthetic cardiac valves, previous bacterial endocarditis, complex congenital heart disease, and pulmonary shunts.
  - Antibiotic regimens for endocarditis prophylaxis are directed toward *Streptococcus* viridans, the most common cause of endocarditis for dental, oral, respiratory tract,

or esophageal procedures, and the recommended standard prophylactic regimen is a single dose of oral amoxicillin administered 1 hour preoperatively.[9]
- Preoperative, intraincisional, prophylactic buffered lidocaine with epinephrine containing clindamycin has been found to be a safe and effective method to reduce postoperative surgical site infections and may help reduce systemic antibiotic overuse.[10]
- Prior to cosmetic peels, some laser therapies, and surgical procedures that remove the top layers of skin such as dermabrasion, patients should be questioned about a history of shingles or herpes.
- Many studies have described the effectiveness of valacyclovir prophylaxis following laser resurfacing and chemical peels.[11] If the patient reports a positive history of shingles or herpes at the surgical site, a prophylactic course of valacyclovir 500 mg twice per day for a week, starting the day of surgery, may be prescribed to reduce the risk of a flare or recurrence. Additional prophylactic dosing regimens may be utilized even for patients with no history of shingles or herpes for higher-risk procedures, given the potential for scarring should an outbreak occurs.

### 1.4. INFORMED CONSENT

- Procedural risk must be clearly explained to patients before any procedure.
- For most surgeries, this may include but is not limited to, pain, swelling, erythema, infection, bleeding, surgical dehiscence, scarring, hyperpigmentation or hypopigmentation, incomplete response, and need for further treatment.
- The health care provider who will be performing the procedure should review the relevant risks and give the patient time to ask any questions or express concerns before written consent is obtained.

### 1.5. SURGICAL PREPARATION

- Surgical preparation begins with careful positioning of the patient.
  - The goal is to maximize patient comfort while providing the surgeon with easy access to the surgical site.
  - Typically, patients are situated in the supine position to maximize comfort unless lesions are located on the back or posterior legs.
  - For even minor biopsies, it is recommended that the patient be reclined to minimize the risk of vasovagal reaction and injury from falling.

### 1.6. ANTISEPTICS

- Antiseptics have a broad spectrum and are important for infection control.
  - For minor procedures such as punch and shave biopsies, isopropyl alcohol preparation and clean nonsterile gloves can be used.
  - Invasive procedures such as surgical excisions and repairs of defects after Mohs micrographic surgery (MMS) should be cleaned with either povidone-iodine or chlorhexidine scrub.
  - Both of these agents have good coverage of Gram-positive and Gram-negative bacteria plus viruses.
  - Chlorhexidine gluconate can cause ototoxicity and keratitis, so it is necessary to avoid contact with eyes and the external auditory canal.
  - Iodine is safe to use around the eyes and ears but must be allowed to dry to become effective.

- Side effects of iodine include skin irritant and allergic contact dermatitis.
- Sterile towels should also be placed around the field, and patients should be reminded to keep their hands away from the sterile field.[12]

## 1.7. ANESTHESIA

- Most cutaneous surgical procedures can be performed under local anesthesia.
- One of the most common local anesthetic used in dermatologic surgery is 1% lidocaine with epinephrine 1:100,000.
- It is important to inquire and document whether the patient has an allergy or adverse reaction to local anesthetic.
- Other options for local anesthesia for minor procedures such as biopsy include diphenhydramine hydrochloride 12.5 mg/mL, intradermal injection of normal saline, and/or cryoanesthesia with ice.[13] Topical anesthetics, such as EMLA cream (a eutectic mixture of lidocaine 2.5% and prilocaine 2.5%) or LMX4 (lidocaine 4% cream), can be used prior to laser therapy and prior to infiltration with local anesthesia but are insufficient to address pain associated with biopsy or dermatologic surgery.
- Female patients must be asked if they are pregnant or breastfeeding.
  - During pregnancy, lidocaine is a category B medication and is considered safe, but timing of the procedure should be taken into consideration so as to minimize risk to the patient and fetus. Because epinephrine alone is pregnancy category C, some physicians will use plain lidocaine on women who are pregnant. Commercially available preparations of lidocaine with epinephrine, 1:100,000 list pregnancy category B on the package insert.
  - Lidocaine concentrations in milk are low, and ingested lidocaine is poorly absorbed by the infant. Lidocaine is not expected to cause any adverse effects in breastfed infants. Therefore, no special precautions are required.[14]
- Local anesthetic agents act by blocking the sodium and potassium channels of nerve cells to prevent depolarization.
  - Unmyelinated C-type nerve fibers conduct pain and temperature signals and are most effectively blocked by local anesthesia.
  - Pressure sensations are transmitted by myelinated A-type fibers that are less effectively blocked by local anesthesia.
    - For this reason, patients commonly report being able to feel pressure but no pain during procedures.
- Most local anesthetics lead to vasodilation and increased bleeding at the surgical site. Epinephrine is a vasoconstrictor and is added to reduce surgical site bleeding, prolong the effectiveness of local anesthetics, and reduce systemic toxicity to local anesthetics by decreasing systemic absorption.
  - Although the anesthetic effects of lidocaine occur within minutes, the full vasoconstrictive effect of epinephrine takes approximately 15 minutes.
  - Without epinephrine, the half-life of lidocaine in healthy individuals is approximately 90 to 120 minutes (1.5-2 hours). This means that it takes 1.5 to 2 hours for the body to reduce the concentration of lidocaine in the bloodstream by half. Lidocaine without epinephrine provides a duration of local anesthesia lasting approximately 30 to 60 minutes.
  - With epinephrine, the half-life of lidocaine remains roughly the same at 90 to 120 minutes, as epinephrine primarily affects the local action of lidocaine rather than its systemic metabolism. However, with epinephrine, the duration of anesthesia is prolonged to approximately 2 to 6 hours, depending on the area of administration.

- Maximum dosing of lidocaine without epinephrine is a 4.5 mg/kg of body weight.[15] The absolute maximum is typically 300 mg total in adults regardless of body weight. This lower dose limit is due to the risk of systemic absorption and potential toxicity, which can include symptoms such as central nervous system effects (dizziness, seizures) and cardiovascular effects (arrhythmias, hypotension).
- Maximum dosing of lidocaine with epinephrine is 7 mg/kg of body weight with an absolute maximum of 500 mg total in adults.[15] The addition of epinephrine (usually at a concentration of 1:100,000 or 1:200,000) allows for a higher maximum dose.
- Use of epinephrine is contraindicated in untreated hyperthyroidism and pheochromocytoma. It should be used cautiously in hypertensive patients because it can lead to increases in blood pressure.
- Although a true allergy to epinephrine is uncommon, patients often describe physiologic symptoms of epinephrine sensitivity including mild tremors and racing heart rate or palpitations.
- The combination of lidocaine 1% with 1:100,000 epinephrine has a very low pH and is painful during injection.
- The pain can be mitigated by adding sodium bicarbonate to neutralize the solution; however, this must be freshly prepared because the basic pH reduces the water solubility and shelf life of the anesthetic.
- Other techniques for reducing pain and burning during injection include injecting slowly, warming the solution to room temperature before injection, using a small-gauge needle (30 g), and placing subsequent needlesticks in areas that are already numb.
- Lidocaine is an amide anesthetic and is metabolized by liver enzymes.
- In patients with reported anesthesia allergies, careful history must be taken to elucidate the actual cause and determine reasonable alternatives.[13]
  - Clindamycin can be added to buffered lidocaine with epinephrine to reduce postoperative surgical site infections and reduce systemic antibiotic overuse.[10]

## 2. Procedural Techniques

- There are several commonly performed procedures in cutaneous surgery.

### 2.1. SHAVE BIOPSY

- A shave biopsy involves removal of a relatively shallow piece of skin with a 15-blade scalpel or a flexible blade such as the DermaBlade (see Chapter 1, Fig. 1-2).
- Suturing is not performed, and the area heals by secondary intention.
- This is an effective procedure for accurately diagnosing benign and malignant neoplasms as well as some skin rashes.
- This technique is most appropriate for raised lesions including papules and plaques.
- An accurate prebiopsy differential diagnosis will be helpful for providing the pathologist with an adequate tissue.
  - A relatively superficial tissue sample (into superficial dermis) is usually satisfactory for diagnosis of a basal cell carcinoma.
  - To make the diagnosis of a squamous cell carcinoma, a deeper biopsy (with adequate dermal sampling to assess for invasion) is necessary. This allows visualization and differentiation of in situ versus invasive squamous cell carcinoma.

- When performing the shave biopsy procedure in the correct upper dermal tissue plane, there should be a slight feeling of reduced resistance, and the resulting defect should have spots of pinpoint bleeding indicating a depth of the upper cutaneous vascular plexus.
- Shave biopsies extending deep into the dermis often lead to atrophic or indented scarring.
- A concern about performing shave biopsies for diagnosis of pigmented lesions is that the biopsy could transect the deeper component of a melanoma.
  - When this happens, only a provisional Breslow depth thickness can be assigned. This affects prognosis and treatment because deeper melanomas are staged differently and may require further testing and treatments such as sentinel lymph node biopsies (see Chapter 8 "Malignant Skin Lesions" regarding melanoma staging).
  - Despite this risk, recent studies have suggested that the deep shave biopsy is a safe and effective technique for diagnosis of melanocytic lesions.[16]
- Many rashes can be diagnosed with shave biopsy.
  - Broad shave biopsies are considered the preferred biopsy technique to diagnose mycosis fungoides and cutaneous T-cell lymphoma.
- Once the shave biopsy is taken, hemostasis can be acquired either with electrodessication or with aluminum chloride.
  - It is important to note that commercially available preparations of aluminum chloride often contain alcohol and are flammable.
  - If bleeding continues after application of the solution, it must be completely cleaned off before subsequent use of heat or electric cautery to avoid risk of fire.
- Shave biopsies heal by second intention, and wound care consists of petrolatum and a daily bandage change until healed.
  - Typical shave biopsies heal in about 1 to 2 weeks but may take longer to heal on the lower extremities.

## 2.2. PUNCH BIOPSY

- Punch biopsies are an important technique in the diagnosis of neoplasms and rashes (see Chapter 1, Fig. 1-3).
- Rashes involving the dermis and subcutaneous tissues are best diagnosed with punch biopsies so the pathologist has the ability to look at the epidermis, entire dermis, and upper subcutaneous fat.
- This is helpful for the diagnosis of vasculitis, panniculitis, drug hypersensitivities, and alopecia.
- A punch excision can be performed to completely remove a pigmented lesion down to the subcutaneous fat and with a small rim of normal tissue.
- Punch biopsies are helpful for assessing whether a neoplasm such as a basal cell carcinoma has recurred within or underneath a scar from prior treatment.
- The technique of a punch biopsy first involves choosing the correct size.
  - Most rashes are diagnosed with a 4-mm punch tool.
  - Punch excision to remove a neoplasm is done with the smallest sized punch tool necessary to completely remove the lesion.
    - By applying pressure with one edge of the punch biopsy tool and pushing the skin toward that edge, it is possible to fit a slightly larger lesion into a smaller punch.
- Once the lesion or area of rash to be biopsied is within the punch, firm downward pressure while rotating the punch biopsy tool in one direction will cut through the epidermis and dermis and into the subcutaneous fat.

- Once dermal release is achieved and the punch biopsy tool is retracted, the circular plug of tissue will typically rise above the surrounding skin.
  - This elevation can be increased by placing downward pressure on the surrounding skin.
  - After gently lifting one edge of the plug of tissue with forceps, the plug of tissue can be easily cut free from its attachment to the subcutaneous fat with surgical scissors.
  - Care must be taken not to crush the tissue with the forceps during this process, or the cellular and tissue architecture will be distorted, and crush artifact will be present on histology.
- Sutures are typically used to close the punch biopsy defect.
  - When using punch biopsy tools 5 mm or less in size, it is common for only epidermal sutures to be placed.
  - When punch biopsies of 6 mm or greater are performed, the defect may be closed in a layered manner with an absorbable deep suture plus epidermal sutures.
- Placing surgical scar lines in the natural relaxed skin tension lines results in improved cosmetic outcomes.
  - By slightly stretching the skin perpendicular to the relaxed skin tension lines, the punch biopsy defect will become a slight oval shape with the long axis in the direction of the relaxed skin tension lines and allow the scar to be in the appropriate orientation.

### 2.3. SNIP REMOVAL

- For some pedunculated lesions such as skin tags, warts, seborrheic keratoses, and dermatosis papulosa nigra, snip excision with curved or straight iris surgical scissors is the preferred technique.
- The sharpest part of the scissor blades is typically located centrally along the scissor blades instead of the tips.
- Pedunculated lesions may have a vascular connection at the pedicle and may bleed after removal.
  - Hemostasis can be achieved with either aluminum chloride or electrodessication.
  - It is often useful to inject local anesthetic such as lidocaine with epinephrine into skin tags with a substantial pedicle. This reduces pain during removal and allows for electrodessication if control of bleeding is necessary.

### 2.4. EXCISION

- Standard excision is performed for diagnosis and treatment of skin neoplasms and pigmented lesions (Fig. 11-1).
- It is used to treat symptomatic benign lesions such as epidermoid cysts and cutaneous malignancies such as basal cell carcinomas, squamous cell carcinomas, and melanoma.
  - Appropriate surgical margin depends on cancer type.
  - For standard excision of basal cell carcinoma and well-differentiated squamous cell carcinoma without high-risk features, in low-risk anatomic areas, a clinical margin of approximately 4 mm is commonly used to achieve pathologic clearance (see Chapter 8 "Malignant Skin Lesions" for further details).[17,18]
  - In squamous cell carcinoma with a diameter larger than 2 cm or with moderate to poor differentiation, a larger margin ranging from 6 to 10 mm is recommended

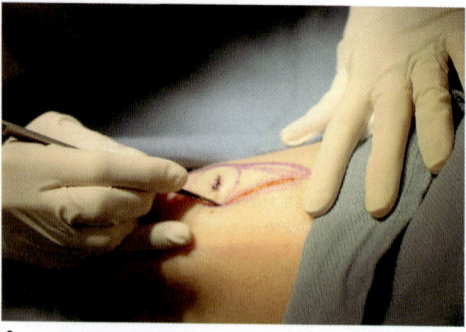

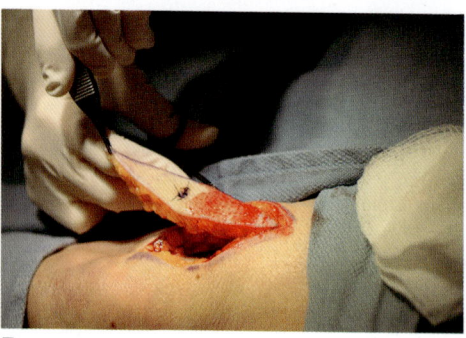

**Figure 11-1.** Elliptical excision. **A.** Margins and cones of redundant tissue are marked and incised. **B.** Specimen is excised to the appropriate tissue depth.

for considertion.[19] However, these tumors are best treated with MMS discussed later in this chapter.
- Margins for excisions of melanomas are set forth by the National Comprehensive Cancer Network® (NCCN®) and include 5- to 10-mm margins for melanoma in situ and 1- to 2-cm clinical margins for thin melanomas.[20]
- Excisions are designed with an elliptical or fusiform shape approximately three times as long as the defect is wide to allow for linear closure with minimal puckering at the ends.
- Scars should be oriented along relaxed skin tension lines when possible.
- For most body areas, a 15-blade scalpel is the most appropriate tool for performing excisions.
  - Exceptions to this include the use of a smaller 15c blade for more precise control around the eyelids and a larger 10 blade for excisions on thick skin such as the back.
- Cutting the skin with the scalpel blade at a 90° angle is common for standard excisions, though for thick skin of the back sometimes it is beneficial to "bevel out" slightly and take a few millimeter wider margins under the epidermis.
  - This helps ensure that you take satisfactory margins in the deeper tissue and may help in approximating the epidermis during suturing.

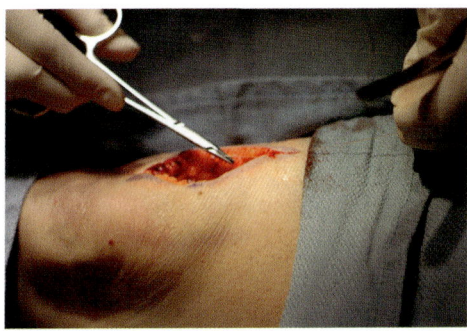

C

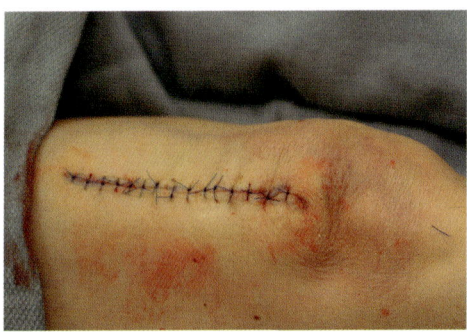

D

**Figure 11-1.** (Continued) **C.** Buried absorbable sutures reapproximate wound edges. **D.** Simple interrupted sutures reapproximate the epidermis. (Courtesy of M. Laurin Council, MD.)

- Different types of malignancies also require different depths of excision.
  - Treatment of basal cell carcinomas and squamous cell carcinomas typically require excising down to the level of the mid-to-deep subcutaneous fat.[17,18]
  - Treatment of melanoma in situ requires excising down to the deep subcutaneous fat.[20]
  - Treatment of invasive melanoma requires excision down through the subcutaneous fat to the fascia overlying muscles.[20]

## 2.5. SURGICAL REPAIRS

- Repairing postexcision defects requires several steps including undermining, hemostasis, and suturing.
- Undermining is sometimes necessary for allowing the edges of the defect to slide over the exposed tissue.
- The recommended depth of undermining depends on the location.
  - On the cheeks, the proper level is the upper subcutaneous fat to ensure that nerves and vessels, which run in deeper tissue planes, are protected.
  - On the scalp, the ideal plane is below the galea because this is a relatively avascular plane.

- On the trunk and extremities, undermining is often performed in the deep subcutaneous fat or fascia.
- Blunt-ended surgical scissors are typically used for undermining to reduce risk of damage to nerves and vessels.
  - On the back, it may be safe to carefully use the 10 blade to quickly undermine since there are minimal important structures at risk for damage.
- Hemostasis with electrocoagulation or heat cautery is typically done after undermining to control bleeding from small, severed vessels.
- Once undermining is complete and hemostasis achieved, suturing is performed to close the defect and complete the repair.
- The first step in suturing is to place deep dermal sutures with absorbable materials, typically poliglecaprone 25, polyglactin 910, or polydioxanone.
- Size of the suture depends on the location, with 5-0 suture typically used for the face/neck, 4-0 for the scalp and extremities, and 3-0 for thicker areas under tension such as the back.
- The deep dermal sutures should both bring the dermal edges of the wound together in good approximation and contribute to eversion of the epidermal wound edges.
- Once the deep layer of sutures is completed, the epidermal sutures can be placed either as simple interrupted sutures or a running suture.
- Either nonabsorbable sutures (polypropylene or nylon) or absorbable sutures (fast absorbing gut) can be utilized for epidermal closure.
- Simple interrupted sutures are more time consuming to place but are very good at approximating the wound edges and useful for wounds under tension.
- Running top stitches are both quick to perform and useful for approximating and everting the wound edges.
- On cosmetically sensitive areas where "track marking" from top sutures is a concern and the wound is under low tension, a running subcuticular suture may be placed.
- Nonabsorbable sutures should be removed in 1 week for facial locations and in 10 to 14 days for extremities and trunk.

## 2.6. MOHS MICROGRAPHIC SURGERY

- It is important to understand the appropriate use criteria and advantages of MMS in the treatment of cutaneous neoplasms such as basal cell carcinoma and squamous cell carcinoma.
- Mohs surgery, named for Dr. Frederic Mohs, is based on the principle that these cutaneous malignancies are contiguous tumors without skip areas.
- The treatment offers the highest cure rates for certain tumors because the technique allows visual confirmation of clear peripheral and deep margins.
- While traditional permanent tissue processing takes days before the slides can be analyzed, with the Mohs technique, fresh tissue is frozen, cut, stained, and ready for microscopic analysis in approximately 1 hour.
- If positive margins are found, additional tissue is removed in a second "stage," and the process is repeated.
- This allows the surgeon to take numerous "stages" as needed to clear the tumor on the day of surgery and ensures that the tumor is fully removed before the defect is repaired.
- The process is considered tissue sparing because conservatively sized pieces of tissue can be excised with each stage.
  - In permanent processing, tissue is cut vertically. This is similar to how a loaf of bread is sliced, and the majority of the margins are not being visualized.

- For MMS, the tissue is cut horizontally or "en face." This can be conceptualized by visualizing the lesion as a pie with the bulk of the tumor making up the pie filling and the surrounding deeper peripheral tissues as the crust.
- The stage is taken by cutting with a 45° bevel so that the tissue can be laid flat on glass microscope slides.
- This allows for microscopic examination of 100% of the margins with the peripheral epidermis around the edges and the deep margins in the middle.
- This technique is especially beneficial for treatment of lesions on cosmetically and functionally important areas such as the face and hands because minimal margins can be taken for tumor clearance.
- It is also beneficial for high-risk tumors with aggressive histologic appearance and recurrent tumors because the rate of recurrence with standard excision or other treatment modalities is much higher than with the MMS technique.

## 2.7. CRYOSURGERY

- Cryosurgery involves applying an extremely cold agent either through a spray or directly via a cotton-tipped applicator.
- The most commonly used agent is liquid nitrogen, which has a boiling point of −196 °C (−320 °F).
- Benign lesions such as verruca, condyloma, seborrheic keratoses, and prurigo nodules and premalignant lesions such as actinic keratoses may be treated with cryotherapy.
- The mechanism of action of cryosurgery involves the transfer of heat away from the skin to the cryogen.
  - This leads to the formation of intracellular and extracellular ice crystals.
  - A fast freeze leads to more intracellular ice crystal formation and increased tissue damage.
  - Cell injury also occurs during the thawing phase because of the occurrence of vascular stasis.
    - A rapid freeze followed by a slow thaw maximizes tissue damage.
- Cryotherapy results in inflammation of the treated area and blister formation may occur due to separation of the basement membrane.
- Different cell types have different susceptibilities to cryotherapy.
  - The most sensitive cell types are melanocytes, which are damaged at −4 to −7 °C.
    - For this reason, hypopigmentation is a common side effect of cryosurgery and should always be discussed before treatment, especially in patients with darker skin pigmentation.
- Keratinocytes are damaged at −20 to −30 °C.
  - Benign and premalignant lesions listed above typically fall into this category, and treatment times range from approximately 5 to 10 seconds of constant liquid nitrogen spray for one or two cycles.
  - One study reported that two cycles of liquid nitrogen were more effective at treating verruca on the feet, but one cycle was equivalent and better tolerated for treating verruca on the hands.[21]
- Fibroblasts of the dermis are usually damaged at −30 to −35 °C.
- Treatment of malignant tumors such as basal cell carcinomas and squamous cell carcinomas has been described but requires measurement of core tissue temperature of −50 °C.[22]

## 2.8. ELECTRODESICCATION AND CURETTAGE

- This is a treatment option for benign and malignant cutaneous neoplasms.
- In electrodesiccation, a high-voltage electric current is generated at the metal tip of the device.
- By directly applying this metal tip to the lesion, heat is delivered, and the tissue is rapidly dried leading to superficial destruction.
- Once the tissue has been heated and dried, a curette can be used to scrape off the upper portions of the lesion.
- Benign seborrheic keratoses can be treated with one cycle of electrodessication and curettage, resulting in a smooth base of superficially eroded skin that should heal with minimal scarring.
- When treating malignancies such as basal cell carcinoma, the curette is first used to scrape off the tumor.
  - This is effective because the tumor cells do not hold together like normal tissue. With firm pressure from the semi-sharp curette edge, the tumor scrapes off, while the underlying normal tissue remains intact.
- Once the tumor is removed with the curette, the base and a few millimeters margin are treated with electrodessication.
- Three passes of curettage and electrodessication are typically performed for the treatment of low-risk malignancies in low-risk locations.[17,18,23]
- Electrodesiccation and curettage are typically utilized for the treatment of small (<1 cm) malignancies on the trunk and extremities.
- Facial areas are typically avoided due to the risk of atrophic or hypopigmented scarring.
- The main types of cancers treated are low-risk superficial or nodular basal cell carcinomas and occasionally squamous cell carcinoma in situ.
- It is not an effective treatment for deeply invasive squamous cell carcinoma or melanoma.
- Cure rates for low-risk basal cell carcinomas, including superficial and nodular subtypes, range from 90% to 95%.
- Cure rates for low-risk squamous cell carcinomas, including squamous cell carcinoma in situ, range from 85% to 90%.
- Lesions are allowed to heal by second intention with petrolatum and a bandage.

## 2.9. DEROOFING FOR MODERATE TO SEVERE HIDRADENITIS SUPPURATIVA

- Deroofing refers to a minimally invasive surgical technique that involves the removal of the top layer of skin in refractory inflamed sinus tracts in patients with moderate or severe hidradenitis suppurativa (Hurley stages II and III).[24]
- Deroofing is performed under local anesthesia, stepwise as follows:
  - Identify sinus tracts and infiltrate the surrounding and affected area with lidocaine. Depending on the size of the lesion, dilute lidocaine or even tumescent anesthesia may be considered.
  - Use a blunt probe to define the borders of the sinus tract and to evaluate for any communicating sinus tracts.
  - Remove the roof of the identified tracts, using a probe as a guide.
  - Enter through the skin or sinus opening using electrocautery or with a scalpel or scissors.

- Reflect the skin overlying the probed areas back and remove the skin to expose the base of the lesion. Explore the exposed base and walls of the lesion with the probe again to assess for hidden tracts; take care not to create false tracts.
  - Débride the surgical wound using electrocautery or curettage to remove remaining inflammatory debris or biofilm. Coat the wound with petroleum jelly and gauze and allow the wound to heal by secondary intention.
  - Educate the patient on wound care, which includes once per day gentle cleansing with soap and water, followed by application of a moist dressing.
- Deroofing offers many benefits compared to alternative surgical interventions for the treatment of hidradenitis suppurativa. For example, deroofing requires only a probe, curette, and electrocautery device, making the procedure more cost effective than standard excisions.[25]
- Moreover, no specialized equipment, such as lasers or surgical instruments, is required for deroofing, which makes deroofing a treatment strategy all clinical dermatologists and dermatologic surgeons should consider regardless of practice setting.

## 3. Wound Dressings

- The main functions of wound dressings are to provide pressure for hemostasis, to maintain a moist environment that promotes healing, and to provide protection from mechanical trauma and infection.
- A moist healing environment leads to more rapid re-epithelialization.
  - It is important to prevent a wound from drying out and forming an eschar.
- Small procedures such as shave and punch biopsies can be dressed with petrolatum and a bandage.[26]
- For surgical excisions and larger procedures, the typical postsurgical wound dressing consists of a generous amount of petrolatum covered by folded clean cotton gauze held tightly in place with paper tape.
  - Petrolatum is recommended instead of over-the-counter antibiotic ointments because a significant proportion of the population either has or will develop an allergic contact dermatitis to these products.
  - Studies have shown equivalent healing using petrolatum compared to topical over-the-counter antibiotic preparations, with lower risk of allergic contact dermatitis.[27]
- There are other occlusive dressings that include films, foams, hydrogels, alginates, and hydrocolloids. These are all semipermeable but have different advantages.
  - Films are translucent and provide a barrier to outside bacteria but may lead to an accumulation of exudate.
  - Foams are very absorbent and comfortable but cannot be used on dry wounds and are opaque.
  - Hydrogels are soothing, cooling, and moisturizing but may have a higher risk of infection.
  - Alginates are the most highly absorbent but require a secondary dressing and may have an undesirable appearance and odor.
  - Hydrocolloids are useful for chronic ulcers and burns but risk leading to maceration of surrounding skin.[28,29]

## 4. Wound Healing

- Breakdown of the epidermal barrier occurs following injury, burns, and surgical procedures.
- These processes activate mechanisms to allow for repair and healing.
- Wound healing occurs in phases consisting of the inflammatory phase, proliferative phase, and the remodeling phase.
  - The acute inflammatory phase takes place 1 to 2 days after surgery and is characterized by cellular and vascular responses.
    - Damage to endothelial cells, blood vessels, and collagen leads to platelet activation and release of growth factors as well as platelet plug formation for initiation of hemostasis.
    - Neutrophils are the first leukocytes to migrate to the site of injury. They function to eliminate bacteria and break down proteins in the wound bed.
    - Macrophages are critical for repair and wound healing. They eliminate pathogens and tissue debris, destroy remaining neutrophils, and induce new blood vessel growth.
    - Many chemical mediators are also important for the inflammatory phase including histamine, serotonin, and prostaglandins.
  - The proliferative phase reestablishes a barrier through re-epithelialization and blood flow through angiogenesis.
    - Fibroblasts migrate into the wound between 2 and 3 days and produce the dermal matrix.
    - Myofibroblasts contribute to wound contraction.
  - In the remodeling phase, collagen is synthesized and present.
    - Initially, type III collagen is the major component, but over time type I collagen predominates.
    - After 1 month, the wound tensile strength approaches 40% of original strength.
    - By 1 year, it reaches its maximum strength, which is only 80% of the original.[28,30]

## 5. Surgical Complications

- Common surgical complications include bleeding, hematoma, dehiscence, and infection.
- Bleeding usually occurs in the first 48 hours following a procedure.[31]
  - As the vasoconstrictive effect of the epinephrine wears off, there is increased small-vessel bleeding and the blood clots that form initially may move or be displaced.
  - The bleeding risk is reduced with a tight pressure dressing held in place for 24 to 48 hours.
  - While a small quantity of bleeding is tolerable, if the bleeding soaks through the bandage, the patient should attempt to hold firm pressure for at least 20 minutes.
  - Applying pressure with an ice pack may also help.
  - If the bleeding continues, the patient should seek evaluation for possible exploration of the wound.[8,32]
- If bleeding occurs under the skin and accumulates, a hematoma forms (Fig. 11-2).
  - Initially, the collection is soft, and if patients present early enough, the hematoma can be easily evacuated or drained. Antibiotics should be administered following drainage.

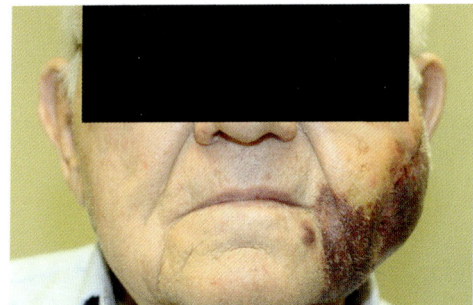

**Figure 11-2.** Hematoma. (Courtesy of M. Laurin Council, MD.)

- If the hematoma goes undetected and untreated for several days, it will organize and harden.
- At this point, if it is not compromising the integrity of the surgical closure, it is often best to allow the body to resorb the hematoma, which will take several weeks.
- The risk of infection may be increased with the presence of a resorbing hematoma so the administration of oral antibiotics and close clinical follow-up is beneficial.
- Surgical site infections most commonly occur during postoperative days 5 to 14 (Fig. 11-3).
  - Increased pain, redness, and drainage or pus are common signs of infection.
  - Antibiotics should be started based on the most likely causative organisms. The wound should be cultured to identify the organism and determine sensitivities.

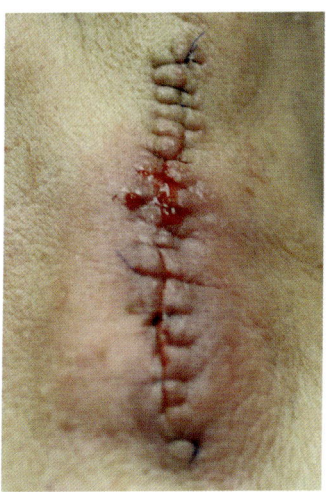

**Figure 11-3.** Infection. (Courtesy of M. Laurin Council, MD.)

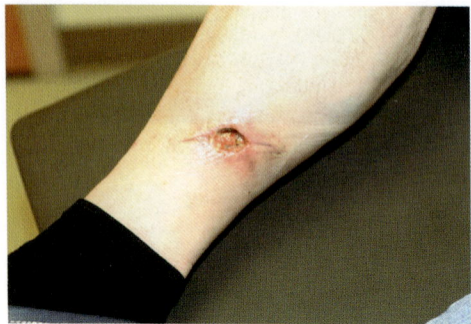

**Figure 11-4.** Dehiscence. (Courtesy of M. Laurin Council, MD.)

- Cephalexin has good coverage of normal skin pathogens and is often started empirically while the cultures are pending.[33]
- In cases where there is concern for Gram-negative infection such as *Pseudomonas*, ciprofloxacin may be used.[8]
- Sometimes it is challenging to determine whether a surgical site is infected or if there is an allergic contact dermatitis reaction.
  - Usually, allergic contact dermatitis will be itchy rather than painful and redness will be present around the surrounding areas where antibiotic ointment or adhesives have been applied.
- Dehiscence is when the wound edges separate. This most commonly occurs at the time of suture removal but may also occur before or after (Fig. 11-4).
  - Risk factors for dehiscence include excessive wound tension, infection, and wound edge necrosis.
  - Areas of dehiscence will heal from the bottom up by second intention and may later require scar revision.[32]

# REFERENCES

1. Plümer L, Seiffert M, Punke MA, et al. Aspirin before elective surgery-stop or continue? *Dtsch Arztebl Int.* 2017;114(27-28):473-480. doi:10.3238/arztebl.2017.0473. PMID: 28764836; PMCID: PMC5545631.
2. Devereaux PJ, Mrkobrada M, Sessler DI, et al. Aspirin in patients undergoing noncardiac surgery. *N Engl J Med.* 2014;370(16):1494-1503. doi:10.1056/NEJMoa1401105. PMID: 24679062.
3. Connelly CS, Panush RS. Should nonsteroidal anti-inflammatory drugs be stopped before elective surgery? *Arch Intern Med.* 1991;151(10):1963-1966. PMID: 1929684.
4. Hurst EA, Yu SS, Grekin RC, Neuhaus IM. Bleeding complications in dermatologic surgery. *Semin Cutan Med Surg.* 2007;26(4):189-195.
5. Schiffer CA, Anderson KC, Bennett CL, et al. Platelet transfusion for patients with cancer: clinical practice guidelines of the American Society of Clinical Oncology. *J Clin Oncol.* 2001;19(5):1519-1538.
6. Weyer C, Siegle RJ, Eng GG. Investigation of hyfrecators and their in vitro interference with implantable cardiac devices. *Dermatol Surg.* 2012;38(11):1843-1848.
7. Ebner JA, Maytin EV. Cutaneous wound healing. *Dermatologic Surgery.* Elsevier; 2009:81-100. doi:10.1016/b978-0-7020-3049-9.00006-3
8. Hurst EA, Grekin RC, Yu SS, Neuhaus IM. Infectious complications and antibiotic use in dermatologic surgery. *Semin Cutan Med Surg.* 2007;26(1):47-53.

9. Wilson W, Taubert KA, Gewitz M, et al. Prevention of infective endocarditis: guidelines from the American Heart Association: a guideline from the American Heart Association Rheumatic Fever, Endocarditis, and Kawasaki Disease Committee, Council on Cardiovascular Disease in the Young, and the Council on Clinical Cardiology, Council on Cardiovascular Surgery and Anesthesia, and the Quality of Care and Outcomes Research Interdisciplinary Working Group. *Circulation.* 2007;116(15):1736-1754. doi:10.1161/CIRCULATIONAHA.106.183095. Erratum in: *Circulation.* 2007;116(15):e376-e377. PMID: 17446442.
10. Soleymani T, Brodland DG, Zitelli JA. A retrospective case series evaluating the efficacy of pre-operative, intra-incisional antibiotic prophylaxis in Mohs micrographic surgery: an effective method to reduce surgical-site infections and minimize systemic antibiotic use. *J Am Acad Dermatol.* 2020;83(5):1501-1503. doi:10.1016/j.jaad.2020.05.146. PMID: 32502584.
11. Beeson WH, Rachel JD. Valacyclovir prophylaxis for herpes simplex virus infection or infection recurrence following laser skin resurfacing. *Dermatol Surg.* 2002;28(4):331-336.
12. Rogues A. Infection control practices and infectious complications in dermatologic surgery. *J Hosp Infect.* 2007;65(3):258-263.
13. Koay J, Orengo I. Application of local anesthetics in dermatologic surgery. *Dermatol Surg.* 2002;28(2):143-148.
14. Drugs and Lactation Database (LactMed®) [Internet]. *Lidocaine.* National Institute of Child Health and Human Development; 2006 [Updated 2024 Sep 15]. https://www.ncbi.nlm.nih.gov/books/NBK501230/
15. Rosenberg PH, Veering BT, Urmey WF. Maximum recommended doses of local anesthetics: a multifactorial concept. *Reg Anesth Pain Med.* 2004;29(6):564-575; discussion 524. doi:10.1016/j.rapm.2004.08.003. PMID: 15635516.
16. Mendese G, Maloney M, Bordeaux J. To scoop of not to scoop: the diagnostic and therapeutic utility of the scoop-shave biopsy for pigmented lesions. *Dermatol Surg.* 2014;40(10):1077-1083.
17. National Comprehensive Cancer Network® (NCCN®). *Clinical Practice Guidelines in Oncology (NCCN Guidelines®) for Basal Cell Skin Cancer V.3.2024.* © National Comprehensive Cancer Network, Inc.; 2024 All rights reserved. Accessed October 8, 2024.
18. National Comprehensive Cancer Network® (NCCN®). *Clinical Practice Guidelines in Oncology (NCCN Guidelines®) for Squamous Cell Skin Cancer V.3.2024.* © National Comprehensive Cancer Network, Inc.; 2024. All rights reserved. Accessed October 8, 2024.
19. Brodland DG, Zitelli JA. Surgical margins for excision of primary cutaneous squamous cell carcinoma. *J Am Acad Dermatol.* 1992;27(2 Pt 1):241-248.
20. National Comprehensive Cancer Network® (NCCN®). *Clinical Practice Guidelines in Oncology (NCCN Guidelines®) for Cutaneous Melanoma V.3.2024.* © National Comprehensive Cancer Network, Inc.; 2024. All rights reserved. Accessed October 8, 2024.
21. Berth-Jones J, Bourke J, Eglitis H, et al. Value of a second freeze-thaw cycle in cryotherapy of common warts. *Br J Dermatol.* 1994;131(6):883-886.
22. Kokoszka A, Scheinfeld N. Evidence-based review of the use of cryosurgery in treatment of basal cell carcinoma. *Dermatol Surg.* 2003;29(6):566-571.
23. Rodriguez-Vigil T, Vázquez-López F, Perez-Oliva N. Recurrence rates of primary basal cell carcinoma in facial risk areas treated with curettage and electrodesiccation. *J Am Acad Dermatol.* 2007;56(1):91-95.
24. Allison D, Sterner J, Parker J, Martin K. Surgical deroofing for hidradenitis suppurativa. *Cutis.* 2022;110(3):147-149. doi:10.12788/cutis.0597. PMID: 36446109.
25. Van der Zee HH, Prens EP, Boer J. Deroofing: a tissue-saving surgical technique for the treatment of mild to moderate hidradenitis suppurativa lesions. *J Am Acad Dermatol.* 2010;63(3):475-480. doi:10.1016/j.jaad.2009.12.018. PMID: 20708472.
26. Pickett H. Shave and punch biopsy for skin lesions. *Am Fam Physician.* 2011;84(9):995-1002. PMID: 22046939.
27. Saco M, Howe N, Nathoo R, Cherpelis B. Topical antibiotic prophylaxis for prevention of surgical wound infections from dermatologic procedures: a systematic review and meta-analysis. *J Dermatolog Treat.* 2015;26(2):151-158.
28. Menaker GM, Mehlis AL, Kasprowicz S. Dressings. In: Bolognia J, Jorizzo JJ, Schaffer JV, et al., eds. *Dermatology.* 3rd ed. Elsevier Saunders; 2012:2365-2379.
29. Thomas S. Hydrocolloid dressings in the management of acute wounds: a review of the literature. *Int Wound J.* 2008;5(5):602-613.
30. Sun BK, Siprashvili Z, Khavari PA. Advances in skin grafting and treatment of cutaneous wounds. *Science.* 2014;346(6212):941-945.
31. Strickler AG, Shah P, Bajaj S, et al. Preventing and managing complications in dermatologic surgery: procedural and postsurgical concerns. *J Am Acad Dermatol.* 2021;84(4):895-903. doi:10.1016/j.jaad.2021.01.037. PMID: 33493570; PMCID: PMC9491026.

32. Alam M, Ibrahim O, Nodzenski M, et al. Adverse events associated with Mohs micrographic surgery: multicenter prospective cohort study of 20,821 cases at 23 centers. *JAMA Dermatol.* 2013;149(12):1378-1385.
33. Stevens DL, Bisno AL, Chambers HF, et al. Infectious Diseases Society of America. Practice guidelines for the diagnosis and management of skin and soft tissue infections: 2014 update by the Infectious Diseases Society of America. *Clin Infect Dis.* 2014;59(2):e10-e52. doi:10.1093/cid/ciu444. Erratum in: *Clin Infect Dis.* 2015;60(9):1448. doi:10.1093/cid/civ114. Dosage error in article text. PMID: 24973422.

# 12. Aesthetic Dermatology

Morgan Nguyen, MD, Ali Malik, MD, and Basia Michalski-McNeely, MD

## 1. Introduction

The popularity of minimally invasive aesthetic procedures has increased as more patients seek nonsurgical methods to achieve facial rejuvenation and body optimization. A cosmetic consultation begins with a thorough assessment of a patient's physical features in the context of their aesthetic concerns and a careful discussion regarding goals of treatment and patient expectations.

Many aesthetic treatments aim to address the four "R's": (1) Resurfacing (chemical peels, dermabrasion, ablative, and nonablative lasers), (2) Redraping (pulling and lifting facial surgical procedures), (3) Relaxing (chemodenervation with neurotoxins), or (4) Replacement/Recontouring (the use of filling agents such as hyaluronic acid (HA) filler for superficial and deep soft tissue augmentation).

## 2. Neurotoxins

### 2.1. BACKGROUND

Botulinum toxin (BoNT) injections have become a cornerstone in both cosmetic and medical dermatology.[1,2] Initially developed to relax involuntary muscle spasms, BoNT injections have expanded to include a wide range of therapeutic applications, from treating excessive sweating (hyperhidrosis) to alleviating chronic migraines.

The notable expansion of the clinical use and applications of BoNT injections can be most readily linked to improved understanding of the mechanism of action and pharmacodynamics of BoNT. Commercial BoNT injections are formulated from strains of *Clostridium botulinum*, a spore-forming bacteria that produces *botulinum toxin*, a lethal neurotoxin.[1] In high doses, BoNT can lead to botulism, a serious paralytic condition, but in its commercial form for dermatologic use, it is heavily diluted to safe, therapeutic levels. This controlled dosage allows for localized muscle relaxation without the risk of systemic toxicity.

BoNT acts by blocking the presynaptic release of the neurotransmitter acetylcholine at the neuromuscular junction[1] (Fig. 12-1). This results in chemical denervation of the respective muscle fibers, thereby inducing localized paralysis and muscle atrophy. There are multiple serotypes of BoNT that affect neural function; these serotypes differ in their cellular mechanism of action and clinical profile and each represent a distinct commercially available formulation of BoNT (Table 12-1).[1,3]

### 2.2. CLINICAL PRESENTATION AND APPLICATIONS

The primary use of BoNT injections by dermatologists is the treatment of dynamic facial rhytids. Relaxing active muscles of the face with BoNT injections can functionally smooth or "flatten" hyperdynamic wrinkles. BoNT injections

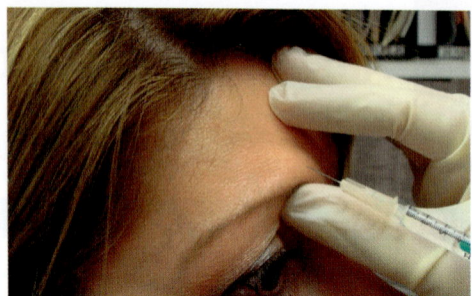

**Figure 12-1.** Injections for glabellar complex. Injection technique for botulinum toxin in the glabellar complex involves using the nondominant hand to stabilize the patient and syringe for precise injection placement. (Reprinted with permission from Council ML. *Guide to Minimally Invasive Aesthetic Procedures*. Wolters Kluwer; 2020. Figure 2.4.

are most commonly used to smooth lines of the forehead (from movement of the frontalis muscle), between the eyebrows (from movement of the glabellar complex consisting primarily of the corrugator and procerus muscles), as well as "crow's feet" and lines around the eye (from movement of the orbicularis oculi).[1,2] Deep folds or grooves in other regions of the face can also be treated with BoNT injections.

Although BoNT injections are primarily used to address rhytids, they can also be used to temporarily change facial anatomy, such as by correcting facial asymmetry or volume loss. For example, injecting BoNT into the masseter muscles can slim the lower face, offering a more contoured appearance to patients with masseter hypertrophy or a square jawline. Additionally, BoNT injections can be used to lift the brows or correct facial asymmetry, enhancing facial harmony and balance. These cosmetic applications are often complemented by the use of dermal fillers, such as HA, to add volume and further refine facial features by strategically adding volume to specific areas of the face, such as the cheeks, lips, and tear troughs.

## 2.3. EVALUATION

Clinical assessment of BoNT injection begins with a thorough physical examination. This includes assessing the patient's facial anatomy, muscle strength, and areas of concern. Dermatologists should observe dynamic lines by asking patients to perform facial expressions, such as raising their eyebrows or frowning, to highlight the areas where BoNT might be beneficial. For example, when a patient is asked to raise their eyebrows, hyperdynamic lines on the forehead may become more prominent and allow dermatologists to identify areas that may benefit from treatment with BoNT injections. This interactive approach helps pinpoint precise injection sites and allows dermatologists to tailor the treatment based on the patient's unique anatomy and aesthetic goals.

The total volume of units administered to each region of the face should be calculated to maximize the effect of BoNT injection treatment, while minimizing potential negative side effects, such as pain or swelling at sites of injection, asymmetry,

## TABLE 12-1 Commercially Available Botulinum Toxin Formulations

| | OnaA | AboA | DAXI | IncoA | PraboA |
|---|---|---|---|---|---|
| **Trade name** | Botox | Dysport Azzalure | Daxxify | Xeomin Bocouture | Jeuveau |
| **Active substance** | BoNT-A + complex | BoNT-A + complex | BoNT-A | BoNT-A | BoNT-A + complex |
| **Units per vial** | 50 or 100 | 300 or 500 | 50 or 100 | 100 | 100 |
| **Clinical indications** | Rhytids, axillary hyperhidrosis, chronic migraines, blepharospasm, cervical dystonia, strabismus, blepharospasm, overactive bladder, temporomandibular dysfunction | Rhytids, cervical dystonia, blepharospasm | Rhytids | Rhytids, blepharospasm, cervical dystonia, chronic sialorrhea | Glabellar lines |

or temporary weakness in surrounding muscles. The number of BoNT units required for adequate treatment varies depending on patient factors such as muscle strength, sex, and previous exposure to BoNT.

## 2.4. TREATMENT

Dosing and injection technique of BoNT injections differs based on the planned treatment area (Figs. 12-1 to 12-6). Generally speaking, men are thought to require higher doses than women. For example, although the package insert of onabotA recommends 20 BoNT units for treatment of glabellar lines, with 4 units distributed in five sites between the eyebrows, dermatologists may use higher dose ranges in clinical practice, such as 10 to 30 units for women and 20 to 60 units for men.[2] For treatment of forehead lines, the onabotA package insert recommends 4 units into five forehead line sites (20 units total), although many dermatologists suggest lower starting doses.[2] Forehead line injections should be administered simultaneously with or shortly following glabellar treatment to maintain neutral eyebrow position.

## 2.5. POSTTREATMENT CARE AND PATIENT COUNSELING

Proper posttreatment care is essential for optimal outcomes and patient satisfaction. After BoNT injections, patients should avoid lying down or massaging the treated area for at least 4 hours to prevent migration of the toxin to unintended muscles. Strenuous exercise, alcohol consumption, and exposure to heat (such as saunas or steam rooms) should also be avoided for 24 hours postinjection to reduce the risk of swelling and bruising.

Patients are typically informed that results will start to appear within 3 to 5 days, with the full effect visible by 2 weeks. The effects of BoNT injections generally last 3 to 4 months, after which patients may return for maintenance treatments. Dermatologists should set realistic expectations with patients, emphasizing that

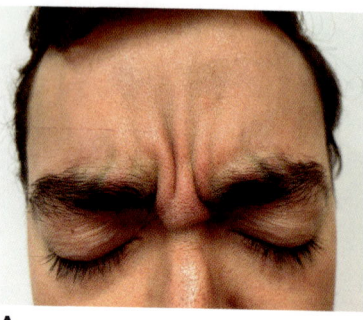
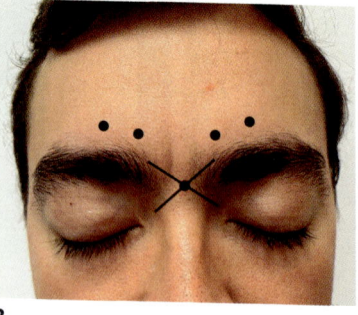

**A**  **B**

**Figure 12-2.** Injections for glabellar frown rhytids. A man during movement **(A)** and at rest **(B)** with five planned injection points. Patients with this degree of muscular activity would require higher starting doses such as 25 units onabotA or 60 units abobotA. (Reprinted with permission from Council ML. *Guide to Minimally Invasive Aesthetic Procedures*. Wolters Kluwer; 2020. Figure 2.6.)

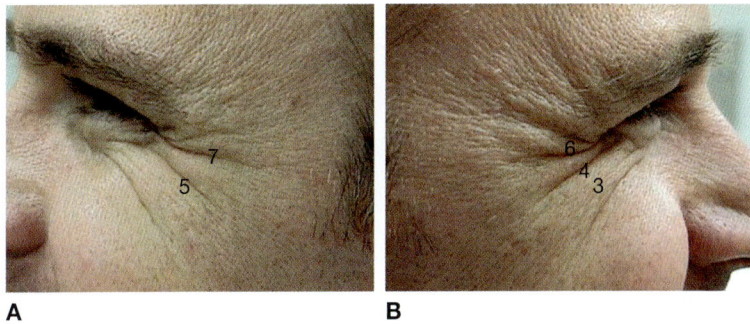

**Figure 12-3.** Injections for lateral canthal rhytides or "crow's feet." It is important to observe natural variations in muscle activity, not only between patients but also in the same patient. As seen in this man, the pattern of movement differs between the left (**A**) and right (**B**) sides. *Numerals* indicate the number of onabotA units used at each injection point. (Reprinted with permission from Council ML. *Guide to Minimally Invasive Aesthetic Procedures.* Wolters Kluwer; 2020. Figure 2.7.)

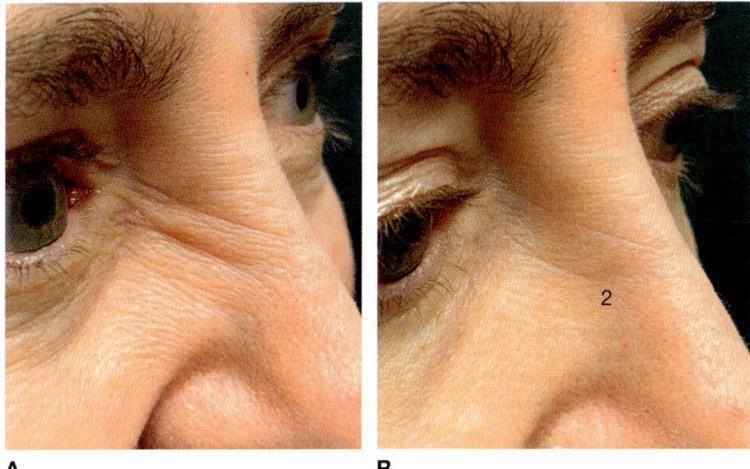

**Figure 12-4.** Injections for nasal rhytides or "bunny lines." A woman with movement (**A**) and at rest (**B**). *Numeral* indicates the number of onabotA units injected which is placed medial to the nasofacial sulcus in order to minimize diffusion into the levator labii superioris and unwanted lip ptosis. (Reprinted with permission from Council ML. *Guide to Minimally Invasive Aesthetic Procedures.* Wolters Kluwer; 2020. Figure 2.8.)

BoNT does not offer permanent results and that follow-up treatments are necessary to maintain the desired appearance.

By following a structured approach to BoNT injections—encompassing pretreatment, tailored dosing, meticulous injection technique, and comprehensive postcare guidance—dermatologists can achieve both safe and effective outcomes for their patients.

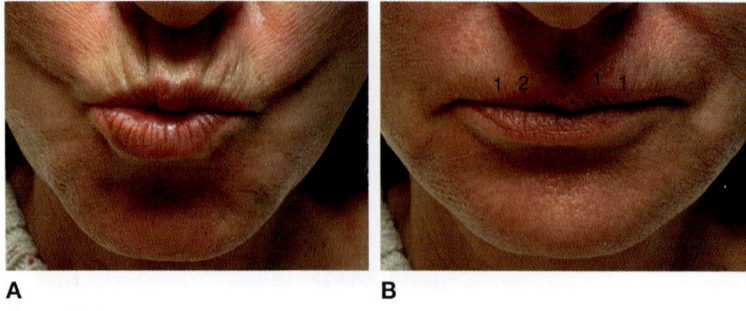

**Figure 12-5.** Injections for perioral rhytides. A female pursing her lips (**A**) and at rest (**B**). Five units total of onabotA were injected into the upper lip just above the vermilion border. Note that the pattern and dosing are based on the individual's muscle activity. (Reprinted with permission from Council ML. *Guide to Minimally Invasive Aesthetic Procedures*. Wolters Kluwer; 2020. Figure 2.9.)

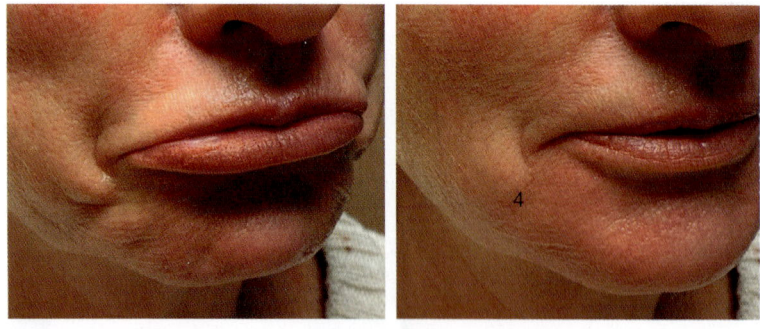

**Figure 12-6.** Injections for frown lines or "marionette lines." A female frowning (**A**) and at rest (**B**). Four units of onabotA were injected into each depressor anguli oris muscle. A more lateral injection helps avoid effect on the more medial depressor labii inferioris. (Reprinted with permission from Council ML. *Guide to Minimally Invasive Aesthetic Procedures*. Wolters Kluwer; 2020. Figure 2.10.)

## 3. Soft Tissue Fillers

### 3.1. BACKGROUND

Injectable soft tissue fillers have become a staple in dermatologic practice for addressing facial volume loss and enhancing facial symmetry.[4,5] As we age, natural facial fat and collagen diminish, leading to sagging, wrinkling, and a less-defined facial contour. Dermal fillers, primarily composed of HA, calcium hydroxyapatite, and poly-L-lactic acid, offer a nonsurgical solution to counteract these effects by restoring volume, enhancing facial features, and smoothing wrinkles. HA, a glycosaminoglycan that supports the extrafibrillar matrix of the dermis, is particularly favored due to its biocompatibility, safety profile, and natural appearance, as it mimics the HA already present in our skin's extracellular matrix, promoting hydration and elasticity.

Several characteristics of dermal fillers make them suitable for clinical use: (1) biocompatibility and a low incidence of adverse effects, (2) ease of preparation, storage, and injection, and (3) affordability and long-lasting effects. Additionally, fillers vary widely in their viscoelastic properties, which impacts their behavior under the skin. The degree of HA crosslinking largely determines a filler's consistency, longevity, and lift capacity. The G prime (G′) of a filler is a measure of its stiffness or viscosity; fillers with high G′ maintain their shape and provide more structural support, whereas those with low G′ are softer, more fluid, and better suited for fine lines and delicate areas.[6] Fillers are often chosen based on their rheological properties for different treatment areas. For example, high G′ HA fillers are typically used in areas that require significant lift and structure, such as the cheeks and chin, while low G′ HA fillers are ideal for subtle volume enhancement in areas like the lips, periorbital region, and for fine lines around the mouth.

### 3.2. CLINICAL PRESENTATION AND EVALUATION

During the initial consultation, dermatologists should help guide patients toward understanding the degree and significance of their individual volume deficit(s) and discuss relevant aspects of facial asymmetry while reinforcing the importance of realistic, grounded patient expectations. In order to most adequately assess facial volume loss, patients should be comfortably seated in an upright seated position with adequate lighting. Absolute contraindications to filler injection include active infection at sites of injection and known allergy or hypersensitivity to injectable materials.[4]

Selection of a dermal filler depends on various factors, including the size, depth, and location of volume deficiency as well as the cost and longevity of the injectable product; as such, dermatologists should provide information regarding the various commercially available injectable products that may be most beneficial to individual patients. Formulations of different fillers have unique characteristics and indications that may make them more appropriate for specific patients. For example, HA-based filler products with a low G′ are soft and gel-like, last between 6 and 12 months, and are often used to treat fine lines and rhytids.[6] In contrast, HA-based filler products with a higher G′ are more viscous and typically last longer.[6] Soft tissue fillers with a low G′ are best for areas of fine lines or rhytids such as around the mouth or "necklace" lines on the neck, while soft tissue fillers with a high G′ are best to treat deep lines and areas that require significant volume restoration such as the midface or cheeks.

### 3.3. TREATMENT

Prior to initiation of treatment with HA-based fillers, dermatologists should ensure that hyaluronidase, a soluble protein enzyme that can dissolve HA-based fillers, is readily available in clinic and maintained in an adequate supply to address any immediate complications or patient dissatisfaction with results.[4,5] Proper patient preparation includes discussing potential risks, side effects, and aftercare instructions, as well as ensuring patients understand the anticipated outcomes.

Various injection techniques are employed depending on the filler type, target area, and desired effect. Injection techniques most commonly include serial puncture (sequential deposition of small amounts of filler along a rhytid or fold), linear threading (retrograde injection of filler during needle withdrawal following full needle insertion into a dermal or subcutaneous plane), fanning (injections of filler in multiple passes in different but evenly spaced directions without needle withdrawal), and cross-hatching or radial injection (evenly spaced linear injections in a gridlike pattern).[4] These techniques are selected based on the treatment area and the depth of injection required for optimal aesthetic results. Superficial injections are typically used for fine lines, while deeper injections provide lift and volume for larger areas.

Common injection-related sequelae, such as transient pain, edema, and bruising, can occur following dermal filler injection; additional sequelae may include hypersensitivity or allergic reactions, granuloma formation, contour irregularities, and vascular compromise, which can result in necrosis or even blindness.[4,5] Correct filler depth is essential as inappropriately superficial placement of fillers may result in the formation of visible papules or nodules, beading, and/or blue-gray discoloration, known as the Tyndall effect. When complications arise, hyaluronidase can be injected to dissolve HA-based fillers, correcting overfill or misplaced product. For non-HA fillers, such as calcium hydroxyapatite or poly-L-lactic acid, more invasive measures may be required if complications occur, including corticosteroid injections or surgical excision in rare cases.

By understanding the characteristics of each filler and the appropriate injection techniques, dermatologists can achieve desirable aesthetic outcomes and minimize the risk of complications, ensuring patient satisfaction and safety.

## 3.4. ASEPTIC TECHNIQUE AND PRECAUTIONS

With the increasing demand for aesthetic procedures, the rate of complications, such as infections, is also on the rise. To minimize risks, stringent aseptic techniques are essential, especially for procedures involving skin penetration, such as filler and neurotoxin injections. Prior to treatment with injectables, patients should be instructed to arrive at the clinic with a clean, makeup-free face. If they come with makeup, it should be gently removed. Both the patient and practitioner should ensure that hair is kept away from treatment areas, using hairbands if necessary, to lower the chance of contamination. Dermatologists should disinfect the treatment area, and this process should be repeated with each change in the injection area when using a cannula. Common antiseptics for skin preparation include isopropyl alcohol, povidone-iodine, and chlorhexidine.[7] Proper hand hygiene is crucial for maintaining aseptic conditions; hands should be cleaned with liquid soap and warm water or with an alcohol-based hand sanitizer (minimum 70% alcohol) if water is not available and hands are not visibly soiled. Needles should be disposed of immediately in a sharps container without recapping. Dermatologists are also required to adhere to standard infection control guidelines, which include avoiding wrist and hand jewelry, keeping fingernails short, clean, and polish free, and covering minor cuts with waterproof dressings.

Dental procedures, which often involve stretching and pressure on different areas of the face, may cause dermal fillers to shift. Additionally, dental work can introduce bacteria into the bloodstream, potentially leading to infections around the filler area. To ensure dermal fillers maintain their intended effect, it is recommended to avoid dental work for about 2 weeks following filler placement.[7]

Patients with distant infections or other local conditions—such as influenza, sinusitis, periodontal disease, ENT infections, dental abscesses, or recent dental surgery—should delay aesthetic treatments until these conditions are fully resolved. Clinical evidence suggests that typically mild infections may spread to filler sites, potentially causing delayed hypersensitivity reactions and late-onset nodules.[7] Some dental surgeons have reported cases of facial swelling following dental infections or procedures performed close to areas with injectable fillers.

# 4. Chemical Peels

## 4.1. BACKGROUND

Chemical peels, or chemoexfoliation, involve the application of a chemical agent to the skin to induce controlled destruction of the epidermis and potentially the dermis. This process leads to exfoliation, removal of superficial skin lesions, and regeneration and remodeling of skin tissues. The practice of chemical peels for aesthetic enhancement dates back to ancient Egypt where people applied animal oils, salt, alabaster, and sour milk to their skin to achieve their cosmetic goals.[8] Cosmetic peel techniques have since been refined, with a wide range of proprietary formulations now available, and use of chemical peels by dermatologists continues to increase.

The primary objective of chemical peels is to remove a uniform layer of skin to eliminate damaged cells and stimulate rejuvenation through wound healing. Caustic agents in peels cause exfoliation through keratocoagulation, protein denaturation, and disruption of intercellular adhesive proteins.[8] This epidermal sloughing improves pigmentation and texture and removes unwanted epidermal growths. The resulting wound triggers the release of pro-inflammatory cytokines and chemokines, initiating the inflammatory cascade. This inflammation subsequently promotes collagenesis, reorganization of dermal connective tissue, and keratinocyte regeneration, leading to epidermal and dermal thickening that can improve the appearance of wrinkles and acne scars. Chemical peels are categorized by depth of injury—superficial, medium, or deep—each with varying effects on tissue remodeling.

## 4.2. TYPES OF PEELS

Superficial peels target different levels of the epidermis; medium depth peels reach through the entire epidermis into the papillary dermis; and deep peels extend into the reticular dermis. The depth of each peel is influenced by the type and concentration of the chemical used, application method, number of applications, and the chemical's active time on the skin.[8] The depth of injury is directly correlated with healing time, complication risk, and aesthetic outcomes.

Superficial peels are the most common type of chemical peel due to their affordability, minimal downtime, safety profile, low discomfort, and suitability for all skin types and various body areas. While commonly used on the face, superficial peels can also treat areas such as the hands, arms, neck, chest, and back. Deeper peels are generally avoided on the body due to a higher risk of scarring. Superficial peels are effective for treating pigmentation issues (eg, melasma, postinflammatory pigment alteration, ephelides, and lentigines), acne (comedones, inflammatory acne, acne excoriee), and minor textural concerns. However, they are less effective for full-thickness epidermal lesions (like seborrheic and actinic keratoses), deeper wrinkles, and scars. Multiple treatments are often required to achieve the desired results. While complications are generally limited, they can include post-inflammatory pigment alteration, prolonged redness, infection, and heightened sensitivity to environmental factors.[8] Improper application of superficial peels can lead to more severe complications like scarring.

Medium-depth peels penetrate to the papillary or upper reticular dermis, which allows users to address aesthetic concerns including pigmentation issues (such as melasma and lentigines) and epidermal growths (like seborrheic and actinic keratoses). Treatment through the level of the papillary dermis also stimulates collagen production, which can help reduce superficial wrinkles and scarring. Initially, trichloroacetic acid 50% was used for medium-depth peels, but it had unpredictable results and posed risks like uneven penetration, postinflammatory pigment alteration, and scarring.[8] Combination peels are now preferred for medium-depth treatments, as they offer a more controlled and safer approach. With combination peels, the initial treatment disrupts the epidermis, enabling deeper and even penetration of 35% trichloroacetic acid. Results from a medium-depth peel can last months to years, though repeat treatments are typically discouraged within a 6-month timeframe.

Deep chemical peels reach the reticular dermis and are effective for treating deeper wrinkles and scarring. Phenol (carbolic acid) remains the primary agent used for deep chemical peeling.[8] At a concentration of 88%, phenol alone typically provides medium-depth peeling by causing keratocoagulation, which limits further penetration. When combined with croton oil, an epidermolytic agent, phenol achieves the necessary depth for a deep peel. The Baker-Gordon formula originally combined phenol, distilled water, croton oil, and an emulsifier called Septisol©. Septisol© contained triclosan and is no longer available due to regulatory restrictions.[8] Research is ongoing to identify an alternative emulsifying agent for this formula. Due to the risk of cardiac arrhythmias during phenol-based peels, intraoperative cardiac monitoring is necessary.

## 4.3. EVALUATION

Counseling patients before a chemical peel is essential to ensure they have realistic expectations, understand the procedure, and follow necessary pre- and posttreatment instructions. Effective counseling minimizes risks, enhances satisfaction, and promotes optimal results. The first step in counseling is to explain the goals and potential outcomes of a chemical peel. Patients should understand that chemical peels improve skin texture, tone, pigmentation, and, to some extent, fine lines and acne scars. However, they are not a replacement for more intensive antiaging treatments like laser therapy or surgery.

Prior to the peel, assess the patient's medical history for any conditions or medications that could interfere with healing or increase the risk of complications. Patients with a history of cold sores, active skin infections, or conditions like rosacea may need special precautions. It is also crucial to discuss any history of scarring or abnormal wound healing, as this can affect the choice of peel. Certain medications, such as retinoids, may increase sensitivity to peeling agents and should be discontinued approximately 7 to 10 days before treatment. Post-peel, retinoids can typically be resumed after the skin has fully healed and any peeling or sensitivity has resolved. This usually takes 1 to 2 weeks for superficial peels, 2 to 3 weeks for medium-depth peels, and at least 4 to 6 weeks for deep peels.

To maximize the peel's effectiveness and reduce complications, provide clear pretreatment guidelines. Patients should avoid sun exposure and use a broad spectrum sunscreen for at least 2 weeks before the procedure, as sunburned or tanned skin can increase the risk of adverse reactions.

## 4.4. TREATMENT

Before starting a chemical peel, it is essential to have all required supplies on hand and easily accessible. The chosen chemical peeling agent and its concentration should be verified and correctly labeled. Patients should cleanse their face with a gentle skin cleanser, and their hair should be secured away from the treatment area using a headband or cap. For facial peels, position the patient in a reclined position at a 30°

to 45° angle, ensuring their eyes are closed. Clean the treatment area with alcohol or acetone applied on gauze to degrease the skin. A fan can help disperse any fumes that may cause discomfort.

To prevent accidental spillage, the peeling solution should not be passed over the patient. Extra caution is necessary to avoid drips or spills near the eyes, and the patient's eyes should remain closed during the entirety of the procedure. An eyewash bottle with saline solution should be on hand in case of accidental exposure. Applying white petrolatum to sensitive areas is optional for added protection. Certain areas, like the medial canthus and nasojugal folds, can trap peeling solution, potentially causing deeper injury than desired.[8] To avoid this, apply petrolatum to the medial and lateral canthi, which also prevents tears from neutralizing the solution or allowing tears to "wick" into the eyes. Clean gauze or cotton-tipped applicators should be used to control any tearing.

When ready to apply the chemical peel, dip a cotton-tipped applicator, gauze, or brush into the peeling solution and begin application from the forehead, moving systematically across the face to ensure even coverage. Watch for signs of frosting (white haze) on the skin, which indicates the depth of peel penetration. Stop application when the desired level of frosting is achieved. If any area appears too sensitive or begins to react intensely, you may neutralize the peel or take extra care to limit further penetration in that area. Some chemical peels require neutralization, while others self-neutralize.[8] Follow the protocol specific to the peel type, using a neutralizing agent or cool water as needed. If the peel needs rinsing, use water or a neutralizing solution with gauze or cotton pads, ensuring complete removal of the peeling agent.

### 4.5. POSTOPERATIVE CARE

Postoperative care is critical for supporting proper wound healing, minimizing complications, and aiding recovery. The post-peel period often includes redness, swelling, and exfoliation, commonly known as "downtime." The intensity and duration of symptoms depend on the peel's depth: 1 to 7 days for superficial peels, 7 to 10 days for medium-depth peels, and 10 to 14 days for deep peels. During this time, patients should receive clear aftercare instructions. Patients should wash the treated area twice daily with a gentle skin cleanser, avoiding scrubbing or peeling the skin. A bland emollient should be applied immediately after washing and reapplied as needed. Sun avoidance is essential following a peel, and in unavoidable situations, a physical sunblock should be applied. Other skincare products and topical treatments should be avoided until the healing process is complete. Patients may experience "tight skin" and mild itching during recovery; cool compresses and bland emollients can offer relief. Persistent itching, increasing redness, discharge, or pain are signs of a potential complication, and patients should be evaluated promptly if these occur. Once healing is complete, a post-peel skincare regimen can begin. A suitable maintenance program, which should include daily use of a broad spectrum sunscreen, is vital to sustaining results.

## 5. Laser and Energy-Based Devices

### 5.1. BACKGROUND

"LASER" stands for "light amplification by stimulated emission of radiation." During laser surgery, optical energy is absorbed by the skin and heats tissue. Laser light has four major interactions with the skin: reflection, scattering, transmission, and absorption.[9] Chromophores are molecules that absorb laser light; visible and near infrared light target melanin and hemoglobin, while far infrared light targets water. Lasers have four components: (1) a medium (gas, liquid or solid), (2) a source of energy to excite the medium, (3) mirrors to amplify, and (4) a delivery mechanism. Lasers can be a continuous beam of light or pulses of light; most all lasers in dermatology emit pulsed light.

Common lasers used in dermatology include the pulsed dye laser (PDL), neodymium-doped yttrium aluminum garnet (Nd:YAG), Alexandrite, erbium-doped yttrium aluminum garnet (Er:YAG), and carbon dioxide laser. Additionally, intense pulsed light (IPL) is a commonly used energy-based light device. For all lasers, it is important to know the clinical end points for sufficient treatment. It is also important to review safety hazards when working with lasers. These include eye injury, fire, cutaneous burns, and generation of "plume" materials from targeted photolysis. Always wear proper protective eyewear, ensuring the glasses are appropriate for the specific wavelength of the laser.

## 5.2. CLINICAL PRESENTATION

Common cosmetic complaints treated by lasers include vascular lesions, tattoos, lentigines, striae, hair removal, and textural changes.

## 5.3. EVALUATION

When a patient presents to discuss laser treatment, identify the patient's chief concern and then select a laser with the appropriate properties and target chromophore. Each laser has variety of indications depending on its wavelength (Table 12-2). The PDL (585-595 nm) is used to treat vascular lesions, including telangiectasias, port-wine stains, hemangiomas, poikiloderma of Civatte, and rosacea.[10] The potassium titanyl phosphate laser (532 nm) treats some vascular lesions, often with less bruising than the PDL. The Nd:YAG laser (1,064 nm) penetrates deeper, exhibiting less absorption by melanin and is used to treat deeper vascular lesions.

Ablative lasers ($CO_2$ and Er:YAG) and fractionated lasers are used for skin resurfacing to improve the appearance of rhytids or acne scarring. The infrared wavelength for both $CO_2$ and Er:YAG targets water as the predominant chromophore. Fully ablative $CO_2$ laser is the gold standard for photorejuvenation, rhytid reduction, and tissue tightening. However, the Er:YAG laser creates less thermal damage than $CO_2$ lasers and is generally better tolerated. Fully ablative lasers result in complete loss of epidermis due to vaporization of tissue; fractionated lasers deliver hundreds of microscopic zones of injury with intervening normal skin. Fractionated lasers yield similar effects as fully ablative lasers with less downtime and fewer side effects.

IPL is a filtered flash lamp device and not a true laser. IPL systems range from visible to near-infrared light (500-1,300 nm); this wide wavelength spectrum can be filtered for specific targets, making IPL one of the most versatile devices in aesthetic dermatology. The target chromophores include hemoglobin, melanin, and water; the wavelength of light emitted by IPL is chosen so it reaches both the correct depth and optimal absorption by target chromophore. Food and Drug Administration approved indications for IPL are benign cutaneous lesions, hair reduction, inflammatory conditions, pigmented lesions, scars, and vascular lesions. The most common dermatologic use of IPL are vascular lesions (rosacea, port wine stains), pigmented

| TABLE 12-2 | Select Laser Devices and Associated Indications | | |
|---|---|---|---|
| Laser or Light-Based Device | Wavelength (nm) | Chromophore | Indication(s) |
| Potassium titanyl phosphate | 532 | LP: hemoglobin | Port wine stain, telangiectasias, scars |
| | | QS/PS: melanin, red tattoo ink | Epidermal pigmented lesions, tattoos |
| QS, frequency doubled Nd:YAG | 532 | Melanin | Lentigines, nevi, melasma |
| Nd:YAG | 1,064 | Melanin | Hair removal, venous lake |
| Pulsed dye (PDL) | 585-600 | Hemoglobin | Port wine stain, telangiectasias, scars |
| Alexandrite | 755 | Melanin, tattoo ink | Epidermal pigmented lesions, vascular lesions, hair removal, tattoos (QS; black, blue, green) |
| Er:YAG | 2,940 | Water | Texture, photoaging (eg, acne scarring, deep rhytids) |
| Carbon dioxide | 10,600 | | Texture, photoaging (eg, acne scarring, deep rhytids) |

LP, long pulsed; QS, q-switched; PS, pico-second device; Nd-YAG, neodymium-doped yttrium aluminum garnet; Er:YAG, erbium-doped yttrium aluminum garnet.

lesions (lentigines), acne vulgaris, photodamaged skin, and skin, and poikiloderma of Civatte.[11] For a majority of indications, several IPL treatments are required, often spaced 4 to 6 weeks apart. Cooling of the skin during treatment is important to protect the epidermis; this is often achieved by aqueous gel, contact cooling, or forced chilled air. A common side effect is "striping" which is due to insufficient overlap of pulses and presents as untreated skin between treatment areas; this is minimized by performing multiple passes with the IPL device.[12]

### 5.4. TREATMENT

The most commonly used devices for vascular lesions (including port-wine stains, hemangiomas, telangiectasias, poikiloderma, and cherry angiomas) are the 532 nm potassium titanyl phosphate, 595 nm PDL, and 1,064 nm Nd:YAG lasers. The chromophore is oxyhemoglobin and the clinical endpoint is purpura.

Tattoo removal often utilizes Q-switched, pigment-specific nanosecond or picosecond lasers. These devices damage intracellular lysosomes containing tattoo ink and cause release of tattoo pigment, which is removed by the lymphatics.[10] Green tattoo pigment is removed by a 755-nm Q-switched Alexandrite, red by 532 nm Nd:YAG and blue and black pigments by ruby, alexandrite and/or Nd:YAG. Yellow and orange pigments are more difficult to target. The clinical end point is immediate whitening of epidermis.

Melanin has a broad absorption spectrum and can therefore be targeted with several different lasers. The frequency-doubled Nd:YAG (532 nm) is an effective choice for epidermal pigmented lesions (eg, lentigines and ephelides). The Q-switched ruby and alexandrite lasers are more effective at treating deeper pigmented lesions (eg, nevus of Ota).[11]

Acne scarring is commonly treated by ablative lasers, with more improvement often seen with the $CO_2$ laser. Elevated or distensible acne scars are more amenable to laser treatment than ice pick scars.

Laser hair removal (LHR) delivers laser energy to the bulge region of the hair follicle, which destroys follicular stem cells with minimal injury to surrounding tissue.[12] Underlying etiologies of excess hair growth should be evaluated before proceeding with LHR. The best wavelengths for LHR are 600 to 1,100 nm. In general, the 755 nm alexandrite or 800 nm diode lasers are appropriate for lighter skin phototypes (I-III), while the 1,064 nm Nd:YAG is a good option for darker skin phototypes (IV-VI).

# 6. Sclerotherapy

## 6.1. BACKGROUND

Reticular and varicose veins of the lower legs result from impairment of the venous system. Poor venous return can be due to incompetence of venous valves or from primary muscle pump failure, resulting in venous reflux. Sclerotherapy is the treatment of choice for skin-level superficial veins, telangiectasias, and small reticular veins.

## 6.2. EVALUATION

All patients interested in sclerotherapy should undergo a thorough history and pretreatment physical examination while standing to identify their highest point of venous reflux.[13] When treating patients, it is imperative to choose the minimal volume and lowest concentration of sclerosing agent to achieve best results with fewest complications.

## 6.3. TREATMENT

There are three main categories of sclerosing agents: hyperosmotic agents, chemical irritants, and detergent sclerosants.[14] Hyperosmotic agents damage the endothelial cell wall via dehydration. Osmotic agents include hypertonic saline, hypertonic saline-dextrose, and nonchromated glycerin. Chemical irritants, which include chromated glycerin and polyiodide iodide, damage cell wall via corrosion. Detergent sclerosants damage cell wall by altering surface tension around endothelial cells. Detergent sclerosants include sodium tetradecyl sulfate, polidocanol, and sodium morrhuate. The only Food and Drug Administration–approved agents for sclerotherapy are sodium tetradecyl sulfate, sodium morrhuate, and polidocanol (all detergent sclerosants). Sodium tetradecyl sulfate and polidocanol are the recommended sclerosing solutions for reticular veins (2-4 mm), nonsaphenous varicose veins (3-8 mm), and saphenous varicose veins (>5 mm); concentrations of these agents increase in conjunction with vein size. Posttreatment compression stockings (preferably 30-40 mm Hg) and ambulation are recommended for optimal healing and results.

# 7. Hair Restoration

## 7.1. BACKGROUND

Hair loss, or alopecia, can be broadly categorized into nonscarring and scarring processes. Nonscarring androgenetic alopecia is a common age-related process, which affects up to 80% of men and 50% of women.[15] Treatment modalities include medications like topical or oral minoxidil, oral finasteride, oral dutasteride, or oral spironolactone, or procedures like hair transplantation or injection of platelet-rich plasma (PRP).

## 7.2. CLINICAL PRESENTATION

Androgenetic alopecia is due to miniaturization of terminal hairs; reduction of hair follicle size is partially driven by androgens.

## 7.3. EVALUATION

Evaluate the patient's scalp to determine the type and etiology of hair loss. Female pattern hair loss is characterized by a progressive widening of the central part line. Male pattern hair loss involves frontotemporal hairline regression and thinning of vertex scalp. Physical and psychosocial examinations prior to hair transplantation surgery are important to ensure the areas of concern can be properly addressed through the planned procedure. The ideal patient has high density, large-caliber hair, and hair loss stabilized with medical interventions.[16]

## 7.4. TREATMENT

Medical therapies for androgenetic alopecia can be employed prior to or alongside interventional treatments for hair loss. Common medications include topical or oral minoxidil, finasteride, dutasteride, or spironolactone.

Hair transplantation involves transplanting hair follicles from the unaffected area of the patient's scalp to the balding area. Androgenetic alopecia is an ongoing process and will continue despite a hair transplant, though the latter can help improve density and overall cosmesis. Candidate selection for hair transplantation includes evaluation of age, hair shaft caliber, donor hair density, degree of baldness, and hair color.[16] The primary methods of harvesting donor hair are elliptical donor harvesting and follicular unit extraction. Both can result in high-quality transplant results. Elliptical donor harvesting involves elliptical incision of occipital scalp (donor site) and subsequent creation of grafts; follicular unit extraction involves removal of follicular units (groupings of one to four hair follicles) with punch tool or needles.

PRP injections are an emerging therapy for hair loss. Most existing literature supports its use in nonscarring alopecia, such as androgenetic alopecia, although its utility for scarring alopecias is being explored. PRP can be used as an adjunctive treatment for androgenetic alopecia, in combination with existing treatments like minoxidil and finasteride. The initial treatment series is three to four monthly injections followed by maintenance injections every 3 to 6 months. Platelet-rich plasma contains an increased concentration of platelets (~1,000,000 platelets/µL); the platelets themselves contain alpha granules, which secrete several growth factors upon platelet degranulation. These growth factors include platelet-derived growth factor, epidermal growth factor, transforming growth factor beta, fibroblast growth factor, and insulin-like growth factor.[15] While the precise mechanism of PRP injections is unknown, it is hypothesized that PRP may induce perifollicular angiogenesis, stimulate proliferation of dermal papillary cells, and prolong the anagen growth phase—all leading to increased hair growth and density. There are several PRP processing techniques, but the fundamental method involves: (1) collecting 10 to 60 mL of whole blood from the patient on day of treatment, (2) adding anticoagulants, (3) centrifuging the sample to separate cell types, (4) collecting the superficial buffy coat for pure PRP, and (5) activation of PRP by adding calcium gluconate, calcium chloride, or thrombin.[1] Variables to PRP preparation include commercial versus manual processing, number of centrifuge spins, procuring pure versus leukocyte-rich PRP, platelet concentration, type of activating agent, exogenous versus endogenous activation, and depth of injection. It has yet to be determined which combination of collection techniques yields the greatest clinical results. In addition to hair loss, PRP injections have also been proposed to help improve appearance of photodamaged skin, facial volume, and acne scars.[1]

## 8. Microneedling

### 8.1. BACKGROUND

Microneedling is an aesthetic treatment in which small needles make microscopic punctures in the skin with the goal of stimulating dermal remodeling. Microscopic injury to the epidermis and dermis is proposed to stimulate new vessel formation, release dermal growth factors, and stimulate fibroblasts with subsequent collagen deposition. These effects lead to improved aesthetic appearance once healed. Microneedling is often in use either in conjunction with or in place of nonablative lasers for the treatment of acne scarring, facial rhytids, and skin tightening.[17] It can also be used to improve drug delivery in the treatment of alopecia. Microneedling devices have needles, tips, or pins that are rolled or stamped over the skin. There are two main categories of devices: manual needle rollers and electric-powered pens. Both create microscopic wounds in the epidermis and dermis. The manual needle rollers involve multidirectional skin penetration on a fixed drum-shaped roller. The electric-powered pens penetrate the skin vertically, offer greater precision for smaller areas, and are assumed to have decreased infection risk due to disposable needles.

### 8.2. CLINICAL PRESENTATION

Microneedling is often employed for the treatment of atrophic acne scars, skin rejuvenation and reduction of fine rhytids (especially perioral), and alopecia. In regard to acne scarring, rolling and boxcar scars are more effectively treated by microneedling than ice pick scars. Microneedling may be an especially attractive option resurfacing in patients with darker Fitzpatrick skin types (IV-VI) as it has been shown to have decreased risk of dyspigmentation compared to laser treatments and chemical peels.[18] In addition to acne scars, microneedling has also been used to treat striae, burn scars, and postsurgical scarring.

### 8.3. EVALUATION

Evaluation before microneedling treatment should involve history and physical examination to develop a safe treatment plan. Counseling involving treatment indications, alternatives, and risks/benefits is essential. Common indications for microneedling are reviewed in Section 7.1. Alternatives include nonintervention, chemical peels, and nonablative or ablative laser resurfacing. Risks include infection, scarring, and dyspigmentation. Risk for hyperpigmentation increase with excessive sun exposure; patients should be counseled to avid tanning prior to procedure. The main benefit is improved cosmetic appearance; as this can be subjective, it is important to review realistic outcome goals with the patient and usual need for several treatments to reach desired effect. Some clinicians recommend pretreatment prophylaxis with valacyclovir for patients with history of herpes simplex infection.

### 8.4. TREATMENT

Treatment with microneedling starts with preparing the face for treatment. Position the patient supine, remove makeup, consider topical anesthetic, clean skin with aseptic material, and ensure clinician is wearing proper protective equipment like gloves. If patient is at increased risk of adverse side effects, consider doing test spot in a discrete area prior to treating the entire face. Recommended steps for treatment include: (1) applying gliding gel to protect epidermis and (2) holding the microneedling device perpendicularly to treatment area and guiding it across the face in three passes of alternating direction (horizontal, vertical, and oblique).[19] Treatment is continued until clinical end point of pinpoint bleeding is observed. Recovery is expedient with transient erythema and swelling, often resolving in 72 hours.

## 9. Conclusion

A wide array of minimally invasive cosmetic procedures are available to the practicing dermatologist to address the needs of an aesthetic patient. After concluding this chapter, the reader should be able to assess common concerns brought by the cosmetic patient, including volume loss, facial rhytids, facial dyschromia, excess or loss of hair, and/or visible veins and telangiectasias. As in all patient-physician relationships, the approach to the aesthetic patient is one that centers on shared decision making.

## REFERENCES

1. Carruthers A, Carruthers J, de Almeida TA. Chapter 159: Botulinum toxin. In: Bolognia JL, Schaffer JV, Cerroni L, eds. *Dermatology*. 4th ed. Elsevier; 2018:2661-2672.
2. Glaser K, Glaser DA. Chapter 2: Botulinum toxin. In: Council ML, ed. *Guide to Minimally Invasive Aesthetic Procedures*. 1st ed. Lippincott Williams & Wilkins; 2021:144-168.
3. Solish N, Carruthers J, Kaufman J, Rubio RG, Gross TM, Gallagher CJ. Overview of daxibotulinumtoxin A for injection: a novel formulation of botulinum toxin type A. *Drugs*. 2021;81(18):2091-2101. doi:10.1007/s40265-021-01631-w
4. Jones D, Bacigalupi R, Beleznay K. Chapter 158: Injectable soft tissue augmentation. In: Bolognia JL, Schaffer JV, Cerroni L, eds. *Dermatology*. 4th ed. Elsevier; 2018:2649-2659.
5. Schneider S, Sundaram H, Council ML. Chapter 3: Soft tissue augmentation. In: Council ML, ed. *Guide to Minimally Invasive Aesthetic Procedures*. 1st ed. Lippincott Williams & Wilkins; 2021:144-168.
6. Al-Ghanim K, Richards R, Cohen S. A practical guide to selecting facial fillers. *J Cosmet Dermatol*. 2023;22(12):3232-3236. doi:10.1111/jocd.15867. PMID: 37395390.
7. Murthy R, Eccleston D, Mckeown D, Parikh A, Shotter S. Improving aseptic injection standards in aesthetic clinical practice. *Dermatol Ther*. 2021;34(1):e14416. doi:10.1111/dth.14416. PMID: 33068030; PMCID: PMC7900975.
8. Rholdon F, Council ML. Chapter 5: Chemical peels. In: Council ML, ed. *Guide to Minimally Invasive Aesthetic Procedures*. 1st ed. Lippincott Williams & Wilkins; 2021:81-100.

9. Sakamoto FH, Avram MM, Anderson RR. Chapter 136: Lasers and other energy-based technologies: principles and skin interactions. In: Bolognia JL, Schaffer JV, Cerroni L, eds. *Dermatology*. 4th ed. Elsevier; 2018:2676-2686.
10. Zachary CB, Kelly KM. Chapter 137: Lasers and other energy-based therapies. In: Bolognia JL, Schaffer JV, Cerroni L, eds. *Dermatology*. 4th ed. Elsevier; 2018:2687-2709.
11. Martin ED, Labadie JG, Alam M. *ASLMS Laser Primer: Lasers and Other Energy-Based Technologies in Dermatology*. 1st ed. American Society for Laser Medicine & Surgery, Inc.; 2022.
12. Wang JV, Saedi N. Chapter 4: Laser and light devices in aesthetic medicine. In: Council ML, ed. *Guide to Minimally Invasive Aesthetic Procedures*. 1st ed. Lippincott Williams & Wilkins; 2021:67-80.
13. Clarey D, Wysong A. Chapter 8: Vascular treatments of the lower extremity. In: Council ML, ed. *Guide to Minimally Invasive Aesthetic Procedures*. 1st ed. Lippincott Williams & Wilkins; 2021:144-168.
14. Goldman MP, Weiss RA. Chapter 155: Phlebology and treatment of leg veins. In: Bolognia JL, Schaffer JV, Cerroni L, eds. *Dermatology*. 4th ed. Elsevier; 2018:2972-2989.
15. Avram M, Shyam N. Chapter 6: Hair loss: established treatments and emerging therapies. In: Council ML, ed. *Guide to Minimally Invasive Aesthetic Procedures*. 1st ed. Lippincott Williams & Wilkins; 2021:102-118.
16. Avram MR, Keene SA, Stough DB, Rogers NE, Cole JP. Chapter 157: Hair restoration. In: Bolognia JL, Schaffer JV, Cerroni L, eds. *Dermatology*. 4th ed. Elsevier; 2018:3002-3015.
17. Voller L, Gupta R, Hussain N, et al. Chapter 10: Miscellaneous aesthetic procedures. In: Counciler ML, ed. *Guide to Minimally Invasive Aesthetic Procedures*. 1st ed. Lippincott Williams & Wilkins; 2021:102-118.
18. Cohen BE, Elbuluk N. Microneedling in skin of color: a review of uses and efficacy. *J Am Acad Dermatol*. 2016;74:348-355. doi:10.1016/j.jaad.2015.09.024
19. Alster TS, Graham PM. Microneedling: a review and practical guide. *Dermatol Surg*. 2018;44:397-404. doi:10.1097/DSS.0000000000001248

# 13 Skin of Color Dermatology

Muithi Mwanthi, MD, PhD
and Damien Abreu, MD, PhD

## 1. Introduction to Skin of Color Dermatology

Dermatology is a uniquely placed medical specialty that addresses skin conditions and diseases that have a higher prevalence or profound impact on persons with respect to skin and hair types. Skin conditions are often visible and significantly influence social identity and interaction. Skin of Color (SOC) Dermatology is a vital field focusing on all aspects of skin health in a diverse population. According to SOC Society, "Individuals with SOC have diverse racial and ethnic backgrounds, and include those of the following ancestries: African, Asian, Hispanic/Latine, Native American, Pacific Islander, as well as individuals with mixed races and/or ethnicities."[1] The scope of SOC Dermatology is broad, encompassing biological diversity, variations in skin tone, and diverse ethnic and cultural practices that affect how skin conditions present and are managed.[2] Biological differences in the epidermis and its appendages, the dermal-epidermal junction (DEJ), and the dermis contribute to variations in skin conditions in SOC populations. However, there are significant knowledge gaps in the cutaneous genetics of SOC populations and how these differences can inform targeted treatments.[3] Dermatologic inequities are worsened by factors such as underrepresentation of SOC in clinical research, few inclusive clinical guidelines, limited access to clinical specialists, lack of knowledge regarding SOC-specific presentations of skin diseases, inadequate clinical training in SOC dermatology, as well as social and cultural determinants of health.[3-5] The goal of SOC Dermatology is to improve the understanding of medical and procedural aspects of skin disease to ensure equitable care for all patients.

Patients of color seek dermatologic care for certain conditions more frequently than White patients, including eczematous dermatitis, hair concerns, vitiligo, and keloids.[6,7] SOC centers in the United States have been established, focusing their research and clinical efforts to address inequities in skin conditions that are common or impactful in these populations.[8,9] This chapter will explore frequently seen and impactful conditions in patients of color, as outlined in Table 13-1, to further the goal of equitable dermatological care.

## 2. Normal Pigmentation Variants

It is crucial to identify benign pigmentary variations in patients with SOC to avoid misdiagnosis. The entities below represent a selection of such variants.

### 2.1. PIGMENTARY DEMARCATION LINES/VOIGT-FUTCHER LINES[36]

- These pigmented boundary lines are bilateral and symmetrical, appearing from infancy into adulthood more prominently in patients of color. Additional lines streak down the arms, inner thighs, upper chest, spine, and face, creating a recognizable pattern (Fig. 13-1A).

| TABLE 13-1 | Selected Skin Conditions With Increased Frequency and Impact in Patients of Color | |
|---|---|---|
| Condition | Population Most Affected | Relative Frequency |
| Acne postinflammatory hyperpigmentation | Black and Latine patients | ~65% (Black) and ~53% (Latine) vs ~20% (Whites)[10] |
| Atopic dermatitis | Black, Latine, Asian, and Native American children | 2%-10% absolute higher prevalence[11] |
| Melasma | Asian, Latine, and mixed-race women | ~150%, 127%, and 142% higher risk[12] |
| Discoid lupus erythematosus | Black and Latine patients | ~1,200% (23.5 vs 1.8) and ~300% (8.2 vs 1.8) higher prevalence[13-15] |
| Hidradenitis suppurativa | Black and biracial women and girls | 211% and 129% higher prevalence (296 and 218 vs 95)[16,17] |
| Central centrifugal cicatricial alopecia | Black women | 3%-17% prevalence (Black) vs rare in White women[a] |
| Acne keloidalis nuchae/folliculitis keloidalis nuchae | Black men | ~1.6%-14% prevalence (Black); rare in White men[a] |
| Pseudofolliculitis barbae | Black men | ~45%-85% prevalence vs <20% in White men[18,a] |
| Traction alopecia | Black women | ~8%-33% prevalence (Black) vs rarer in Whites[19] |
| Keloids | Black and Asian populations | ~300% and 250% higher[20,21,a] |
| Dermatofibrosarcoma protuberans | Black patients | ~2 times greater incidence compared to Whites[22,23] |
| Atopic dermatitis persistence | Black children | Persistence into teenage years[24] |
| Cutaneous T-cell lymphoma mortality | Black patients | 54%-100% higher vs White patients[25,26] |
| Sarcoidosis mortality | Black patients | ~1,200% higher age-adjusted mortality[27] |
| Melanoma late diagnosis | Black, Latine, and Asian and Pacific Islanders patients | 150%-160% higher vs White patients[28-30] |
| Melanoma 5-y mortality | Black patients | 200%-210% higher vs White patients[30,31] |
| Vitiligo | Black, Latine, and Asian populations | Greater psychosocial burden in darker skin tones[32-35] |

[a]Lack of well-designed, population-based studies.

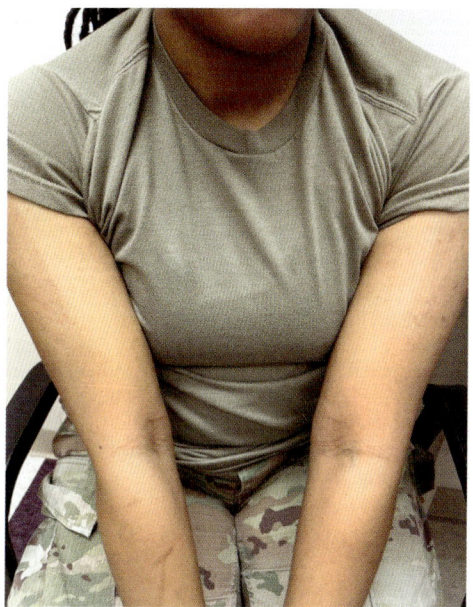

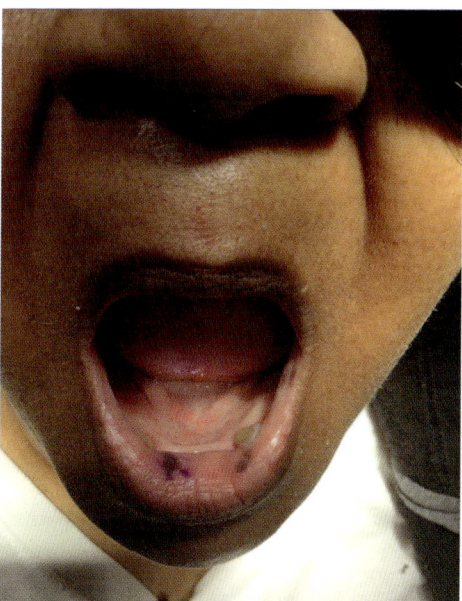

**Figure 13-1. A.** Voigt-Futcher lines. Exaggerated pigmentary demarcation lines between the medial and lateral arms. **B.** Labial melanotic macules. Brown macules on mucosal lower lip.

## 2.2. MUCOSAL PIGMENTATION

### 2.2.1. Complexion-Associated Melanosis[37]
- This represents acquired ocular pigmentation typically appearing as flat, noncystic lesions with ill-defined margins and a "cobblestone" texture. This condition is usually bilateral and symmetrical and may also affect the palpebral conjunctiva.

### 2.2.2. Oral Mucosal Melanosis[38,39]
- These benign nonsyndromic pigmented macules and patches on lips gingival and buccal mucosa can be seen more often in patients of color (Fig. 13-1B).

## 2.3. MULTIPLE LINEAR MELANONYCHIA[40,41]

- Longitudinal nail pigmentation in dark-skinned individuals can manifest as one or, more commonly, multiple bands across one or more digits. There may be a family history and occur mostly from melanocyte activation (Fig. 13-2A and B). This benign presentation should be distinguished from nail unit melanocyte neoplasms (nevi and melanomas) (Fig. 13-2C and D).

## 2.4. MELANOCYTOSIS VARIANTS

### 2.4.1. Dermal Melanocytosis[42]
- These benign skin lesions appear at birth or in the first weeks of life as blue-gray, blue-green, or blue-black patches. They are commonly found in the lumbosacral or sacrogluteal regions (Fig. 13-3A) and are particularly prevalent among infants of African and Asian descent. While many of these lesions regress in childhood, those with nonsacral distributions may persist into adulthood (Fig. 13-3B).

### 2.4.2. Oculodermal Melanocytosis[43]
- These benign dark blue-gray or brown patches of hyperpigmentation frequently appear on the face as nevus of Ota or Hori's nevus or on the shoulder or neck as nevus of Ito. They can be present at birth or develop later, during puberty.

### 2.4.3. Scleral Melanocytosis
- A benign condition characterized by dark pigmentation on the sclera of the eye due to an increased number of melanocytes (Fig. 13-4). It is typically congenital but can also develop later in life and does not affect vision.

# 3. Erythema[44-50]

- Erythema, one hallmark of skin inflammation, can be difficult to detect in individuals with darker skin tones. This can lead to underdiagnosis, misdiagnosis, or a lack of appreciation for the true severity of skin conditions in patients of color. The challenge in detecting erythema in darker skin also impacts clinical trials, where an overreliance on redness can underestimate inflammation and potentially exclude patients of color.[50]
- Instead of the typical pink or red, erythema may appear dark brown or violaceous in darker skin. Pink lesions might look violaceous, gray, or even dark brown (Fig. 13-5A and B).

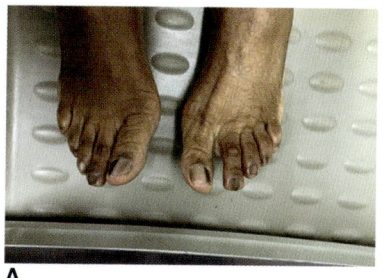

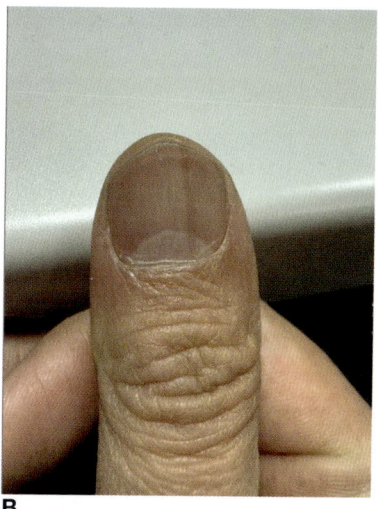

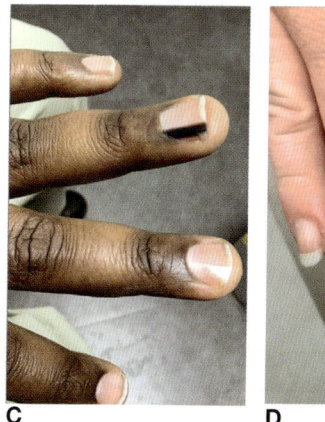
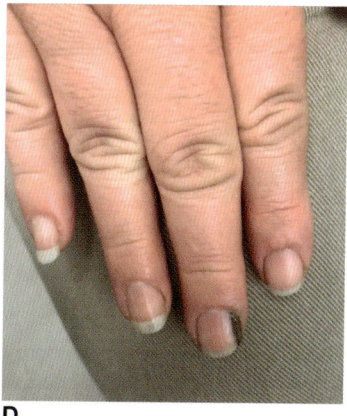

**Figure 13-2. A.** Multiple longitudinal melanonychia. **B.** Longitudinal melanonychia. Brown longitudinal band on toes and right thumb more common in SOC from melanocyte activation. **C, D.** Longitudinal melanonychia. Dark longitudinal bands in SOC on left fourth digit and right third digit found on nail matrix biopsy to be benign melanocytic neoplasms (melanocyte proliferation).

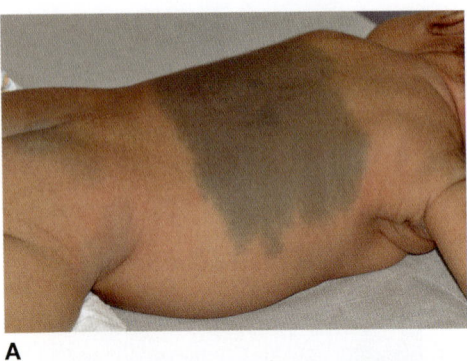

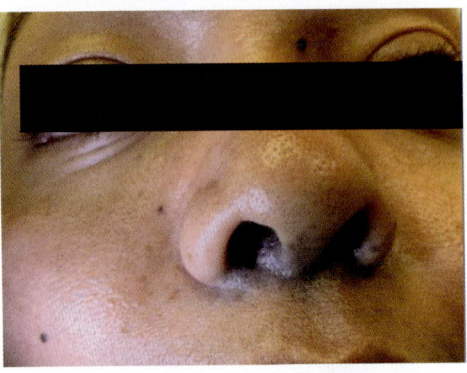

**Figure 13-3.** Dermal melanocytosis. **A.** Blue-grey patches on the thoracic, upper lumbar, and sacrogluteal skin of a newborn. Photograph is provided courtesy of Susan Bayliss, MD. **B.** Blue-black pigmented patches on the nasal alar and columella since childhood in an adult female.

- In patients with darker skin, many conditions cause changes in skin color (darkening or lightening), which can obscure the perception of erythema and mask other clinical features, including hives and purpura. Hyperpigmented skin might be mistakenly identified as benign postinflammatory hyperpigmentation (PIH) instead of actively inflamed skin.
- Experienced clinicians must examine SOC under proper lighting, understand the varied presentations of erythema, and consider palpable skin changes when making clinical decisions.

# 4. Postinflammatory Pigmentary Alteration

## 4.1. POSTINFLAMMATORY HYPERPIGMENTATION[51,52]

- PIH is a reactive darkening of the skin (mixed epidermal and dermal melanosis) following inflammation from internal or external causes. It significantly affects individuals with darker skin tones more than those with lighter skin.

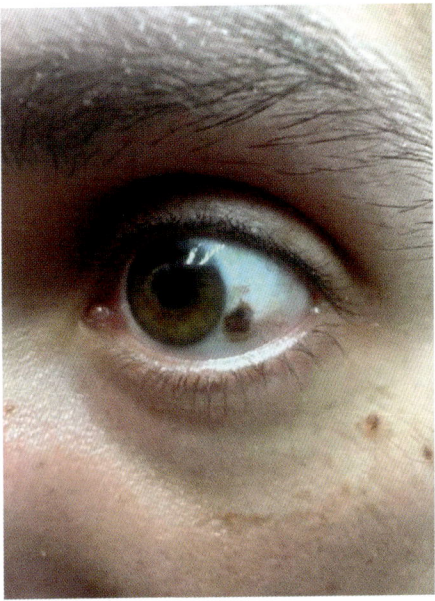

**Figure 13-4.** Conjunctival nevus/scleral melanocytosis. Well-defined dark brown papule on conjunctiva of left eye.

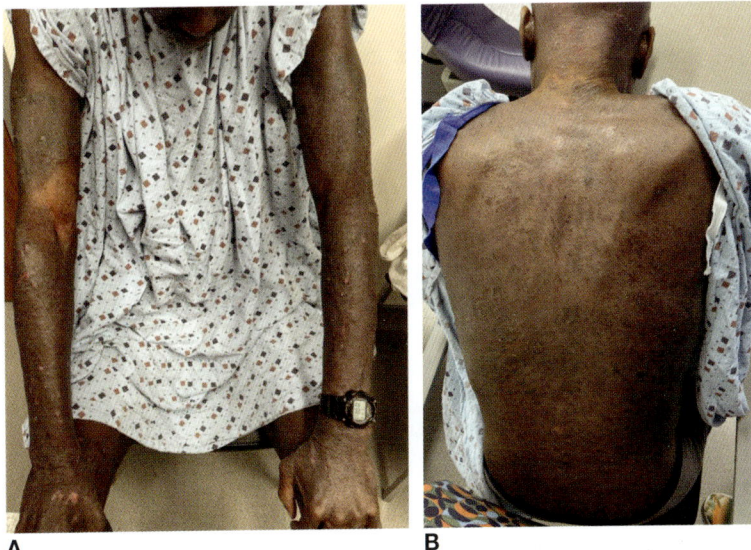

**Figure 13-5. A.** Erythrodermic atopic dermatitis (extremities). Confluent hyperpigmented and edematous plaques with excoriation and erosions. Mild erythema is seen at the border with unaffected skin in the right antecubital. **B.** Erythrodermic atopic dermatitis (back). Confluent hyperpigmented, violaceous, and edematous plaques with excoriation, erosions, and crust.

- Inflammation leads to excessive melanin production and abnormal distribution in skin cells (keratinocytes), the DEJ, and the dermis. Inflammation can also disrupt the DEJ, allowing immune cells (macrophages) to engulf and retain pigment in the dermis for extended periods.
- Presentation: Typically appears as asymptomatic tan or darker macules and patches in the areas where inflammation occurred (Fig. 13-6A-C). There is often a history

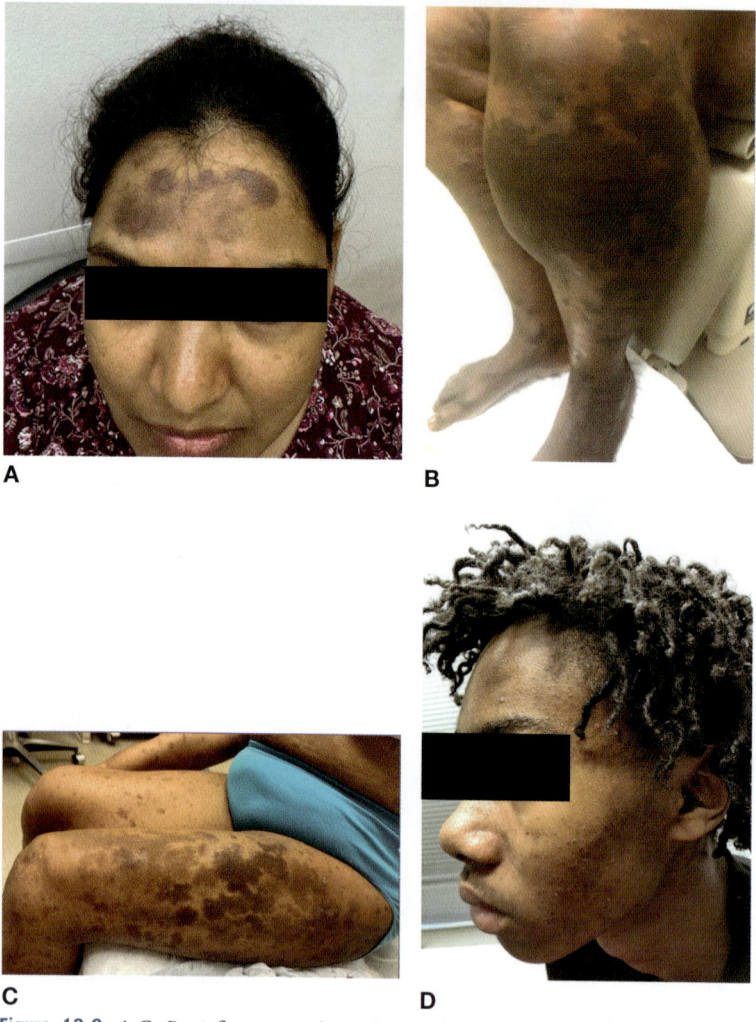

**Figure 13-6. A-C.** Postinflammatory hyperpigmentation: well-demarcated hyperpigmented patches on the face and lower extremities resulting from actinic lichen planus, generalized lichen planus, and psoriasis. **D.** Acne with postinflammatory hyperpigmentation: open and closed comedones, hyperpigmented macules and papules, and papules on cheeks, temple, and forehead.

of a skin injury or condition. Examination with a Wood's lamp can highlight the borders of epidermal hyperpigmentation but not dermal PIH.
- Resolution: Epidermal PIH may take months to years to resolve without treatment, while dermal PIH may persist for years.
- Management:
  - Patient education about PIH is crucial.
  - Prevention and treatment of the underlying inflammatory condition are essential.
  - Strict photoprotection of exposed skin areas is vital. Patients of color may need specific guidance on sunscreen and product recommendations.[53-55]
  - Camouflage with makeup or tinted sunscreen may be necessary for long-standing PIH.
- Medical treatment[52,56]: Medical treatment is for those seeking faster resolution.
  - First-line: Hydroquinone-based topical agents.
  - Other effective options: Topical retinoids and azelaic acid (especially for acne-induced PIH), cysteamine, thiamidol, and oral tranexamic acid (newer treatments).
  - Procedures used cautiously: Chemical peels, microdermabrasion, microneedling, and lasers (Table 13-2) must be used with care in patients of color to avoid causing more PIH.

### TABLE 13-2 Selected Applications of Lasers in Skin of Color

| Condition | Laser | Wavelength | Study Type |
| --- | --- | --- | --- |
| **Postinflammatory hyperpigmentation (PIH)**[a] | Q-Switched neodymium-doped yttrium aluminum garnet (Nd:YAG) laser | 1,064 nm | Case series[57] |
| | Picosecond Alexandrite laser | 755 nm | Case series[58] |
| | Intense pulse light | Various | Case series[59] |
| **Melasma** | Q-switched Nd:YAG laser | 1,064 nm | Randomized controlled trial (RCT)[60] |
| | Fractional diode laser | 1,927 nm | RCT (<50)[61,62] |
| | Fractional 1,064-nm picosecond laser | 1,064 nm | Cohort[63] |
| | Other Pico lasers | | Cohorts reviewed[64] |
| **Vascular lesions** | Pulse dye laser | 595 nm | Cases[65] |
| | Broadband light devices | Different wavelengths | |
| **Acne scarring** | Erbium-glass fractionated nonablative laser | 1,540-1,550 nm | Cohort, trial, RCT (<50)[66-70] |
| | Fractional $CO_2$ laser | 10,600 nm | Cohort[69,71] |
| | Er:YAG laser (fractional ablative mode) | 2,940 nm | Cohort[69,72] |

(*continued*)

| TABLE 13-2 | Selected Applications of Lasers in Skin of Color (*continued*) | | |
|---|---|---|---|
| Condition | Laser | Wavelength | Study Type |
| | Nonablative fractional erbium laser | 1,340 nm | RCT[73] |
| | Picosecond lasers | 755 nm, 1,064 nm | Cohort, RCT[74,75] |
| **Hidradenitis suppurativa** | Nd:YAG | 1,064 nm | RCT (<50)[76] |
| | Alexandrite laser | 755 nm | RCT (<50)[77] |
| | $CO_2$ ablative laser | 10,600 nm | [b] |
| **Pseudofolliculitis barbae and acne keloidalis nuchae** | Nd:YAG laser (long-pulse) | 1,064 nm | RCT (<50)[78,79] |
| | $CO_2$ ablative laser | 10,600 nm | Cohort[80] |
| **Keloids** | Fractional $CO_2$ ablative laser | 10,600 nm | Cohort, RCT (<50), meta-analysis[81-83] |
| | Nd:YAG laser | 1,064 nm | Cohort[84] |
| | Pulsed dye laser | 595 nm | RCT (<50)[85] |
| **Dermatosis papulosa nigra** | Fractional $CO_2$ ablative laser | 10,600 nm | Case series[86] |
| | Nd:YAG laser (1,064 nm) | 1,064 nm | Case reports[87] |
| | Potassium titanyl phosphate (KTP) | 532 nm | RCT (<50)[88] |

[a]Mostly in the context of acne-induced PIH.
[b]Skin phototype not reported in available retrospective studies.

## 4.2. POSTINFLAMMATORY HYPOPIGMENTATION

- Postinflammatory hypopigmentation (PIHo) is a partial or complete loss of skin color following inflammatory skin conditions or skin injury (from irritants or procedures).
- Skin injury and inflammation can disrupt melanosome transfer or result in melanocyte death.
- Presentation: Usually presents as asymptomatic lighter macules and patches in the areas of previous inflammation. Complete depigmentation is rare.
- Resolution: Hypopigmented lesions tend to improve over weeks or months, while completely depigmented patches may not improve.
- Pityriasis alba is a common and prominent pediatric form of PIHo on the cheeks of both atopic and nonatopic individuals, especially in patients of color.[89]

# 5. Adult and Pediatric Dermatology in Skin of Color

## 5.1. ACNE VULGARIS

- Acne vulgaris is a common skin condition among pediatric and adult patients of color, often presenting with different clinical and histological characteristics

compared to white skin. Hyperpigmented macules, keloids, and pomade acne from acne are more common and long lasting in SOC.[10]
- The pathogenesis of acne in SOC is similar to that in white skin. Notably, the inflammation from the inflammatory process and acne treatment can cause PIH (Fig. 13-6D).
- A major concern in acne is acne-induced PIH, which is often the primary complaint and requires early and aggressive treatment.[10,56]
- Irritant contact dermatitis from topical treatments is a common, necessitating careful selection and application of topical therapies.
- Management requires understanding these factors and potential differences in presentation and treatment response. Individualized treatment is key, considering skin type, seasonal changes, and specific acne lesions, with a focus on treating both acne and hyperpigmentation early.[56,90]

### 5.2. ATOPIC DERMATITIS

- Atopic dermatitis (AD) is a very common skin condition leading patients of color to seek dermatologic care. AD is more common in childhood, and children of color have a higher prevalence and greater persistence of AD compared to white children.[24,91] They also tend to experience greater disease severity and health care utilization.[44,92]
- AD is an inflammatory condition due to skin barrier dysfunction and immune dysregulation, leading to itching, scratching, dysbiosis, sensitivity to contactants, and sleep and mood disturbances. There may be differences in barrier defects and immune profiles in patients of African and Asian descent compared to White populations.[3,93-95]
- Clinical presentation, symptoms, color, distribution, and morphology of AD can vary across different skin complexions and racial/ethnic backgrounds (Table 13-3).
- Erythema, often used to assess AD severity, is frequently underestimated in SOC, leading to the development of more inclusive assessment tools.[44,50]
- Pruritus (itching) is a major symptom and diagnostic criterion. Patients of color with AD may present with significant itching without prominent primary skin lesions, often exhibiting secondary lesions from scratching like prurigo nodules, which can lead to scarring and dyspigmentation (Fig. 13-5A and B). This "itch-prominent" variant is now a recognized treatment indication for biologics like dupilumab and nemolizumab.
- Pigmentary alterations (PIH and PIHo) are common and significantly impact the burden of AD in patients of color.

### 5.3. ALLERGIC CONTACT DERMATITIS[45]

- Allergic contact dermatitis (ACD) is a common inflammatory skin condition. While its overall prevalence does not differ significantly across demographics, exposure patterns and sensitivity to specific allergens can vary by age, geography, race, or sex.
- Presentation: ACD should be suspected when there is a localized, persistent, or unusual pattern of eczematous dermatitis. Patch testing is crucial but may be underutilized in patients of color with eczema. ACD often occurs alongside AD but is more commonly diagnosed in individuals without AD.
- Patch testing: Relying solely on erythema for a positive patch test result may underestimate ACD frequency in darker skin.[49] Accurate interpretation requires

| TABLE 13-3 | Physical and Histological Features of Atopic Dermatitis That Are Found More Commonly in Patients of Color | |
|---|---|---|
| Common Atopic Dermatitis Features | Darker Skin Tone Features[93-95] | Asian Features[93-95] |
| Pruritus | Skin thickening | Well-demarcated lesions |
| Erythematous plaques | Hyperpigmented, violaceous, gray | Psoriasiform scaling |
| Fine overlying scale | Accentuation of skin lines | Lichenification |
| Flexural distribution | Numerous excoriations | Wrist dermatitis |
| | Perifollicular accentuation/lichenoid | Eyelid dermatitis |
| | Diffuse xerosis | Epidermal hyperplasia |
| | Dennie-Morgan lines | Greater acanthosis |
| | Hyperlinearity of palms | Hyperkeratosis |
| | Prurigo nodularis | |
| | Postinflammatory hyperpigmentation | |
| | Periorbital dark circles | |

palpation, adequate front and side lighting, and awareness of the varied appearance of erythema in all skin tones.[49,50,96] This can make telehealth assessment of patch tests challenging (Fig. 13-7C and D).
- Allergens:
  ○ Nickel is a common sensitizer among most demographics and is seen in patients of color at higher rates than in White patients (Fig. 13-7A and B).
  ○ Colophony, fragrance, and diazolidinyl urea sensitivities were higher in patients of Asian descent compared to White patients.
  ○ Sensitivities to rubber accelerator, some formaldehyde releasers, and fragrances are detected at higher rates in Latin American patients compared to White patients.
  ○ Paraphenylenediamine, rubber accelerators, formaldehyde releasers, Colophony, textile dyes, and bacitracin sensitivities are detected in African American patients at higher rates than White patients.

## 5.4. SEBORRHEIC DERMATITIS[97]

- Seborrheic dermatitis is a chronic inflammatory condition and a frequent reason for dermatologic consultations in patients of color, possibly with a slightly higher incidence in African Americans.
- It primarily affects areas with high sebum production, such as the scalp, ears, nasolabial folds, glabella, and eyebrows, often presenting as erythema, flaking, and hypopigmentation (Fig. 13-8C and D).
- Darker-skinned patients may present with hypopigmentation alone in typical areas of with underlying erythema being difficult to detect. They may also show with arcuate and petaloid lesions (Fig. 13-8A and B).
- It is important to rule out tinea capitis or faciei, especially in pediatric patients where it is common.

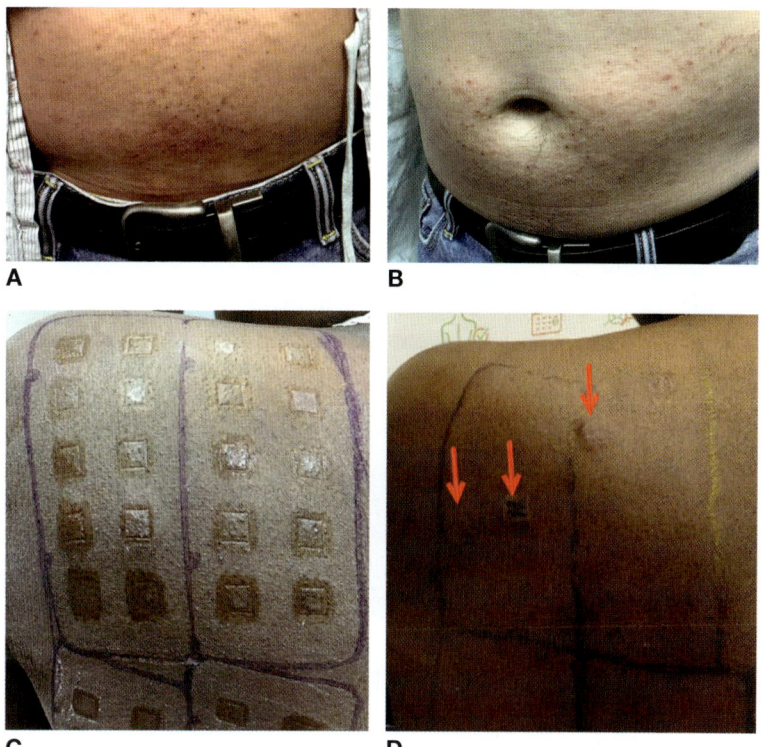

**Figure 13-7.** Allergic contact dermatitis. **A, B.** Nickel dermatitis. Clustered pink and hyperpigmented excoriated papules on lower abdomen near location of belt buckle. **C, D.** Positive patch test in dark skin. ++ and +++ reactions to neomycin, parabens, and cobalt with little erythema.

- The management of seborrheic dermatitis focuses on reducing *Malassezia* overgrowth, penetrating the scale and crust, and treating inflammation and pruritus.
- A tailored treatment plan should consider the patient's hairstyle, hair texture, washing frequency, and hair products. Drying treatments, hair extensions, infrequent washing, pomades, and oil use can worsen symptoms.

### 5.5. HIDRADENITIS SUPPURATIVA[98-100]

- Presentation: Hidradenitis suppurativa (HS) is a chronic inflammatory disorder characterized by painful, purulent, deep-seated nodules with pus and interconnecting tracts, typically in intertriginous areas like the armpits, groin, buttocks, and under the breasts (Fig. 13-9A and B). Chronic scarring from flares can cause lymphedema (Fig. 13-9C). These lesions can significantly impact quality of life due to pain and unpredictable flares.
- In the United States, Black and female patients are disproportionately affected by HS. The reasons for this disparity (biology vs environmental/social factors) are not fully understood.[16,50,101,102]

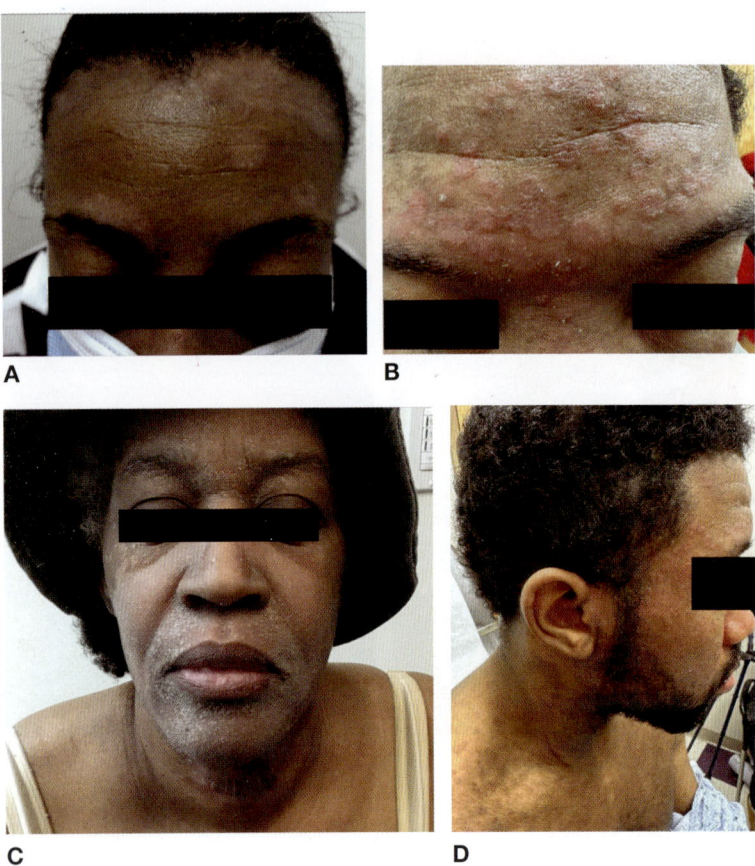

**Figure 13-8. A, B.** Seborrheic dermatitis, petaloid variant. Thin scaly erythematous hypopigmented annular plaques along bilateral eyebrows, forehead, and frontal hairline. **C, D.** Seborrheic dermatitis. Desquamative slightly hypopigmented plaques along hairlines and on sebaceous areas on the face.

- Diagnosis: HS is often diagnosed based on a history of recurrent boils (two or more in a 6-month period) in characteristic locations.[103] Clinical evaluation of HS should include a severity assessment based on objective physical examination findings. Severity is often clinically classified using the Hurley Clinical Staging System.[104]
  - Stage 1: Abscesses without sinus tracts and scarring
  - Stage II: Recurrent abscesses with sinus tracts and scarring
  - Stage III: Diffuse involvement or multiple interconnected sinus tracts and abscesses (Fig. 13-9A and B)
    Additional tools are used in clinical trials but not often in clinical practice more dynamically capture aspects of disease stability and pain than Hurley staging but may still underrepresent the severity in patients of color.[50]
- Management: Requires a multidisciplinary team approach, with proactive management of early stages being crucial to delay or prevent disease progression.

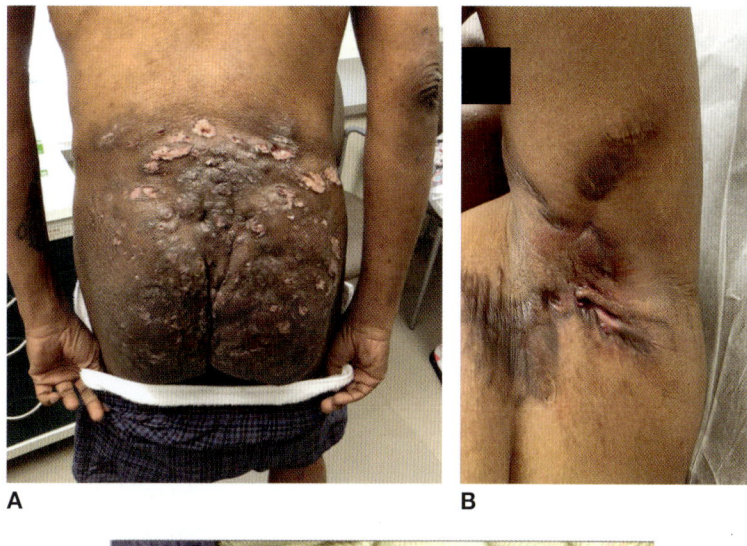

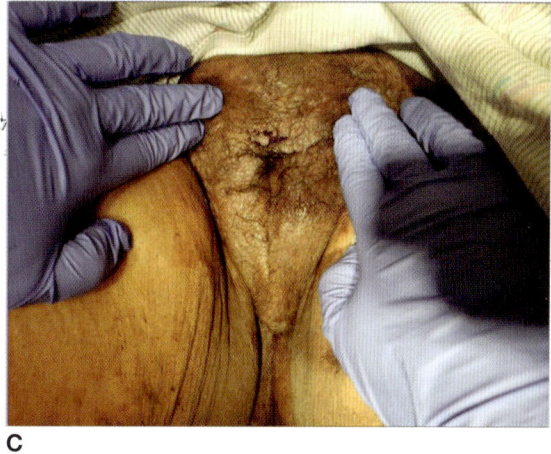

**Figure 13-9. A, B.** Hidradenitis suppurativa. Tender, boggy nodules and interconnected sinuses in the background of firm hyperpigmented cicatricial plaques on bilateral buttocks (**A**) and left axillae (**B**). **C.** Lymphedema from scarring. Skin colored, smooth, edematous, and papillomatous papules on the mons pubis and labia majora.

Shared decision making that considers disease severity, comorbidities, and quality of life is important. Patients with HS have an increased risk of various health issues, including mental health conditions, tobacco use, metabolic syndrome, cardiovascular disease, polycystic ovarian syndrome, sexual dysfunction, inflammatory bowel disease, and spondyloarthritis.[105]

- The dermatologist's primary role is to optimize medical management to minimize flares, using topical, intralesional, and systemic (antibiotics, steroids, biologics) options (Tables 13-4 and 13-5). Once medical therapy has successfully stabilized

## TABLE 13-4 Treatments for Hidradenitis Suppurativa[99]

| Treatment Type | Example(s) | Mechanism/Notes |
|---|---|---|
| **Topical antibiotics** | Clindamycin 1% solution or gel | Anti-inflammatory and antimicrobial; often first-line for mild hidradenitis suppurativa (HS) |
| **Systemic antibiotics** | Tetracyclines (doxycycline > minocycline) | Anti-inflammatory and antibacterial properties; commonly used for moderate HS |
| | Clindamycin + rifampin | Combination therapy for refractory or more severe cases |
| **Hormonal therapy** | Spironolactone, oral contraceptives | Antiandrogen effects may reduce flare frequency |
| **Retinoids** | Isotretinoin, acitretin | Modulate keratinization; mixed evidence of efficacy |
| **Immunosuppressants** | Cyclosporine, systemic corticosteroids | May be helpful in severe, refractory cases |

## TABLE 13-5 FDA-Approved Biologic Treatments for Hidradenitis Suppurativa

| Mechanism of Action | Drug Name (Brand) | Target(s) | Approval Year | Notes |
|---|---|---|---|---|
| Tumor necrosis factor-α inhibitor | **Adalimumab (Humira)**[106] | TNF-α | 2015 | First biologic approved for hidradenitis suppurativa (HS); administered via subcutaneous injection |
| Interleukin (IL)-17A inhibitor | **Secukinumab (Cosentyx)**[107] | IL-17A | 2023 | First IL-17A inhibitor approved for HS; shown to improve HS symptoms |
| IL-17A and IL-17F dual inhibitor | **Bimekizumab (Bimzelx)**[108] | IL-17A and IL-17F | 2024 | First treatment targeting both IL-17A and IL-17F; demonstrated significant efficacy in clinical trials |

the HS, further interventions may be considered to address persistent lesions or scarring. These localized procedures can include intralesional steroid injections, incision and drainage, excisions, or lasers (Table 13-2).
- Common myths about HS: It is not an infection, not contagious, not due to poor hygiene, and not cured by weight loss or smoking cessation alone. While

microbiome and these lifestyle factors can play a role in management, they are not the root cause or sole cure.

## 5.6. CUTANEOUS T-CELL LYMPHOMA[91,92,109-111]

- Mycosis fungoides (MF) is the most common type of cutaneous t-cell lymphoma (CTCL) and can mimic many common inflammatory skin conditions. MF is more common in Black populations compared to White populations but may be less common in Latine and Asian and Pacific Islander populations. Patients of African ancestry are also more likely to present at a younger age, with advanced disease, and have higher mortality.
- MF can present as cutaneous patches, plaques, or tumors. Three common presentations of MF in patients of color include hypopigmented lesions, hyperpigmented lesions, and itchy skin with secondary darkening and lichenification (Fig. 13-10A-D).
- Hypopigmented MF is the most common subtype in children and adults of color, mimicking conditions like pityriasis alba, hypopigmented sarcoidosis, progressive macular hypomelanosis, PIHo, tinea versicolor, and inflammatory vitiligo. However, it generally has a better prognosis, and repigmentation can indicate remission.
- Sézary syndrome, another form of CTCL presenting with erythroderma, abnormal T-cell clones in the blood, and swollen lymph nodes, is also more common in Black patients than White patients.
- Treatment depends on the disease stage and can include topical steroids, topical and oral retinoids, topical and systemic chemotherapeutics, immunosuppressants, narrow band UVB light (NBUVB), psoralens with UVA light (PUVA), extracorporeal photopheresis, radiotherapy, and biologics. Phototherapy may be less effective in hypopigmented MF.[110] There may also be disparities to the use of radiotherapy and extracorporeal photopheresis in certain patients of color.

## 5.7. DISCOID LUPUS ERYTHEMATOSUS[112-114]

- Discoid lupus erythematosus (DLE) is a chronic form of cutaneous lupus erythematosus that can occur alone or be associated with/progress to systemic lupus erythematosus. It is more common in adults and children of color, particularly women of African descent.[13-15]
- Presentation: DLE presents as discrete hypertrophic or atrophic plaques. Active lesions have pink, slow-growing, slightly firm edges, with a scale that extends into hair follicles. Older areas become burned out central hypopigmented atrophic and cicatricial plaques with peripheral hyperpigmented borders. DLE most often affects the head and neck, especially the scalp, face, ears, and hard palate but can also occur on the upper trunk and extremities (Fig. 13-11A-D). Caudal spread of DLE plaques has higher association with systemic lupus. DLE often causes permanent discoloration, scarring, and hair loss (Fig. 13-11A and B).
- Chronic inflammation in DLE increases the risk of cutaneous squamous cell carcinoma (cSCC) in some patients. This DLE-associated cSCC tends to be more aggressive with higher rates of metastasis than UV-induced cSCC.
- The primary treatment goal is to stop the progression of active lesions as scarring and dyspigmentation are often permanent. Regular screening for systemic lupus erythematosus is also important.
- Initial management includes strict sun protection (SPF 30+ sunscreen, protective clothing), medication review for photosensitizers and drug-induced DLE, as well as smoking cessation.

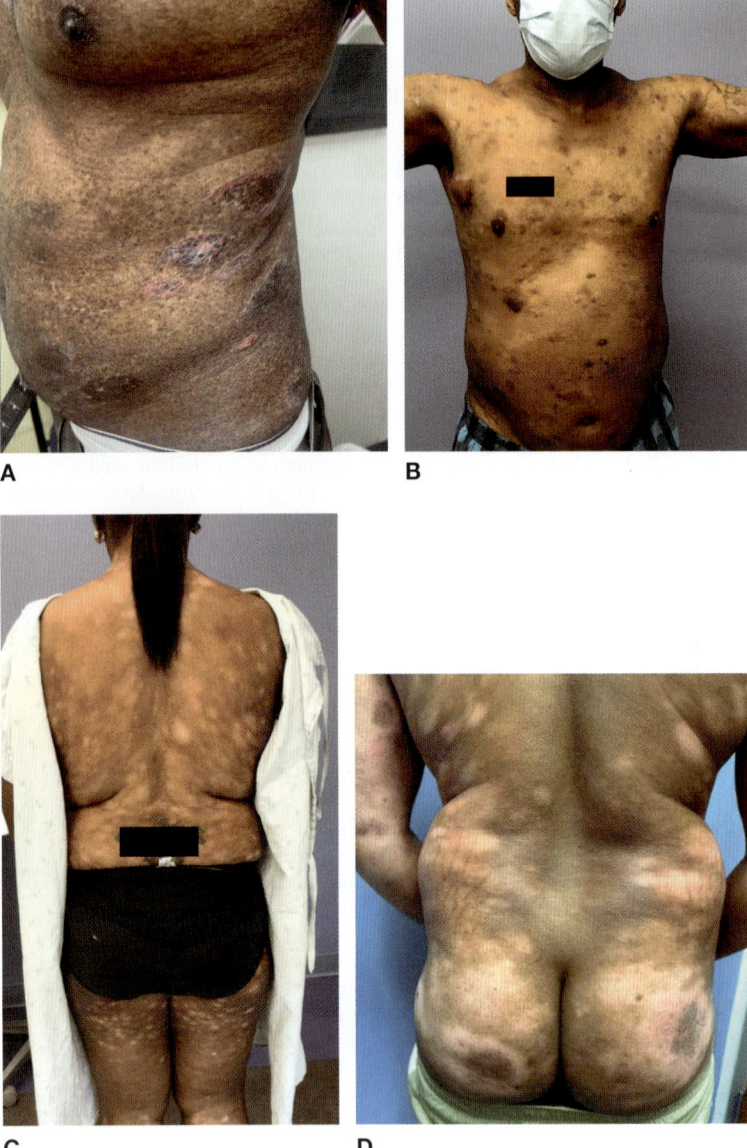

**Figure 13-10.** Cutaneous T-cell lymphoma, mycosis fungoides. **A.** Erythematous, scaly, lichenified, annular plaques on left abdomen, flank, and left hand. **B.** Tumors and polymorphous plaques on the trunk and upper extremities. **C, D.** Cutaneous T-cell lymphoma, hypopigmented mycosis fungoides. Hypopigmented patches, some with central thin hyperpigmented scaly annular plaques with peripheral erythema, scattered on posterior arms, back, legs, and buttocks.

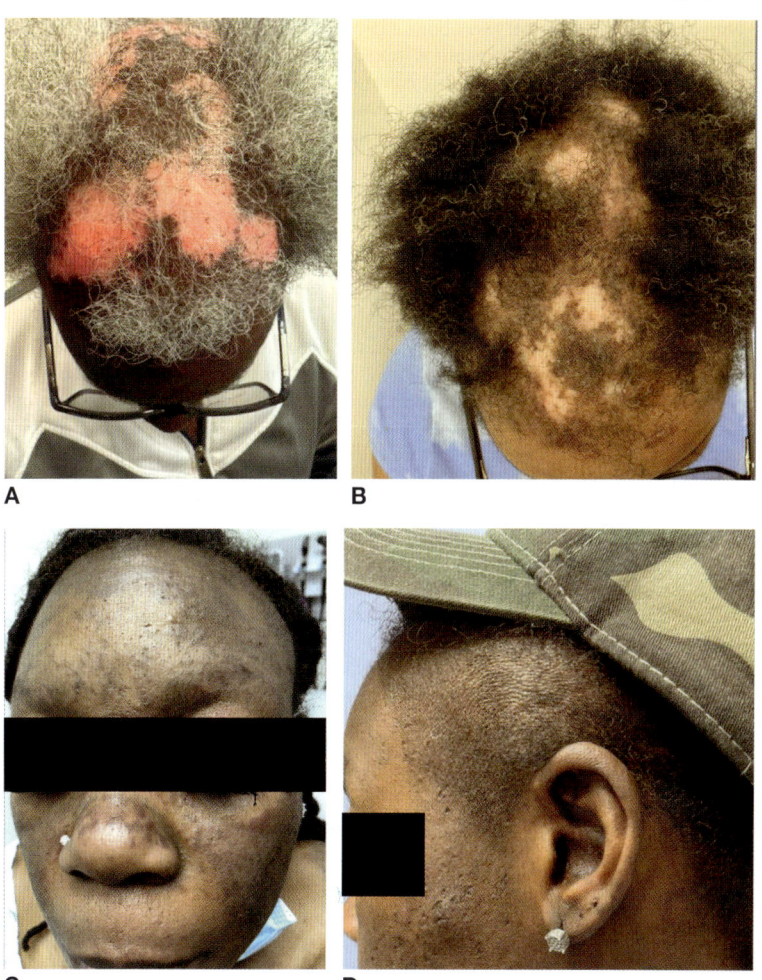

**Figure 13-11. A, B.** Discoid lupus erythematosus. Well-demarcated scaly plaques with central depigmentation and peripheral hyperpigmentation on the frontal and crown scalp. **C, D.** Discoid lupus erythematosus. Well-demarcate plaques with adherent scale, central depigmentation, and peripheral hyperpigmentation cheeks, nose, and concha/triangular fossa of the ear.

- First-line treatment for localized DLE is topical and intralesional corticosteroids, while hydroxychloroquine is first line for widespread or resistant localized disease. Acitretin is also effective but has limited use for women of childbearing age.

### 5.8. CUTANEOUS SARCOIDOSIS[115]

- Sarcoidosis is a multisystem inflammatory disorder characterized by infiltration of noncaseating granulomatous inflammation that invades normal tissue of the lungs,

lymph nodes, liver, heart, eyes, bone marrow, endocrine system, nervous system, and skin. Its cause is unknown but is linked to certain immune system genetics and environmental exposures. It is more common in certain professions.
- Cutaneous sarcoidosis occurs in approximately one-third of all patients and may be the first sign of systemic sarcoidosis. Patients of African ancestry tend to have a higher incidence of cutaneous sarcoidosis, more progressive systemic disease, and greater associated mortality. Systemic sarcoidosis is almost twice as common in females, and early-onset disease or comorbid autoimmune conditions are associated with more severe systemic involvement.[116]
- Presentation: The morphology of skin lesions varies greatly and can be specific to sarcoid infiltration or nonspecific due to the body's immune response to granulomas.
- Specific sarcoidal skin lesions are more closely associated with systemic disease. These lesions include red-brown papules, nodules and plaques, verrucous plaques, subcutaneous nodules, cicatricial plaques, hypopigmented patches, ichthyosiform thin plaques, lupus pernio, nail abnormalities, and hair loss (Fig. 13-12A-E). Lupus pernio (Fig. 13-12A) is more common in Black patients and is associated with more progressive respiratory and systemic disease.[116] Hypopigmented variants of cutaneous sarcoidosis (Fig. 13-12D and E) and sarcoidal alopecia (Fig. 13-12D) as well as hyperpigmentation from sarcoidal inflammation (Fig. 13-12E) are more noticeable in patients of color.[117]
- The most common nonspecific skin lesion is erythema nodosum, often on the lower legs, and associated with fever, arthralgias, and lower leg swelling. It is more common in White patients and corresponds to milder systemic disease and lower mortality.[116]
- Diagnosis: Suspected based on multiple types of lesions in one patient or specific lesions linked to sarcoidosis. Biopsy showing granulomas prompts a systemic evaluation.
- Management: First-line treatments include hydroxychloroquine and topical or intralesional steroids.[118] Systemic steroids, methotrexate, tumor necrosis factor-α inhibitors, and JAK inhibitors are used for more resistant cases. For lupus pernio, advanced treatments like tumor necrosis factor-α inhibitors should be considered due to systemic association.[115]

## 5.9. PSEUDOFOLLICULITIS BARBAE[119]

- Pseudofolliculitis barbae (PFB) is a chronic inflammatory condition of hair follicles in shaved areas, with significantly higher rates in men of African descent, caused by ingrown hairs.
- Shaved hair reentering the skin, genetic factors, and trauma during shaving cause a foreign body reaction.[120]
- Clinical features include follicular or perifollicular bumps in shaved areas (Fig. 13-13A and B), most commonly the neck in men and the chin in women, due to sterile inflammation or secondary infection.[119,120]
- Potential complications include PIH and keloid formation from chronic inflammation.
- A true cure for PFB involves the growth of a beard or permanent hair removal. Effective prevention includes growing beards or optimizing shaving practices.
- Medical letters allowing beard growth at work are often necessary to break the inflammatory cycle.[121] Education of community barbers has been implemented as an effective community outreach measure to identify and reduce morbidity due to PFB.[122]
- Treatments are reviewed in Table 13-6.[123,124]

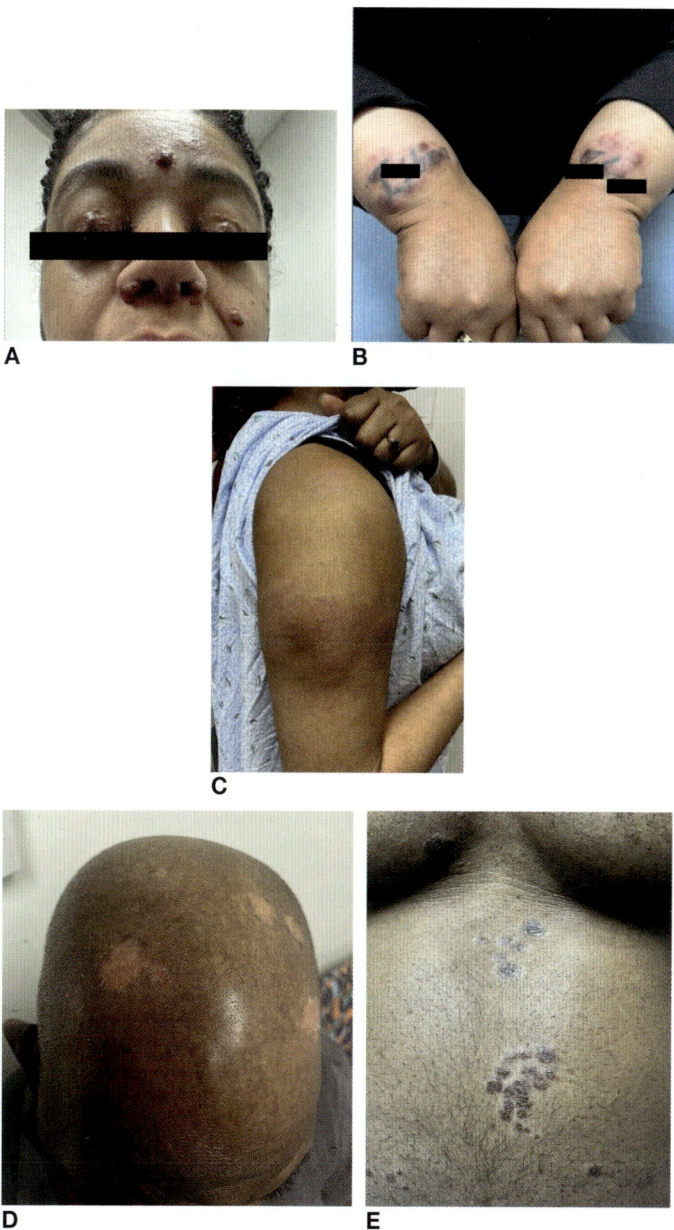

**Figure 13-12. A-F. Cutaneous Sarcoidosis. A, B.** Infiltrative indurated violaceous nodules of **lupus pernio** (nose) and **nodular sarcoid** and **tattoo sarcoid**. **C.** Indurated subcutaneous nodules of **subcutaneous sarcoid** on the upper arm. **D.** Hypopigmented cicatricial hairless plaques of **sarcoidal alopecia** on the scalp. **E.** Violaceous and **hyperpigmented plaques** of sarcoid with rims of hypopigmentation.

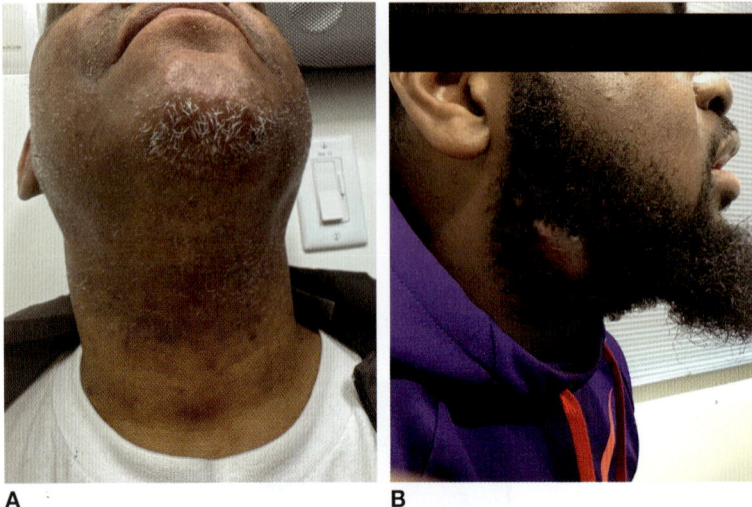

**Figure 13-13.** Pseudofolliculitis barbae. **A.** Multiple hyperpigmented follicular and perifollicular papules chin, anterior neck and lateral neck. **B.** Smooth cicatricial and keloidal plaques on the beard distribution of the right cheek.

## 5.10. ACNE KELOIDALIS NUCHAE/FOLLICULITIS KELOIDALIS NUCHAE[119]

- Acne keloidalis nuchae (AKN) is a follicular disorder mainly affecting the nape of the neck and has characteristics of a primary scarring alopecia (Fig. 13-14A and B).
- AKN is more common in men of African descent with naturally curly and textured hair.
- The exact cause is not fully understood but may be linked to frequent close haircuts and mechanical irritation.
- Management focuses on preventing mechanical irritation and using topical or oral anti-inflammatory treatments. Modifying shaving practices is a key first step. Educating community barbers has also been a successful preventive measure.[125]
- Treatment options are similar to PFB and range from topical and oral anti-inflammatory agents to surgical excision and laser hair removal[126] (Table 13-6).

## 5.11. SCARRING ALOPECIA[113]

- Scarring alopecia involves the destruction of hair follicles and their replacement with scar tissue. Early detection and treatment are vital to prevent permanent hair loss.
- Curly hair is drier and more susceptible to chemical and physical damage. Clinical assessment may underestimate scalp inflammation in patients of color.
- Patients of African descent commonly experience multiple hair disorders simultaneously.

## 5.12. CENTRAL CENTRIFUGAL CICATRICIAL ALOPECIA[127]

- Central centrifugal cicatricial alopecia (CCCA) is a very common cause of hair loss in women of African descent, with a prevalence of 2% to 10% in African American

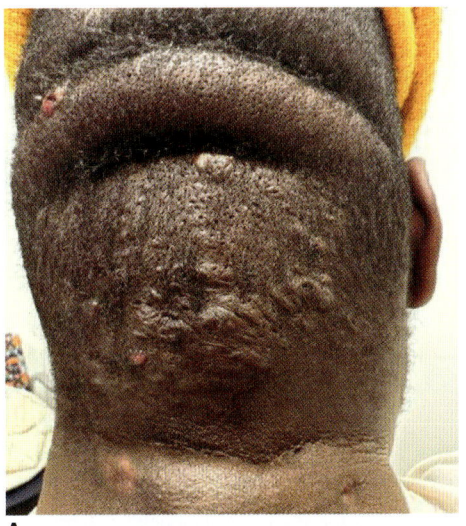

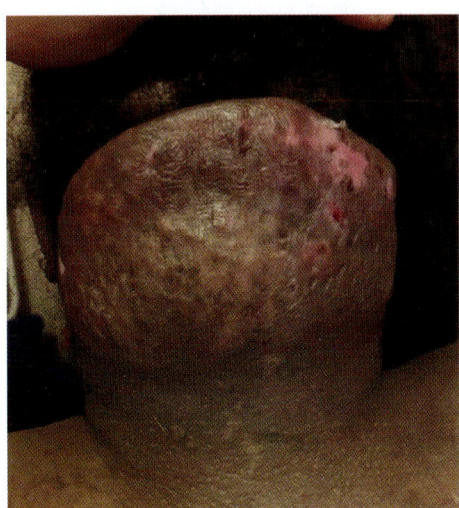

**Figure 13-14.** Acne keloidalis nuchae. Few scattered erythematous papules in the background of multinodular cicatricial plaque (**A**) and smooth eroded large cicatricial plaque (**B**) on the occipital scalp and neck.

women, though it can occur in others with curly hair. It typically presents between the ages of 30 and 40, but pediatric cases have been reported.
- Presentation: Characterized by a focal and expanding area of hair loss on the crown of the scalp, often with burning, itching, and tenderness (Fig. 13-15A and B). Notably, redness may not be obvious. Besides the classic pattern, patchy hair loss in other areas of the scalp and trichorrhexis have been described.[128]

### TABLE 13-6: Treatments Used in Pseudofolliculitis Barbae and Acne Keloidalis Nuchae

| | Pseudofolliculitis Barbae[122-124] | Acne Keloidalis Nuchae[125,126] |
|---|---|---|
| | Behavioral Changes and Shaving Modifications | Behavioral Changes and Shaving Modifications |
| **Topicals** | Corticosteroids (low potency) | Corticosteroids (mid to high potency) |
| | Retinoids | Retinoids |
| | Keratolytics | |
| | Antibiotics | Antibiotics |
| | Benzoyl peroxide | Benzoyl peroxide |
| | Skin lighteners | |
| | Chemical depilatories | |
| | Fusidic acid | Fusidic acid |
| | Urea | Urea |
| **Oral** | Tetracycline antibiotics | Tetracycline antibiotics |
| | Macrolide antibiotics | |
| | Cefadroxil | Cefadroxil |
| | Isotretinoin | Isotretinoin |
| **Intralesional** | Triamcinolone | Triamcinolone |
| **Energy-based devices** | Lasers (Table 13-2) | Lasers (Table 13-2) |
| | Cryotherapy | Cryotherapy |
| | Photodynamic therapy | Targeted UVB |
| | Radiofrequency ablation | |
| **Surgery/procedures** | Excisions | Excisions |
| | Electrosurgery | Electrosurgery |
| | Surgical depilation | Surgical depilation |
| | Dermabrasion | Dermabrasion |
| | Radiation | Radiation |
| **Community intervention** | Barber education | Barber education |

- Pathogenesis: There is increasing evidence of genetic factors and a hereditary predisposition to CCCA, involving premature shedding of the inner root sheath, hair shaft abnormalities, fragility, and excessive fibrous tissue growth.[129,130] Traction from hairstyles, chemical relaxers, and styling practices can worsen the condition. There is also a link between CCCA and type II diabetes mellitus and breast cancer.[127]
- Management[131]: Aims to stop inflammation, control symptoms, and encourage some hair regrowth.
  - Avoiding tight hairstyles and limiting chemical treatments can reduce disease activity.
  - Shampooing every 2 weeks is recommended.

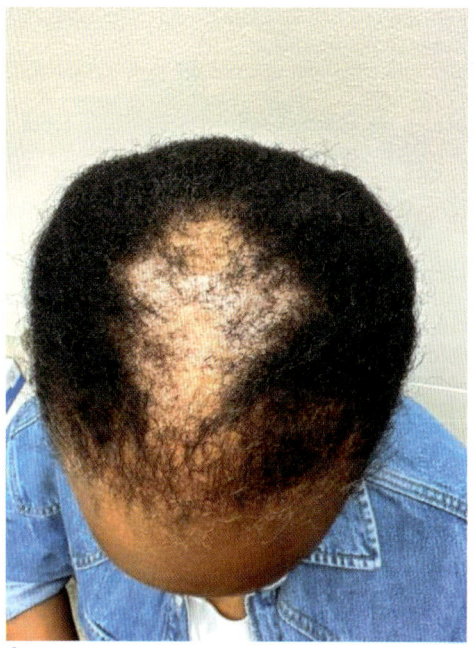

**Figure 13-15. A, B.** Central centrifugal cicatricial alopecia. Shiny large patch of scarring alopecia with increased follicular spacing along central anterior frontal and vertex scalp.

- High potency topical and intralesional steroids with adjunctive topical or oral minoxidil are mainstays of treatment.
- Oral tetracycline antibiotics and occasionally hydroxychloroquine use also have general expert consensus.
- Hair transplantation is considered only when there is no active inflammation.
- Screening for and treating iron or vitamin D deficiencies may be helpful.

## 5.13. TRACTION ALOPECIA[113,132]

- Traction alopecia is a form of mechanical hair loss that is primarily caused by hairstyles with prominent repetitive and prolonged tension of the hair shaft. This hair loss is commonly associated with high-tension braids, locks, adhesive styles, hair wraps, buns, and hair clip use. Traction alopecia is one of the most common types of hair loss in women of African descent at any age.
- Presentation: Affects areas with the most tension, typically the marginal hairline, especially behind the front hairline (Fig. 13-16A and B). Nonmarginal patterns also occur. The acute form may show scalp bumps, pustules, redness, and tenderness with broken hairs and hair casts and is nonscarring. The chronic form shows reduced hair density, scarring, and retained fine hairs (vellus hairs) along the hairline, known as the fringe sign.
- Traction alopecia differs from frontal fibrosing alopecia and trichotillomania by the preserved vellus hairline and does not involve the eyebrows.
- Education about hairstyling is crucial for management. Patients with tight hairstyles, especially with heat-treated or relaxed hair, are at high risk of traction.
- Medical treatments include topical and intralesional steroids and oral antibiotics to reduce inflammation, particularly in the acute phase. Topical or oral minoxidil can also stimulate hair regrowth.
- Hair transplantation may be an option for chronic, stable traction alopecia to restore the frontal hairline.[133]

# 6. Surgical and Procedural Dermatology in Skin of Color

## 6.1. PROCEDURAL CONSIDERATIONS IN PATIENTS OF COLOR[134,135]

- Special considerations are necessary for procedures in patients of color. Before any procedure, it is important to assess for specific risks and if any existing skin conditions might be affected. A history of inflammatory skin diseases should be reviewed, and the risk of koebnerization (new lesions developing at the site of trauma) in conditions like vitiligo, lichen planus, psoriasis, and sarcoidosis should be discussed. Any active skin infection should be treated before surgery. A history of radiation or previous procedures in the treatment area should be noted. The risk of herpes reactivation should be discussed, and medical prophylaxis may be given if needed.
- Patients of color have a higher tendency for dyspigmentation (PIH and PIHo) and keloid formation, which are important considerations in procedural dermatology. Medications that can cause hyperpigmentation or photosensitivity should be reviewed. Pre- and postprocedure prophylaxis with tyrosinase inhibitors, retinoids, topical steroids, and ointments can help reduce PIH.
- Test spots ideally should be performed for cosmetic procedures to assess the suitability of the procedure in individual patients.

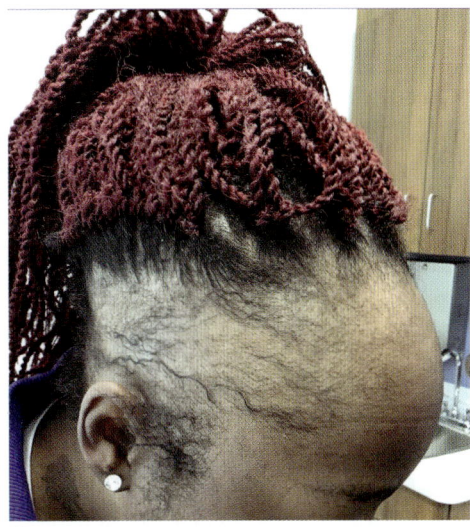

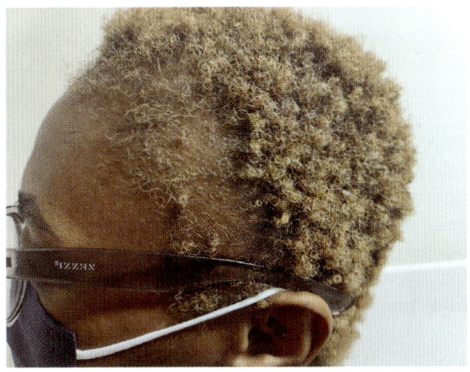

**Figure 13-16. A, B.** Traction alopecia. Patchy bandlike alopecia along the frontotemporal hairline behind the hairline.

- Chemical peels are often used to treat dyspigmentation, photodamage, mild scarring, and skin textural issues. Superficial peels are generally safest in patients of color. The safety of glycolic acid and salicylic acid peels has been shown in this population.
- Microneedling and subcision are used for acne scarring and are often safe in patients of color as they avoid full-thickness destruction of the epidermis.
- Injectables: With injected treatments, it is advisable to limit the number of injections to minimize inflammation and PIH.
- Lasers: Nonablative lasers with longer wavelengths are preferred as they reduce the injury to the skin and absorption by epidermal melanin. Laser use in SOC is reviewed in Table 13-5.

## 6.2. KELOIDS[136]

- Keloids are an abnormal, exaggerated wound healing response that extends beyond the original skin injury or can occur spontaneously as an isotopic response to a previous or existing skin condition. Keloids do not require known cutaneous injury to form.
- Keloids occur on a continuum with normal scar formation and hypertrophic scars but differ from these clinical entities by histopathology and ultrastructural composition.
- Presentation: Keloids appear as cicatricial, often irregularly shaped, and variably pigmented nodules, with a predilection for the upper trunk, ears, hairline, beard line, and surgical sites (Fig. 13-17A and B).[137]
- Pathogenesis: Keloids form when injury to the deeper layer of the skin (reticular dermis) triggers chronic inflammation, leading to excessive growth of fibrous tissue (fibroproliferation), irregular collagen deposition, and reduced collagen breakdown. Keloids can expand, invade, and replace surrounding tissue.
- There is a higher prevalence of keloids in individuals of African or Asian ancestry or Latine ethnicity.[20,21,138]
- Keloids frequently cause pruritus, pain, and burning and can result in movement restriction and disfigurement.[139] Keloids can also ulcerate further exacerbating these effects as well as breed infection (Fig. 13-17A).
- Prevention:
  - Individuals prone to keloids should avoid unnecessary surgeries and piercings.
  - Postsurgical use of silicone sheets, pressure dressings/earrings, and steroid tape has been shown to reduce keloid formation.
- Management:
  - An early multimodal intervention approach is recommended for those with a history or family history of keloids.
  - Surgical excision followed by adjunctive treatment with intralesional steroids is considered the standard of care to reduce the high keloid recurrence rate.
  - Other intralesional treatments like 5-fluorouracil and bleomycin can cause significant hyperpigmentation, especially in patients of color.
  - Topical and intralesional cryotherapy has lower effectiveness and higher recurrence rates than the standard of care.
  - Oral pentoxifylline has shown some benefit in managing postsurgical and multiple symptomatic keloids.[140]
  - Radiotherapy, pulsed dye lasers, neodymium-doped yttrium aluminum garnet (Nd:YAG) lasers, and electron beam radiation are also used as adjunctive therapies. Brachytherapy is becoming more widely adopted.

## 6.3. DERMATOSIS PAPULOSA NIGRA[141]

- Dermatosis papulosa nigra (DPN) are benign, superficial epidermal growths (a variant of seborrheic keratoses) common in patients of African and Asian descent. They may be cosmetically and socially bothersome for some patients.
- Presentation: DPNs clinically appear hyperpigmented papules sometimes filiform or sessile on cheeks and around the eyes, as well as other parts of the face and trunk (Fig. 13-18). They increase with age.
- Management: Treatments are primarily cosmetic, and care must be taken to avoid PIH and PIHo. Electrodessication with or without light curettage can cause

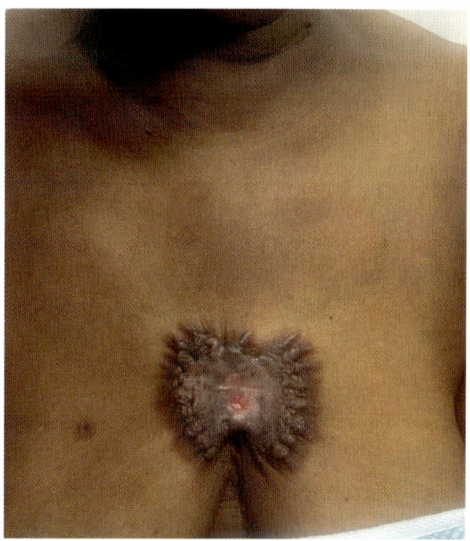

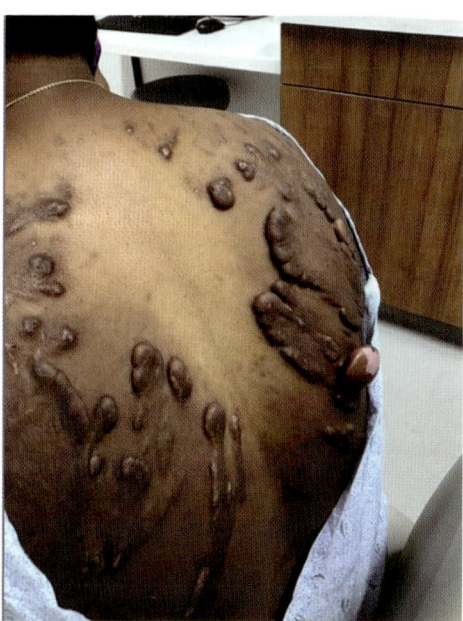

**Figure 13-17. A.** Ulcerated keloid. Smooth firm, ulcerated, and hyperpigmented plaque with infiltrative borders on central chest from median sternotomy. **B.** Generalized keloids. Scattered smooth firm hyperpigmented plaques on back sparing central mid back with no known history of skin injury.

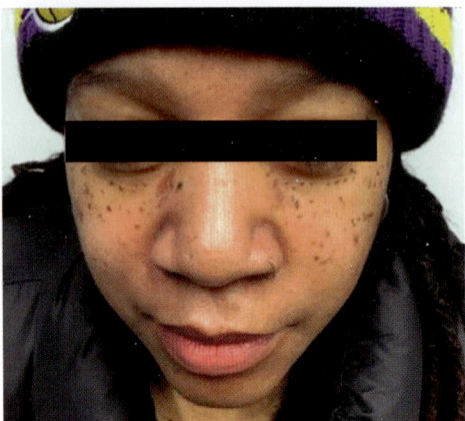

**Figure 13-18.** Dermatosis papulose nigra. Scattered dark brown papules in a periocular distribution.

PIH. Cryotherapy can cause long-lasting PIHo especially in darker skin. Snip excision has a variable risk of recurrence.
- Nonablative lasers offer similar effectiveness to traditional methods and are increasingly used, but precautions are needed to minimize pigment changes and burns, including test spots, epidermal cooling, and topical ointments and steroids.

## 6.4. SKIN CANCER IN PATIENTS OF COLOR

This section briefly reviews common skin cancers for which surgery is the main treatment. Cutaneous lymphoma, managed primarily with medical therapies, was discussed earlier in the chapter.
- **Cutaneous squamous cell carcinoma (cSCC)** is a common skin cancer in patients of color and the most common in those of African and Asian Indian descent. Chronic scarring and inflammation are greater risk factors than UV exposure in Black patients. These often-tender nodules and ulcers tend to occur in non–sun-exposed areas and can be more aggressive with a higher risk of metastasis (Fig. 13-19A and B). cSCC surgical treatment occurs more frequently at advanced stages in patients of color possibly due to delayed recognition and diagnosis.[109]
- **Basal cell carcinoma (BCC)**[109] is the most common skin cancer in patients of Caucasian, Latine, and East Asian descent. BCC is the second most common skin cancer in patients of African and Asian Indian descent although BCC is approximately 20 times more common in White patients than Black patients. Pigmented BCC is an uncommon variant that is the most common type in Black patients and typically occurs on the head and neck (Fig. 13-20A-C). The classic pearly appearance with rolled borders may be harder to see in darker skin, potentially delaying diagnosis and treatment.
- **Melanoma** is less common in patients of color than in White patients. In individuals of African descent, most melanomas occur on the palms, soles (Fig. 13-21), and nail units (acral lentiginous melanoma), and UV radiation is not considered a major risk factor.[142] Mucosal and ocular melanoma subtypes are also common types of melanoma in Black patients. Despite a lower incidence of

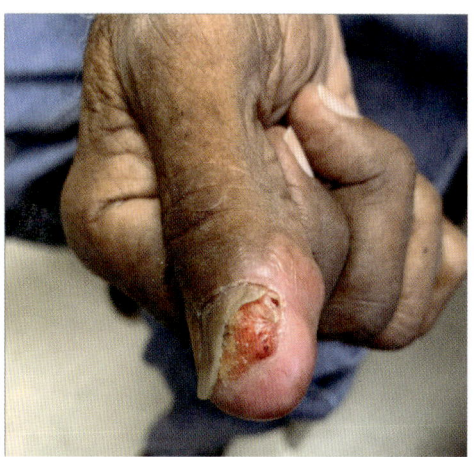

**A**

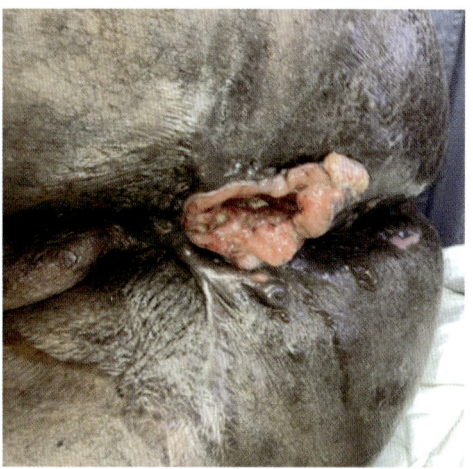

**B**

**Figure 13-19.** Cutaneous squamous cell carcinoma. **A.** Subungual painful scaly keratotic plaque on right thumb. **B.** Pink, ulcerated, indurated, and painful tumor arising in Hurley Stage III HS on the left intergluteal cleft.

melanoma and advances in melanoma treatment, Black melanoma patients have a higher and unimproved mortality rate, possibly due to the biology of these melanoma subtypes, inequities in research and treatment access, and diagnosis at more advanced stages.[109,142,143]

- **Dermatofibrosarcoma protuberans** is a rare, locally invasive mesenchymal tumor more common in individuals of African and Korean descent, typically appearing in middle age as an irregular skin colored or hyperpigmented indurated nodule/s on the trunk or extremities (Fig. 13-22). Standard treatment is wide surgical removal or Mohs surgery.[144]

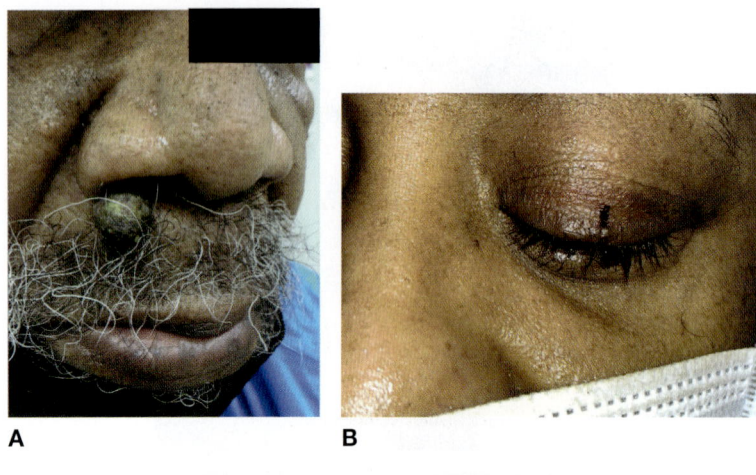

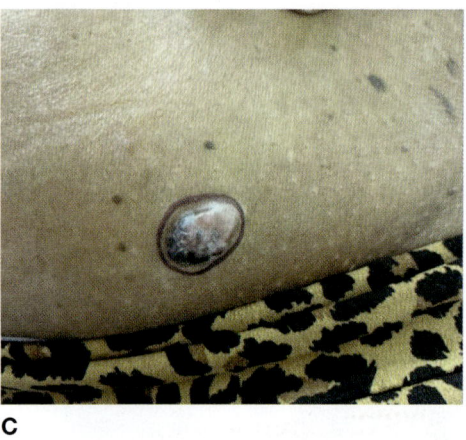

**Figure 13-20.** Pigmented basal cell carcinoma. **A.** Crusted friable nodule on the right upper lip. **B.** Beaded and slightly hyperpigmented papule along the upper left eyelid margin. **C.** Large, smooth, pigmented and firm nodule with telangiectasia on the lower abdomen.

- **Merkel cell carcinoma (MCC)** is an aggressive primary skin neuroendocrine tumor associated with the Merkel cell polyomavirus and UV radiation that shows high rates of metastasis and mortality. MCC often appears as hyperpigmented or ulcerative nodules on the lower extremities in patients of color as opposed to a fast-growing violaceous nodule on the head and neck in White patients (Fig. 13-23). All-cause mortality is higher in non-White patients.[144]
- **Sebaceous carcinoma (SC)** is a malignant sebaceous tumor on the head and neck. While uncommon overall in patients of color, it is the second most common eyelid cancer in those of East Asian ancestry. It typically presents as a painless yellow/pink nodule around the eyelids. Black patients with SC have a higher mortality compared with White patients with SC.[144]

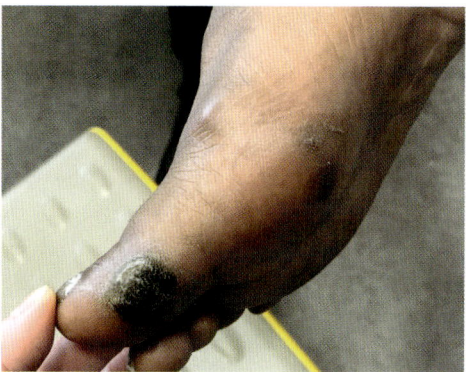

**Figure 13-21.** Acral lentiginous melanoma. Irregular brown and black hyperkeratotic plaque on the medial aspect of the right greater toe.

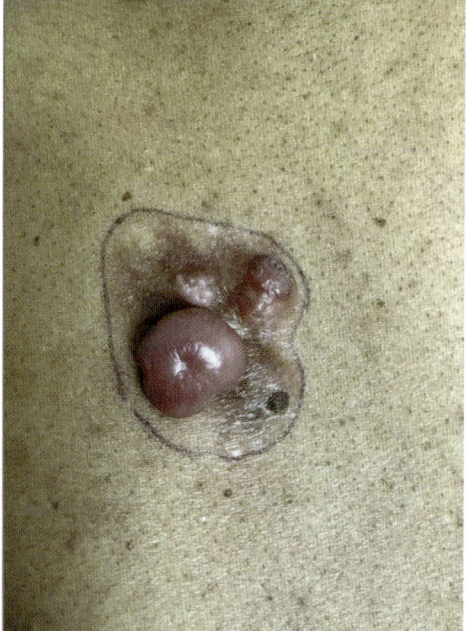

**Figure 13-22.** Dermatofibrosarcoma protuberans. Violaceous and hyperpigmented, multinodular, rubbery plaque on the back.

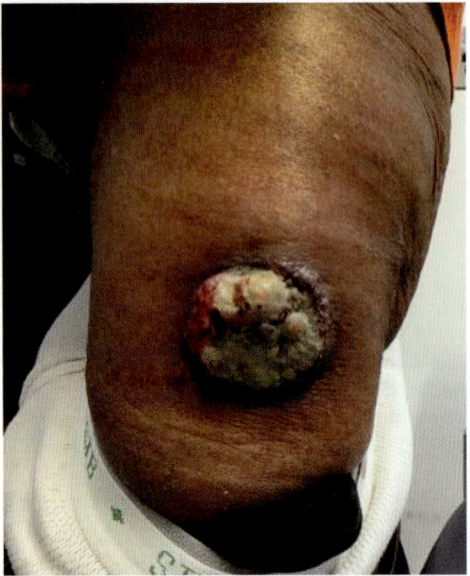

**Figure 13-23.** Merkel cell carcinoma. Friable fungating exophytic ulcerated tumor with erythematous borders on left lateral thigh.

# REFERENCES

1. Society SoC. *Who We Are / About SOCS*. Accessed December 14, 2024. https://skinofcolorsociety.org/who-is-socs/about-socs
2. Taylor SC, Cook-Bolden F. Defining skin of color. *Cutis*. 2002;69(6):435-437.
3. Brown-Korsah JB, McKenzie S, Omar D, Syder NC, Elbuluk N, Taylor SC. Variations in genetics, biology, and phenotype of cutaneous disorders in skin of color—part I: genetic, biologic, and structural differences in skin of color. *J Am Acad Dermatol*. 2022;87(6):1239-1258. doi:10.1016/j.jaad.2022.06.1193
4. Taylor SC. Skin of color: biology, structure, function, and implications for dermatologic disease. *J Am Acad Dermatol*. 2002;46(2 Suppl):S41-S62. doi:10.1067/mjd.2002.120790
5. Beiter K, Culotta N, Hilton D. An inventory of current interventions to improve dermatologic clinical assessment in skin of color and recommendations for continued advancement. *J Am Acad Dermatol*. 2023;88(4):864-866. doi:10.1016/j.jaad.2022.10.051
6. Alexis AF, Sergay AB, Taylor SC. Common dermatologic disorders in skin of color: a comparative practice survey. *Cutis*. 2007;80(5):387-394.
7. Henderson MD, Abboud J, Cogan CM, et al. Skin-of-color epidemiology: a report of the most common skin conditions by race. *Pediatr Dermatol*. 2012;29(5):584-589. doi:10.1111/j.1525-1470.2012.01775.x
8. Rosa-Nieves PM, Schissel M, Wysong A, Hayes K, Wei EX. Impact of skin of color specialty dermatologic clinics on diagnoses and management. *Arch Dermatol Res*. 2024;317(1):1. doi:10.1007/s00403-024-03493-0
9. Tull RZ, Kerby E, Subash JJ, McMichael AJ. Ethnic skin centers in the United States: where are we in 2020? *J Am Acad Dermatol*. 2020;83(6):1757-1759. doi:10.1016/j.jaad.2020.03.054
10. Taylor SC, Cook-Bolden F, Rahman Z, Strachan D. Acne vulgaris in skin of color. *J Am Acad Dermatol*. 2002;46(2 Suppl):S98-S106. doi:10.1067/mjd.2002.120791
11. Gottlieb S, Madkins K, Lio P. An updated scoping review of disparities in pediatric atopic dermatitis. *Pediatr Dermatol*. 2025; doi:10.1111/pde.15914
12. Sharma AN, Kincaid CM, Mesinkovska NA. The burden of melasma: race, ethnicity, and comorbidities. *J Drugs Dermatol*. 2024;23(8):691-693. doi:10.36849/JDD.8233
13. Izmirly P, Buyon J, Belmont HM, et al. Population-based prevalence and incidence estimates of primary discoid lupus erythematosus from the Manhattan Lupus Surveillance Program. *Lupus Sci Med*. 2019;6(1):e000344. doi:10.1136/lupus-2019-000344

14. Ezeh N, Ardalan K, Buhr KA, et al. Cross-sectional characteristics of pediatric-onset discoid lupus erythematosus: results of a multicenter, retrospective cohort study. *J Am Acad Dermatol*. 2022;87(3):559-566. doi:10.1016/j.jaad.2022.04.028
15. Haq Z, Diaz MJ, Abdi P, et al. Epidemiology of discoid lupus erythematosus among adults in the United States: a cross-sectional analysis. *Int J Dermatol*. 2025; doi:10.1111/ijd.17603
16. Garg A, Kirby JS, Lavian J, Lin G, Strunk A. Sex- and age-adjusted population analysis of prevalence estimates for hidradenitis suppurativa in the united states. *JAMA Dermatol*. 2017;153(8):760-764. doi:10.1001/jamadermatol.2017.0201
17. Garg A, Wertenteil S, Baltz R, Strunk A, Finelt N. Prevalence estimates for hidradenitis suppurativa among children and adolescents in the united states: a gender- and age-adjusted population analysis. *J Invest Dermatol*. 2018;138(10):2152-2156. doi:10.1016/j.jid.2018.04.001
18. Gray J, McMichael AJ. Pseudofolliculitis barbae: understanding the condition and the role of facial grooming. *Int J Cosmet Sci*. 2016;38(Suppl 1):24-27. doi:10.1111/ics.12331
19. Raffi J, Suresh R, Agbai O. Clinical recognition and management of alopecia in women of color. *Int J Womens Dermatol*. 2019;5(5):314-319. doi:10.1016/j.ijwd.2019.08.005
20. Davis SA, Feldman SR, McMichael AJ. Management of keloids in the United States, 1990-2009: an analysis of the National Ambulatory Medical Care Survey. *Dermatol Surg*. 2013;39(7):988-994. doi:10.1111/dsu.12182
21. Olopoenia A, Yamaguchi Y, Peeva E, Berman B, Jagun O, George P. Demographics, clinical characteristics, and treatment patterns among keloid patients: United States Electronic Health Records (EHR) Database Study. *Int J Dermatol*. 2024;63(8):e163-e170. doi:10.1111/ijd.17099
22. Kreicher KL, Kurlander DE, Gittleman HR, Barnholtz-Sloan JS, Bordeaux JS. Incidence and survival of primary dermatofibrosarcoma protuberans in the United States. *Dermatol Surg*. 2016;42(Suppl 1):S24-S31. doi:10.1097/DSS.0000000000000300
23. Maghfour J, Genelin X, Olson J, Wang A, Schultz L, Blalock TW. The epidemiology of dermatofibrosarcoma protuberans incidence, metastasis, and death among various population groups: a surveillance, epidemiology, and end results database analysis. *J Am Acad Dermatol*. 2024;91(5):826-833. doi:10.1016/j.jaad.2024.05.088
24. McKenzie C, Silverberg JI. The prevalence and persistence of atopic dermatitis in urban United States children. *Ann Allergy Asthma Immunol*. 2019;123(2):173-178.e1. doi:10.1016/j.anai.2019.05.014
25. Imam MH, Shenoy PJ, Flowers CR, Phillips A, Lechowicz MJ. Incidence and survival patterns of cutaneous T-cell lymphomas in the United States. *Leuk Lymphoma*. 2013;54(4):752-759. doi:10.3109/10428194.2012.729831
26. Bradford PT, Devesa SS, Anderson WF, Toro JR. Cutaneous lymphoma incidence patterns in the United States: a population-based study of 3884 cases. *Blood*. 2009;113(21):5064-5073. doi:10.1182/blood-2008-10-184168
27. Mirsaeidi M, Machado RF, Schraufnagel D, Sweiss NJ, Baughman RP. Racial difference in sarcoidosis mortality in the United States. *Chest*. 2015;147(2):438-449. doi:10.1378/chest.14-1120
28. Wu XC, Eide MJ, King J, et al. Racial and ethnic variations in incidence and survival of cutaneous melanoma in the United States, 1999-2006. *J Am Acad Dermatol*. 2011;65(5 Suppl 1):S26-S37. doi:10.1016/j.jaad.2011.05.034
29. Clairwood M, Ricketts J, Grant-Kels J, Gonsalves L. Melanoma in skin of color in Connecticut: an analysis of melanoma incidence and stage at diagnosis in non-Hispanic blacks, non-Hispanic whites, and Hispanics. *Int J Dermatol*. 2014;53(4):425-433. doi:10.1111/j.1365-4632.2012.05713.x
30. Qian Y, Johannet P, Sawyers A, Yu J, Osman I, Zhong J. The ongoing racial disparities in melanoma: an analysis of the surveillance, epidemiology, and end results database (1975-2016). *J Am Acad Dermatol*. 2021;84(6):1585-1593. doi:10.1016/j.jaad.2020.08.097
31. Culp MB, Lunsford NB. Melanoma among non-Hispanic Black Americans. *Prev Chronic Dis*. 2019;16:E79. doi:10.5888/pcd16.180640
32. Hanson KA, Ezzedine K, Austin J, et al. Demographics and clinical characteristics among patients with distinct psychosocial burden profiles related to vitiligo: results of a latent class analysis. *Dermatol Ther (Heidelb)*. 2025;15(5):1195-1208. doi:10.1007/s13555-025-01401-6
33. Pahwa P, Mehta M, Khaitan BK, Sharma VK, Ramam M. The psychosocial impact of vitiligo in Indian patients. *Indian J Dermatol Venereol Leprol*. 2013;79(5):679-685. doi:10.4103/0378-6323.116737
34. Akl J, Lee S, Ju HJ, et al. Estimating the burden of vitiligo: a systematic review and modelling study. *Lancet Public Health*. 2024;9(6):e386-e396. doi:10.1016/S2468-2667(24)00026-4
35. Strouphauer E, Suhail S, Mulinda C, et al. Prevalence of psychiatric comorbidities and treatment initiation in African American pediatric patients with vitiligo: a retrospective, single-center, case-control study. *JAAD Int*. 2024;17:104-110. doi:10.1016/j.jdin.2024.07.012
36. Zieleniewski Ł, Schwartz RA, Goldberg DJ, Handler MZ. Voigt-Futcher pigmentary demarcation lines. *J Cosmet Dermatol*. 2019;18(3):700-702. doi:10.1111/jocd.12884
37. Oellers P, Karp CL. Management of pigmented conjunctival lesions. *Ocul Surf*. 2012;10(4):251-263. doi:10.1016/j.jtos.2012.08.002

38. Abed SS, Fitzpatrick SG, Bhattacharyya I, Islam MN, Cohen DM. Oral melanoacanthoma: case series of 33 cases and review of the literature. *Head Neck Pathol*. 2023;17(2):364-370. doi:10.1007/s12105-022-01506-w
39. Kaugars GE, Heise AP, Riley WT, Abbey LM, Svirsky JA. Oral melanotic macules. A review of 353 cases. *Oral Surg Oral Med Oral Pathol*. 1993;76(1):59-61. doi:10.1016/0030-4220(93)90295-f
40. Braun RP, Baran R, Le Gal FA, et al. Diagnosis and management of nail pigmentations. *J Am Acad Dermatol*. 2007;56(5):835-847. doi:10.1016/j.jaad.2006.12.021
41. Colin Tan W, Wang DY, Seghers AC, Koh MJA, Nicholas Goh SG, Joyce Lee SS. Should we biopsy melanonychia striata in Asian children? A retrospective observational study. *Pediatr Dermatol*. 2019;36(6):864-868. doi:10.1111/pde.13934
42. Habeshian KA, Kirkorian AY. Congenital pigmentary anomalies in the newborn. *Neoreviews*. 2021;22(10):e660-e672. doi:10.1542/neo.22-10-e660
43. Franceschini D, Dinulos JG. Dermal melanocytosis and associated disorders. *Curr Opin Pediatr*. 2015;27(4):480-485. doi:10.1097/MOP.0000000000000247
44. Adawi W, Cornman H, Kambala A, Henry S, Kwatra SG. Diagnosing atopic dermatitis in skin of color. *Dermatol Clin*. 2023;41(3):417-429. doi:10.1016/j.det.2023.02.003
45. Burli A, Vashi NA, Li BS, Maibach HI. Allergic contact dermatitis and patch testing in skin of color patients. *Dermatitis*. 2023;34(2):85-89. doi:10.1089/derm.2022.29011.abu
46. Khanna R, Desai SR. Diagnosing psoriasis in skin of color patients. *Dermatol Clin*. 2023;41(3):431-434. doi:10.1016/j.det.2023.02.002
47. Nazarian A, Alexis AF. Diagnosis of allergic dermatoses in skin of color. *Curr Allergy Asthma Rep*. 2024;24(6):317-322. doi:10.1007/s11882-024-01148-8
48. Simmons-O'Brien E, Callender VD, Orlinsky D, Hassan S, Okeke CAV, Byrd AS. Exploring the importance of inclusion criteria beyond the color of skin: improvement in facial redness in skin of color subjects: an open-label, single center clinical study utilizing low molecular weight heparan sulfate. *J Am Acad Dermatol*. 2023;88(5):1204-1206. doi:10.1016/j.jaad.2022.12.041
49. Weber B, Karels S, Hylwa S, Neeley A, Ophaug S, Lee K. Are patch testing reactions underrecognized in skin of color? Evaluating the frequency of borderline reactions by Fitzpatrick skin type. *Dermatitis*. 2024; doi:10.1089/derm.2024.0470
50. Mora Hurtado AC, Endo JO. Lack of skin of color reporting in disease severity rating tools used for inflammatory skin conditions: a scoping review. *J Am Acad Dermatol*. 2024;90(2):432-434. doi:10.1016/j.jaad.2023.09.083
51. Wang RF, Ko D, Friedman BJ, Lim HW, Mohammad TF. Disorders of hyperpigmentation. Part I. Pathogenesis and clinical features of common pigmentary disorders. *J Am Acad Dermatol*. 2023;88(2):271-288. doi:10.1016/j.jaad.2022.01.051
52. Ko D, Wang RF, Ozog D, Lim HW, Mohammad TF. Disorders of hyperpigmentation. Part II. Review of management and treatment options for hyperpigmentation. *J Am Acad Dermatol*. 2023;88(2):291-320. doi:10.1016/j.jaad.2021.12.065
53. Callender VD, Ginn LR, Boyd CM, et al. Sunscreen use for photoprotection in skin of color: a literature review. *J Drugs Dermatol*. 2024;23(7):575-577. doi:10.36849/JDD.8250
54. Dumbuya H, Grimes PE, Lynch S, et al. Impact of iron-oxide containing formulations against visible light-induced skin pigmentation in skin of color individuals. *J Drugs Dermatol*. 2020;19(7):712-717. doi:10.36849/jdd.2020.5032
55. Patel S, Watchmaker JD, Dover JS. Darker skin types are underrepresented in sunscreen clinical trials: results of a literature review. *J Am Acad Dermatol*. 2022;87(4):862-864. doi:10.1016/j.jaad.2021.11.009
56. Taylor S, Elbuluk N, Grimes P, et al. Treatment recommendations for acne-associated hyperpigmentation: results of the Delphi consensus process and a literature review. *J Am Acad Dermatol*. 2023;89(2):316-323. doi:10.1016/j.jaad.2023.02.053
57. Zawar VP, Agarwal M, Vasudevan B. Treatment of postinflammatory pigmentation due to acne with q-switched neodymium-doped yttrium aluminum garnet in 78 Indian cases. *J Cutan Aesthet Surg*. 2015;8(4):222-226. doi:10.4103/0974-2077.172196
58. Ren R, Bao S, Qian W, Zhao H. 755-nm Alexandrite picosecond laser with a diffractive lens array or zoom handpiece for post-inflammatory hyperpigmentation: two case reports with a three-year follow-up. *Clin Cosmet Investig Dermatol*. 2021;14:1459-1464. doi:10.2147/ccid.s323872
59. Wu X, Wang X, Cen Q, et al. Intense pulsed light therapy improves acne-induced post-inflammatory erythema and hyperpigmentation: a retrospective study in Chinese patients. *Dermatol Ther (Heidelb)*. 2022;12(5):1147-1156. doi:10.1007/s13555-022-00719-9
60. Bansal C, Naik H, Kar HK, Chauhan A. A comparison of low-fluence 1064-nm q-switched nd: YAG laser with topical 20% azelaic acid cream and their combination in melasma in Indian patients. *J Cutan Aesthet Surg*. 2012;5(4):266-272. doi:10.4103/0974-2077.104915
61. Wanitphakdeedecha R, Sy-Alvarado F, Patthamalai P, Techapichetvanich T, Eimpunth S, Manuskiatti W. The efficacy in treatment of facial melasma with thulium 1927-nm fractional laser-assisted topical tranexamic acid delivery: a split-face, double-blind, randomized controlled pilot study. *Lasers Med Sci*. 2020;35(9):2015-2021. doi:10.1007/s10103-020-03045-8

62. Vanaman Wilson MJ, Jones IT, Bolton J, Larsen L, Fabi SG. The safety and efficacy of treatment with a 1,927-nm diode laser with and without topical hydroquinone for facial hyperpigmentation and melasma in darker skin types. *Dermatol Surg*. 2018;44(10):1304-1310. doi:10.1097/dss.0000000000001521
63. Wong CSM, Chan MWM, Shek SYN, Yeung CK, Chan HHL. Fractional 1064 nm picosecond laser in treatment of melasma and skin rejuvenation in Asians. A prospective study. *Lasers Surg Med*. 2021;53(8):1032-1042. doi:10.1002/lsm.23382
64. Sanyal RD, Fabi SG. Energy-based devices for the treatment of facial skin conditions in skin of color. *J Clin Aesthet Dermatol*. 2024;17(6):22-32.
65. Eckembrecher FJ, Eckembrecher DG, Camacho I, Shah H, Jaalouk D, Nouri K. A review of treatment of port-wine stains with pulsed dye laser in fitzpatrick skin type IV-VI. *Arch Dermatol Res*. 2023;315(9):2505-2511. doi:10.1007/s00403-023-02640-3
66. Lee HS, Lee JH, Ahn GY, et al. Fractional photothermolysis for the treatment of acne scars: a report of 27 Korean patients. *J Dermatolog Treat*. 2008;19(1):45-49. doi:10.1080/09546630701691244
67. Mahmoud BH, Srivastava D, Janiga JJ, Yang JJ, Lim HW, Ozog DM. Safety and efficacy of erbium-doped yttrium aluminum garnet fractionated laser for treatment of acne scars in type IV to VI skin. *Dermatol Surg*. 2010;36(5):602-609. doi:10.1111/j.1524-4725.2010.01513.x
68. Leheta TM, Abdel Hay RM, Hegazy RA, El Garem YF. Do combined alternating sessions of 1540 nm nonablative fractional laser and percutaneous collagen induction with trichloroacetic acid 20% show better results than each individual modality in the treatment of atrophic acne scars? A randomized controlled trial. *J Dermatolog Treat*. 2014;25(2):137-141. doi:10.3109/09546634.2012.698249
69. You HJ, Kim DW, Yoon ES, Park SH. Comparison of four different lasers for acne scars: resurfacing and fractional lasers. *J Plast Reconstr Aesthet Surg*. 2016;69(4):e87-e95. doi:10.1016/j.bjps.2015.12.012
70. Alexis AF, Coley MK, Nijhawan RI, et al. Nonablative fractional laser resurfacing for acne scarring in patients with Fitzpatrick skin phototypes IV-VI. *Dermatol Surg*. 2016;42(3):392-402. doi:10.1097/dss.0000000000000640
71. Chan HH, Manstein D, Yu CS, Shek S, Kono T, Wei WI. The prevalence and risk factors of post-inflammatory hyperpigmentation after fractional resurfacing in Asians. *Lasers Surg Med*. 2007;39(5):381-385. doi:10.1002/lsm.20512
72. Cenk H, Sarac G. Effectiveness and safety of 2940-nm multifractional Er: YAG laser on acne scars. *Dermatol Ther*. 2020;33(6):e14270. doi:10.1111/dth.14270
73. Cachafeiro T, Escobar G, Maldonado G, Cestari T, Corleta O. Comparison of nonablative fractional erbium laser 1,340 nm and microneedling for the treatment of atrophic acne scars: a randomized clinical trial. *Dermatol Surg*. 2016;42(2):232-241. doi:10.1097/DSS.0000000000000597
74. Haimovic A, Brauer JA, Cindy Bae YS, Geronemus RG. Safety of a picosecond laser with diffractive lens array (DLA) in the treatment of Fitzpatrick skin types IV to VI: a retrospective review. *J Am Acad Dermatol*. 2016;74(5):931-936. doi:10.1016/j.jaad.2015.12.010
75. Kwon HH, Yang SH, Cho YJ, et al. Comparison of a 1064-nm neodymium-doped yttrium aluminum garnet picosecond laser using a diffractive optical element vs. a nonablative 1550-nm erbium-glass laser for the treatment of facial acne scarring in Asian patients: a 17-week prospective, randomized, split-face, controlled trial. *J Eur Acad Dermatol Venereol*. 2020;34(12):2907-2913. doi:10.1111/jdv.16643
76. Tierney E, Mahmoud BH, Hexsel C, Ozog D, Hamzavi I. Randomized control trial for the treatment of hidradenitis suppurativa with a neodymium-doped yttrium aluminium garnet laser. *Dermatol Surg*. 2009;35(8):1188-1198. doi:10.1111/j.1524-4725.2009.01214.x
77. Sidhom S, Petry SU, Ward R, Daveluy S. Treatment of hidradenitis suppurativa with 755-nm alexandrite laser hair removal: a randomized controlled trial. *JAAD Int*. 2024;16:239-243. doi:10.1016/j.jdin.2024.04.005
78. Amer A, Elsayed A, Gharib K. Evaluation of efficacy and safety of chemical peeling and long-pulse Nd:YAG laser in treatment of pseudofolliculitis barbae. *Dermatol Ther*. 2021;34(2):e14859. doi:10.1111/dth.14859
79. Woo DK, Treyger G, Henderson M, Huggins RH, Jackson-Richards D, Hamzavi I. Prospective controlled trial for the treatment of acne keloidalis nuchae with a long-pulsed neodymium-doped yttrium-aluminum-garnet laser. *J Cutan Med Surg*. 2018;22(2):236-238. doi:10.1177/1203475417739846
80. Kantor GR, Ratz JL, Wheeland RG. Treatment of acne keloidalis nuchae with carbon dioxide laser. *J Am Acad Dermatol*. 1986;14(2 Pt 1):263-267. doi:10.1016/s0190-9622(86)70031-5
81. Arellano-Huacuja A. Effective keloid management using a combinatorial continuous-wave and repeat fractionated ablative CO. *J Cosmet Dermatol*. 2024;23(Suppl 1):7-12. doi:10.1111/jocd.16282
82. Azzam OA, Bassiouny DA, El-Hawary MS, El Maadawi ZM, Sobhi RM, El-Mesidy MS. Treatment of hypertrophic scars and keloids by fractional carbon dioxide laser: a clinical, histological, and immunohistochemical study. *Lasers Med Sci*. 2016;31(1):9-18. doi:10.1007/s10103-015-1824-4
83. Foppiani J, Khaity A, Al-Dardery NM, et al. Laser therapy in hypertrophic and keloid scars: a systematic review and network meta-analysis. *Aesthetic Plast Surg*. 2024;48(19):3988-4006. doi:10.1007/s00266-024-04027-9
84. Rossi A, Lu R, Frey MK, Kubota T, Smith LA, Perez M. The use of the 300 microsecond 1064 nm Nd:YAG laser in the treatment of keloids. *J Drugs Dermatol*. 2013;12(11):1256-1262.

85. Yang Q, Ma Y, Zhu R, et al. The effect of flashlamp pulsed dye laser on the expression of connective tissue growth factor in keloids. *Lasers Surg Med.* 2012;44(5):377-383. doi:10.1002/lsm.22031
86. Ali FR, Bakkour W, Ferguson JE, Madan V. Carbon dioxide laser ablation of dermatosis papulosa nigra: high satisfaction and few complications in patients with pigmented skin. *Lasers Med Sci.* 2016;31(3):593-595. doi:10.1007/s10103-016-1906-y
87. Schweiger ES, Kwasniak L, Aires DJ. Treatment of dermatosis papulosa nigra with a 1064 nm Nd:YAG laser: report of two cases. *J Cosmet Laser Ther.* 2008;10(2):120-122. doi:10.1080/14764170801950070
88. Kundu RV, Joshi SS, Suh KY, et al. Comparison of electrodesiccation and potassium-titanyl-phosphate laser for treatment of dermatosis papulosa nigra. *Dermatol Surg.* 2009;35(7):1079-1083. doi:10.1111/j.1524-4725.2009.01186.x
89. Miazek N, Michalek I, Pawlowska-Kisiel M, Olszewska M, Rudnicka L. Pityriasis alba: common disease, enigmatic entity: up-to-date review of the literature. *Pediatr Dermatol.* 2015;32(6):786-791. doi:10.1111/pde.12683
90. Pathmarajah P, Peterknecht E, Cheung K, Elyoussfi S, Muralidharan V, Bewley A. Acne vulgaris in skin of color: a systematic review of the effectiveness and tolerability of current treatments. *J Clin Aesthet Dermatol.* 2022;15(11):43-68.
91. Mitchell KN, Tay YK, Heath CR, Silverberg NB. Review article: emerging issues in pediatric skin of color, part 2. *Pediatr Dermatol.* 2021;38(Suppl 2):30-36. doi:10.1111/pde.14774
92. McKenzie S, Brown-Korsah JB, Syder NC, Omar D, Taylor SC, Elbuluk N. Variations in genetics, biology, and phenotype of cutaneous disorders in skin of color. Part II: differences in clinical presentation and disparities in cutaneous disorders in skin of color. *J Am Acad Dermatol.* 2022;87(6):1261-1270. doi:10.1016/j.jaad.2022.03.067
93. Brunner PM, Guttman-Yassky E. Racial differences in atopic dermatitis. *Ann Allergy Asthma Immunol.* 2019;122(5):449-455. doi:10.1016/j.anai.2018.11.015
94. Mei-Yen Yong A, Tay YK. Atopic dermatitis: racial and ethnic differences. *Dermatol Clin.* 2017;35(3):395-402. doi:10.1016/j.det.2017.02.012
95. Kaufman BP, Guttman-Yassky E, Alexis AF. Atopic dermatitis in diverse racial and ethnic groups-variations in epidemiology, genetics, clinical presentation and treatment. *Exp Dermatol.* 2018;27(4):340-357. doi:10.1111/exd.13514
96. Nguyen L, Parker L, Hennessy K, Shah N, Cohen G. Comparison of patch testing results of White and Black patients. *J Clin Aesthet Dermatol.* 2024;17(6):55-57.
97. Elgash M, Dlova N, Ogunleye T, Taylor SC. Seborrheic dermatitis in skin of color: clinical considerations. *J Drugs Dermatol.* 2019;18(1):24-27.
98. Alikhan A, Sayed C, Alavi A, et al. North American clinical management guidelines for hidradenitis suppurativa: a publication from the United States and Canadian Hidradenitis Suppurativa Foundations: part I: diagnosis, evaluation, and the use of complementary and procedural management. *J Am Acad Dermatol.* 2019;81(1):76-90. doi:10.1016/j.jaad.2019.02.067
99. Alikhan A, Sayed C, Alavi A, et al. North American clinical management guidelines for hidradenitis suppurativa: a publication from the United States and Canadian Hidradenitis Suppurativa Foundations: part II: topical, intralesional, and systemic medical management. *J Am Acad Dermatol.* 2019;81(1):91-101. doi:10.1016/j.jaad.2019.02.068
100. Jenkins T, Isaac J, Edwards A, Okoye GA. Hidradenitis suppurativa. *Dermatol Clin.* 2023;41(3):471-479. doi:10.1016/j.det.2023.02.001
101. Serrano L, Ulschmid C, Szabo A, Roth G, Sokumbi O. Racial disparities of delay in diagnosis and dermatologic care for hidradenitis suppurativa. *J Natl Med Assoc.* 2022;114(6):613-616. doi:10.1016/j.jnma.2022.08.002
102. Moseley I, Ragi SD, Handler MZ. Racial disparities in the treatment of hidradenitis suppurativa: an analysis of data from the national ambulatory medical care survey. *J Drugs Dermatol.* 2023;22(7):692-693. doi:10.36849/jdd.6803
103. Vinding GR, Miller IM, Zarchi K, Ibler KS, Ellervik C, Jemec GB. The prevalence of inverse recurrent suppuration: a population-based study of possible hidradenitis suppurativa. *Br J Dermatol.* 2014;170(4):884-889. doi:10.1111/bjd.12787
104. Hurley H, Roenigk R, Roenigk H. *Dermatologic surgery, principles and practice.* Marcel; 1989.
105. Garg A, Malviya N, Strunk A, et al. Comorbidity screening in hidradenitis suppurativa: evidence-based recommendations from the US and Canadian Hidradenitis Suppurativa Foundations. *J Am Acad Dermatol.* 2022;86(5):1092-1101. doi:10.1016/j.jaad.2021.01.059
106. Kimball AB, Okun MM, Williams DA, et al. Two phase 3 trials of adalimumab for hidradenitis suppurativa. *N Engl J Med.* 2016;375(5):422-434. doi:10.1056/NEJMoa1504370
107. Kimball AB, Jemec GBE, Alavi A, et al. Secukinumab in moderate-to-severe hidradenitis suppurativa (SUNSHINE and SUNRISE): week 16 and week 52 results of two identical, multicentre, randomised, placebo-controlled, double-blind phase 3 trials. *Lancet.* 2023;401(10378):747-761. doi:10.1016/s0140-6736(23)00022-3
108. Kimball AB, Jemec GBE, Sayed CJ, et al. Efficacy and safety of bimekizumab in patients with moderate-to-severe hidradenitis suppurativa (BE HEARD I and BE HEARD II): two 48-week, randomised,

double-blind, placebo-controlled, multicentre phase 3 trials. *Lancet.* 2024;403(10443):2504-2519. doi:10.1016/s0140-6736(24)00101-6
109. Munjal A, Ferguson N. Skin cancer in skin of color. *Dermatol Clin.* 2023;41(3):481-489. doi:10.1016/j.det.2023.02.013
110. Hinds GA, Heald P. Cutaneous T-cell lymphoma in skin of color. *J Am Acad Dermatol.* 2009;60(3):359-375; quiz 376-8. doi:10.1016/j.jaad.2008.10.031
111. Mosallaei D, Thomas SI, Lobl M, et al. Cutaneous T-cell lymphoma in skin of colour: a review. *Clin Exp Dermatol.* 2025;50(2):279-286. doi:10.1093/ced/llae338
112. Elman SA, Joyce C, Braudis K, et al. Creation and validation of classification criteria for discoid lupus erythematosus. *JAMA Dermatol.* 2020;156(8):901-906. doi:10.1001/jamadermatol.2020.1698
113. Larrondo J, McMichael AJ. Scarring alopecia. *Dermatol Clin.* 2023;41(3):519-537. doi:10.1016/j.det.2023.02.007
114. Jessop S, Whitelaw DA, Grainge MJ, Jayasekera P. Drugs for discoid lupus erythematosus. *Cochrane Database Syst Rev.* 2017;5(5):CD002954. doi:10.1002/14651858.CD002954.pub3
115. Ezeh N, Caplan A, Rosenbach M, Imadojemu S. Cutaneous sarcoidosis. *Dermatol Clin.* 2023;41(3):455-470. doi:10.1016/j.det.2023.02.012
116. Lai J, Almazan E, Le T, Taylor MT, Alhariri J, Kwatra SG. Demographics, cutaneous manifestations, and comorbidities associated with progressive cutaneous sarcoidosis: a retrospective cohort study. *Medicines (Basel).* 2023;10(10): doi:10.3390/medicines10100057
117. Heath CR, David J, Taylor SC. Sarcoidosis: are there differences in your skin of color patients? *J Am Acad Dermatol.* 2012;66(1):121.e1-121.e14. doi:10.1016/j.jaad.2010.06.068
118. Cohen E, Lheure C, Ingen-Housz-Oro S, et al. Which first-line treatment for cutaneous sarcoidosis? A retrospective study of 120 patients. *Eur J Dermatol.* 2023;33(6):680-685. doi:10.1684/ejd.2023.4584
119. Alexis A, Heath CR, Halder RM. Folliculitis keloidalis nuchae and pseudofolliculitis barbae: are prevention and effective treatment within reach? *Dermatol Clin.* 2014;32(2):183-191. doi:10.1016/j.det.2013.12.001
120. Perry PK, Cook-Bolden FE, Rahman Z, Jones E, Taylor SC. Defining pseudofolliculitis barbae in 2001: a review of the literature and current trends. *J Am Acad Dermatol.* 2002;46(2 Suppl):S113-S119. doi:10.1067/mjd.2002.120789
121. Kelly AP. Pseudofolliculitis barbae and acne keloidalis nuchae. *Dermatol Clin.* 2003;21(4):645-653. doi:10.1016/s0733-8635(03)00079-2
122. Rice X, Omar D, Goodwin BP, Adotama P. Barber knowledge and recommendations for pseudofolliculitis barbae. *JAMA Dermatol.* 2024;160(1):111-113. doi:10.1001/jamadermatol.2023.4913
123. Nussbaum D, Friedman A. Pseudofolliculitis barbae: a review of current treatment options. *J Drugs Dermatol.* 2019;18(3):246-250.
124. Ogunbiyi A. Pseudofolliculitis barbae: current treatment options. *Clin Cosmet Investig Dermatol.* 2019;12:241-247. doi:10.2147/CCID.S149250
125. Adotama P, Tinker D, Mitchell K, Glass DA, Allen P. Barber knowledge and recommendations regarding pseudofolliculitis barbae and acne keloidalis nuchae in an urban setting. *JAMA Dermatol.* 2017;153(12):1325-1326. doi:10.1001/jamadermatol.2017.3668
126. Maranda EL, Simmons BJ, Nguyen AH, Lim VM, Keri JE. Treatment of acne keloidalis nuchae: a systematic review of the literature. *Dermatol Ther (Heidelb).* 2016;6(3):363-378. doi:10.1007/s13555-016-0134-5
127. George EA, Matthews C, Roche FC, Taylor SC. Beyond the hot comb: updates in epidemiology, pathogenesis, and treatment of central centrifugal cicatricial alopecia from 2011 to 2021. *Am J Clin Dermatol.* 2023;24(1):81-88. doi:10.1007/s40257-022-00740-w
128. Sow YN, Jackson TK, Taylor SC, Ogunleye TA. Lessons from a scoping review: clinical presentations of central centrifugal cicatricial alopecia. *J Am Acad Dermatol.* 2024;91(2):259-264. doi:10.1016/j.jaad.2024.03.009
129. Aguh C, Dina Y, Talbot CC, Garza L. Fibroproliferative genes are preferentially expressed in central centrifugal cicatricial alopecia. *J Am Acad Dermatol.* 2018;79(5):904-912.e1. doi:10.1016/j.jaad.2018.05.1257
130. Malki L, Sarig O, Romano MT, et al. Variant *PADI3* in central centrifugal cicatricial alopecia. *N Engl J Med.* 2019;380(9):833-841. doi:10.1056/NEJMoa1816614
131. Jackson T, Sow Y, Dinkins J, et al. Treatment for central centrifugal cicatricial alopecia-Delphi consensus recommendations. *J Am Acad Dermatol.* 2024;90(6):1182-1189. doi:10.1016/j.jaad.2023.12.073
132. Larrondo J, McMichael AJ. Traction alopecia. *JAMA Dermatol.* 2023;159(6):676. doi:10.1001/jamadermatol.2022.6298
133. Akingbola CO, Vyas J. Traction alopecia: a neglected entity in 2017. *Indian J Dermatol Venereol Leprol.* 2017;83(6):644-649. doi:10.4103/ijdvl.IJDVL_553_16
134. Desai M, Gill J, Luke J. Cosmetic procedures in patients with skin of color: clinical pearls and pitfalls. *J Clin Aesthet Dermatol.* 2023;16(3):37-40.

135. Alexis AF, Andriessen A, Beach RA, et al. Periprocedural skincare for nonenergy and nonablative energy-based aesthetic procedures in patients with skin of color. *J Cosmet Dermatol*. 2025;24(1):e16712. doi:10.1111/jocd.16712
136. Limmer EE, Glass DA. A review of current keloid management: mainstay monotherapies and emerging approaches. *Dermatol Ther (Heidelb)*. 2020;10(5):931-948. doi:10.1007/s13555-020-00427-2
137. Jagdeo J, Kerby E, Glass DA. Keloids. *JAMA Dermatol*. 2021;157(6):744. doi:10.1001/jamadermatol.2020.4705
138. Ung CY, Warwick A, Onoufriadis A, et al. Comorbidities of keloid and hypertrophic scars among participants in UK biobank. *JAMA Dermatol*. 2023;159(2):172-181. doi:10.1001/jamadermatol.2022.5607
139. Lee SS, Yosipovitch G, Chan YH, Goh CL. Pruritus, pain, and small nerve fiber function in keloids: a controlled study. *J Am Acad Dermatol*. 2004;51(6):1002-1006. doi:10.1016/j.jaad.2004.07.054
140. Tan A, Martinez Luna O, Glass DA. Pentoxifylline for the prevention of postsurgical keloid recurrence. *Dermatol Surg*. 2020;46(10):1353-1356. doi:10.1097/DSS.0000000000002090
141. Maghfour J, Ogunleye T. A systematic review on the treatment of dermatosis papulosa nigra. *J Drugs Dermatol*. 2021;20(4):467-472. doi:10.36849/jdd.2021.5555
142. Thakker S, Jaguan D, Belzberg M, et al. Acral lentiginous melanoma. Part I. Epidemiology, etiology, clinical presentation, and diagnosis. *J Am Acad Dermatol*. 2025; doi:10.1016/j.jaad.2024.10.124
143. Nadelmann ER, Singh AK, Abbruzzese M, et al. Acral melanoma in skin of color: current insights and future directions: a narrative review. *Cancers (Basel)*. 2025;17(3): doi:10.3390/cancers17030468
144. Mosallaei D, Lee EB, Lobl M, Clarey D, Wysong A. Rare cutaneous malignancies in skin of color. *Dermatol Surg*. 2022;48(6):606-612. doi:10.1097/DSS.0000000000003440

# 14. Pediatric Dermatology

Carly Stevens, MD, Liza Siegel, MD, and Susan Bayliss, MD

Skin disorders are one of the most common problems in pediatrics. While there is overlap with adult dermatology, there are often unique disease processes in this age group. Conservative treatment is often recommended.

## Neonatal and Infantile Dermatology

### 1. Neonatal Acne (Cephalic Pustulosis)

#### 1.1. CLINICAL PRESENTATION

- Small pustules and papules on the face (resembles miliaria rubra) (Fig. 14-1). Comedones are absent.
- Transient. Generally develops at 2 to 3 weeks of age and resolves within 6 months.
- May represent an inflammatory reaction to *Malassezia* species.

#### 1.2. TREATMENT

- No treatment is usually necessary; wash face with baby soap. In severe cases, consider ketoconazole cream.

### 2. Aplasia Cutis Congenita

#### 2.1. CLINICAL PRESENTATION

- Absence of skin with scar formation in a localized area, most commonly on the scalp (Fig. 14-2).
- Defects are present from birth.
- Larger or multiple lesions may be associated with other congenital anomalies or genetic syndromes.

#### 2.2. EVALUATION

- MRI should be considered before biopsy.

#### 2.3. TREATMENT

- Small defects often heal on their own, leaving scar tissue and localized alopecia. Larger defects may require skin grafting or other surgical intervention.

---

*The authors would like to acknowledge the first edition authors* Carrie Coughlin, Leo Shmuylovich, Monique Kumar, and Kara Blackwell.

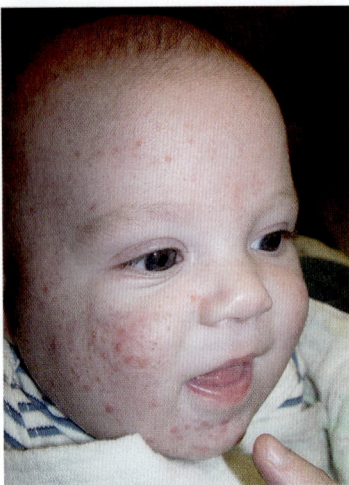

**Figure 14-1.** Acne neonatorum. (Reprinted with permission from White AJ. *The Washington Manual of Pediatrics.* 3rd ed. Wolters Kluwer; 2022:283-304. Figure 15-3.)

# 3. Erythema Toxicum Neonatorum

## 3.1. CLINICAL PRESENTATION

- Scattered yellowish, erythematous papules and pustules may occur anywhere on the body, except palms and soles (Fig. 14-3).
- More common in full-term infants. Generally appears in the first 24 to 48 hours of life and resolves within 1 week.

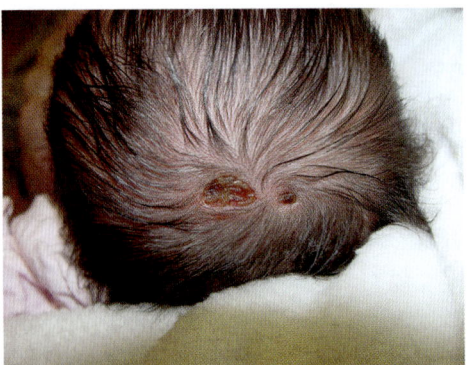

**Figure 14-2.** Aplasia cutis congenita. (Reprinted with permission from White AJ. *The Washington Manual of Pediatrics.* 3rd ed. Wolters Kluwer; 2022:283-304. Figure 15-9.)

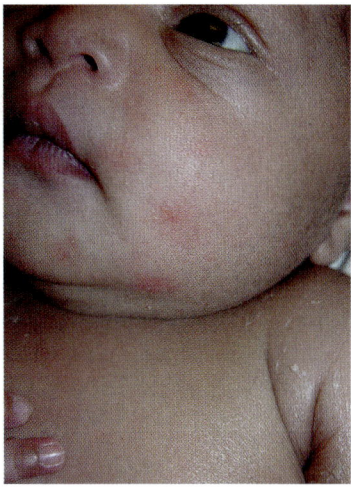

**Figure 14-3.** Erythema toxicum neonatorum. (Reprinted with permission from White AJ. *The Washington Manual of Pediatrics.* 3rd ed. Wolters Kluwer; 2022:283-304. Figure 15-1.)

### 3.2. EVALUATION

- Diagnosis is clinical. Can be confirmed by the presence of eosinophils on a smear of the pustule.

### 3.3. TREATMENT

- Self-limited condition. No treatment needed.

## 4. Milia

### 4.1. CLINICAL PRESENTATION

- 1- to 2-mm pearly white, firm papules found most commonly on the face (Fig. 14-4) but may occur anywhere. Represent tiny inclusion cysts.
- May be present at birth.
- Rarely associated with certain syndromes such as epidermolysis bullosa, orofaciodigital syndrome type 1, and Basan syndrome.

### 4.2. TREATMENT

- Usually resolve without treatment by 2 to 6 months of age. If persistent, lesions can be punctured and expressed.

## 5. Miliaria

- General term describing obstruction of the eccrine ducts at different levels, often secondary to heat and humidity

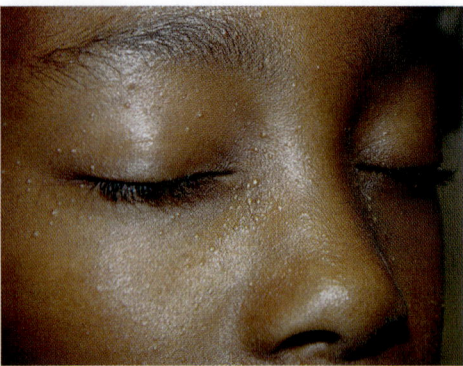

**Figure 14-4.** Milia. (Reprinted with permission from White AJ. *The Washington Manual of Pediatrics*. 3rd ed. Wolters Kluwer; 2022:283-304. Figure 15-4.)

## 5.1. CLINICAL PRESENTATION

- Miliaria crystallina: 1- to 2-mm clear vesicles without erythema in intertriginous areas, neck, and chest. Obstruction is in the most superficial level of the stratum corneum.
- Miliaria rubra ("heat rash"): erythematous papules in the same distribution that result from obstruction deeper in the epidermis, with resulting erythema.

## 5.2. TREATMENT

- Treatment involves correcting overheating conditions.

# 6. Nevus Sebaceous

- Nevus sebaceous is an organoid hamartoma of sebaceous and apocrine glands that is present at birth. It is caused by a postzygotic somatic gene mutation in *HRAS* or *KRAS*.[1]

## 6.1. CLINICAL PRESENTATION

- Alopetic, yellow-colored plaque tends to have a bumpy surface (Fig. 14-5).
- Usually present from birth on the scalp or elsewhere on head and neck. Lesion becomes less prominent after the newborn period but later becomes more papular or verrucous around puberty, when hormone levels increase.

## 6.2. TREATMENT

- Treatment is surgical excision or observation.
  - Surgery is often deferred until puberty when the lesion begins to grow.
  - Plaque can be followed by clinical observation until excision because there is a low risk of developing neoplastic growths within the lesion.[2]

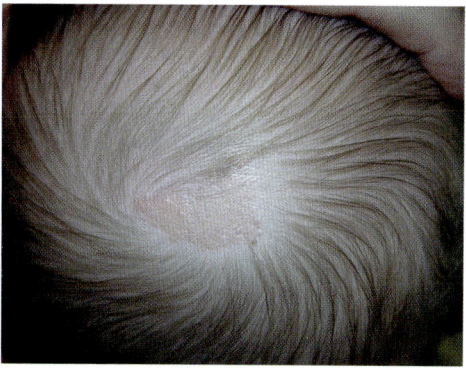

**Figure 14-5.** Nevus sebaceous. (Reprinted with permission from White AJ. *The Washington Manual of Pediatrics*. 3rd ed. Wolters Kluwer; 2022:283-304. Figure 15-8.)

- Most neoplasms within the nevus sebaceous are benign and include syringocystadenoma papilliferum and trichoblastoma.
- Rarely, malignant tumors can be identified such as basal cell carcinoma and squamous cell carcinoma.

## 7. Subcutaneous Fat Necrosis

### 7.1. CLINICAL PRESENTATION

- Localized indurated erythematous plaques or subcutaneous nodules on buttocks, thighs, trunk, face, and/or arms. Lesions may be fluctuant (Fig. 14-6).

### 7.2. EVALUATION

- Subcutaneous fat necrosis is usually diagnosed clinically. Diagnosis can be confirmed by skin biopsy.

### 7.3. TREATMENT

- Patches appear at 1 to 6 weeks of life and generally resolve without treatment in 2 to 6 months. Fluctuant nodules require drainage.

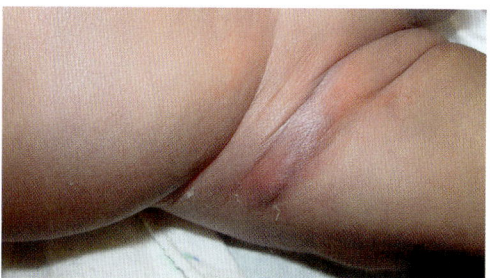

**Figure 14-6.** Subcutaneous fat necrosis.

- Uncommonly, can be associated with significant hypercalcemia as well as localized calcification. Infants should be monitored for hypercalcemia for at least 3 months after appearance of extensive lesions.[3]

## 8. Transient Neonatal Pustular Melanosis

### 8.1. CLINICAL PRESENTATION

- Present at birth. More common in dark-skinned infants.
- Pustular lesions rupture easily with a collarette of scale and leave hyperpigmented macules on the neck, chin, forehead, lower back, and shins (Fig. 14-7), which fades over 6 to 12 months.

### 8.2. TREATMENT

- Self-limited. Pustules resolve within days, but hyperpigmentation may take months to resolve. No treatment needed.

## Pigmented Lesions

## 9. Café Au Lait Macules

### 9.1. CLINICAL PRESENTATION

- Light brown macules (Fig. 14-8) can occur anywhere on the body, ranging from small (<0.5 mm) to large, including segmental patches.

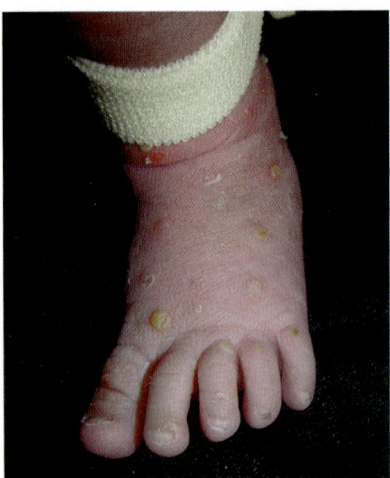

**Figure 14-7.** Transient neonatal pustular melanosis. (Reprinted with permission from White AJ. *The Washington Manual of Pediatrics*. 3rd ed. Wolters Kluwer; 2022:283-304. Figure 15-2.)

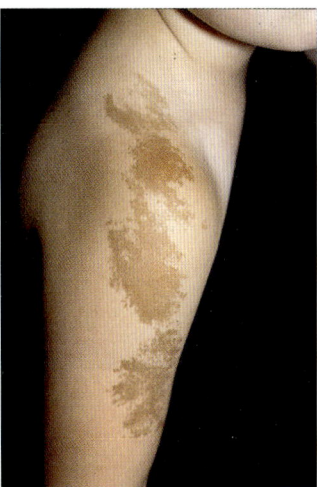

**Figure 14-8.** Café au lait macules. (Reprinted with permission from White AJ. *The Washington Manual of Pediatrics.* 3rd ed. Wolters Kluwer; 2022:283-304. Figure 15-6.)

### 9.2. EVALUATION

- May occur in isolation or with a syndrome
  - Neurofibromatosis 1: The presence of six or more macules greater than 0.5 cm in diameter in prepubertal children or greater than 1.5 cm in postpubertal, as well as inguinal or axillary freckling.
  - Large, very irregular truncal patches may be associated with McCune-Albright syndrome.

### 9.3. TREATMENT

- Treatment is generally not required. Laser therapy with Q-switched lasers can be attempted but is not permanent.

## 10. Congenital Dermal Melanocytosis (Mongolian Spot)

### 10.1. CLINICAL PRESENTATION

- Blue-gray poorly circumscribed macules most commonly in lumbosacral area but can be seen anywhere (Fig. 14-9).
- More common in skin of color; present at birth.
- Lumbosacral lesions tend to lighten in childhood; however, lesions in other locations usually persist.

## 11. Congenital Melanocytic Nevi

### 11.1. CLINICAL PRESENTATION

- Present at birth or become evident in the first year of life.

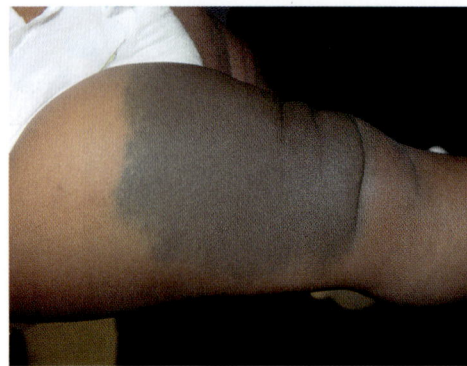

**Figure 14-9.** Congenital dermal melanosis (mongolian spots). (Reprinted with permission from White AJ. *The Washington Manual of Pediatrics.* 3rd ed. Wolters Kluwer; 2022:283-304. Figure 15-5.)

- Brown pigmented macules or plaques may have dark brown or black papules or other irregular pigmentation within the lesions (Fig. 14-10). Lesions can have hypertrichosis. Larger lesions may have ulceration, a cobblestoned surface, nodules, and/or satellite lesions.
- They are found in 1% to 3% of newborn babies.
- These nevi enlarge in proportion to the child's growth and are classified based on their projected final adult size, with the following categories:
  ○ Small congenital melanocytic nevi (CMN): less than 1.5 cm in diameter (projected adult size).
  ○ Medium CMN: 1.5 to 20 cm in diameter (projected adult size).
  ○ Large or giant CMN: greater than 20 cm in diameter (projected adult size).
  ○ Giant CMN can cover a large portion of the body (eg, in a "bathing trunk" or "cape" distribution) and are rare, found in fewer than 1 in 20,000 newborn infants.

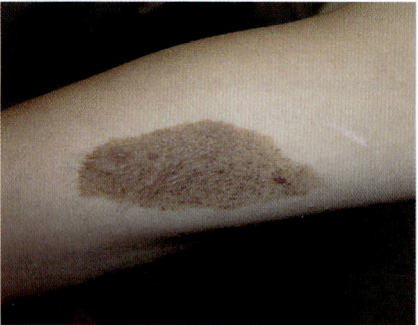

**Figure 14-10.** Congenital melanocytic nevi. (Reprinted with permission from White AJ. *The Washington Manual of Pediatrics.* 3rd ed. Wolters Kluwer; 2022:283-304. Figure 15-7.)

### 11.2. EVALUATION

- The small increased risk of melanoma development within lesions makes close follow-up important. This risk is less than 1% over a lifetime for small and medium CMN and is extraordinarily low before puberty. Risk of melanoma is greatest (~5%) in giant CMN, over a lifetime.
- Children with giant and/or numerous (eg, >20) CMN also have an increased number of melanocytes around their brain, which is referred to as neurocutaneous melanocytosis.
- Magnetic resonance imaging with contrast of the brain and spine is recommended in patients with multiple medium CMN, ≥10 satellite lesions, and giant CMN to rule out neurocutaneous melanosis.[4]

### 11.3. TREATMENT

- CMN are managed on an individual basis depending on their location, size, appearance, and evolution over time. Factors that may prompt surgical excision of a congenital nevus include cosmetic concerns, difficulty in monitoring the lesion, and worrisome changes in its appearance.

## 12. Spitz Nevus

### 12.1. CLINICAL PRESENTATION

- Dome-shaped tan-pink papule appears over a few months and is a subtype of melanocytic nevus. Common in first two decades of life. Usual locations for pediatric Spitz nevi include head, neck, and extremities.

### 12.2. EVALUATION

- Biopsy confirms diagnosis.

### 12.3. TREATMENT

- The management of pediatric Spitz nevi has no clear consensus. Surgical excision may be considered.

## Vascular Lesions

## 13. Capillary Malformation (Port-Wine Stain)

### 13.1. CLINICAL PRESENTATION

- Pink, red, or purple blanchable small to large patch caused by capillary malformations (Fig. 14-11). This is most commonly due to a somatic mutation in GNAQ.[5] Other somatic mutations have been found in GNA11, PIK3R1, and PIK3CA.[5-7]

### 13.2. EVALUATION

- Lesions in hemifacial (involving forehead and/or eyelid) distribution on the face should be evaluated for associated glaucoma and/or Sturge-Weber syndrome.

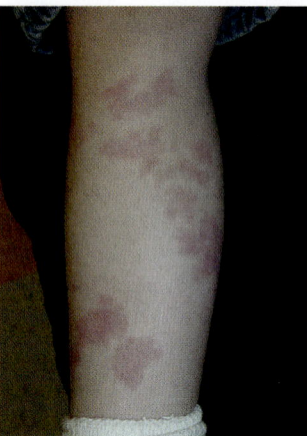

**Figure 14-11.** Capillary malformation (port-wine stain). (Reprinted with permission from White AJ. *The Washington Manual of Pediatrics*. 3rd ed. Wolters Kluwer; 2022:283-304. Figure 15-10.)

Lesions persist and generally become darker and thicker with age. Segmental capillary malformations on an extremity may be associated with overgrowth of the extremity. Patients with multiple capillary malformations should be evaluated for capillary malformation-arteriovenous malformation syndrome.[8]

### 13.3. TREATMENT

- Treatment is not required. If families desire treatment, pulse dye laser can be used to light the lesions. Complete clearance is often not attainable.

## 14. Cutis Marmorata Telangiectatica Congenita

### 14.1. CLINICAL PRESENTATION

- Fixed, blanchable purple, reticular pattern most commonly on unilateral extremity. Focal areas with atrophy and/or ulceration. Considered a vascular malformation
- Does not disappear with rewarming (unlike cutis marmorata)
- May be associated with body asymmetry
- May improve with age but rarely disappears completely

### 14.2. TREATMENT

- No treatment is usually needed and can improve with time. Poorly responsive to pulsed-dye laser treatment.

## 15. Infantile Hemangioma

- Most common vascular tumor of infancy

## 15.1. CLINICAL PRESENTATION

- Superficial: bright red vascular plaques or nodules
- Deep: bluish purple nodules, sometimes with overlying telangiectatic markings (Fig. 14-12)
- Mixed: both deep and superficial components present

## 15.2. COURSE

- Lesions usually are not present at birth, or a precursor lesion may be present.
  - Appear as faint vascular markings initially and then enlarge and develop characteristic appearance over 2 to 4 months.
  - Typically by 6 months, infantile hemangioma (IH) stabilizes in size and appearance and then slowly involutes by 5 years of age. Some leave behind residual markings or fibrous tissue.

## 15.3. COMPLICATIONS AND ASSOCIATIONS

- Ulceration may occur in any hemangioma but is more common on the lip and in the diaper area.
- Depending on the location and size, the IH may cause disfigurement or may interfere with vision, eating, or breathing.
- Disseminated neonatal hemangiomatosis: multiple scattered small hemangiomas. Can be accompanied by internal involvement most commonly found in the liver, followed by brain, mediastinum, and lung, brain, or gastrointestinal tract.[9]
- PHACES syndrome: **p**osterior fossa malformations, **h**emangiomas, **a**rterial anomalies, **c**oarctation of the aorta, **e**ye anomalies, and **s**ternal cleft.
- Segmental facial hemangiomas may be associated with PHACES syndrome or severe GI bleeding.
- Chin and neck hemangiomas may be associated with tracheal involvement.
- Sacral hemangiomas may be associated with tethered cord or spinal dysraphism.
- LUMBAR syndrome: **l**ower body segmental IHs with **u**rogenital anomalies, **u**lceration, **m**yelopathy, **b**ony deformities, **a**norectal malformations, **a**rterial anomalies, and **r**enal anomalies.

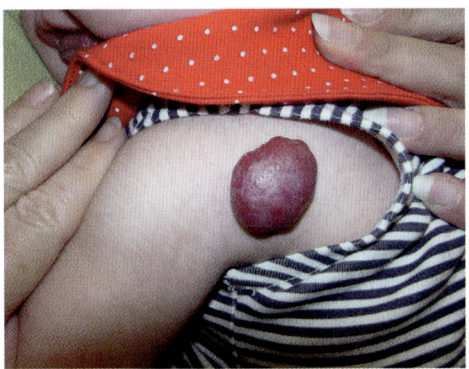

**Figure 14-12.** Hemangioma. (Reprinted with permission from White AJ. *The Washington Manual of Pediatrics*. 3rd ed. Wolters Kluwer; 2022:283-304. Figure 15-12.)

## 15.4. EVALUATION

- Early evaluation is imperative if treatment is needed. Evaluation depends on type and presentation of hemangioma.
  - If periocular, ophthalmologic evaluation is warranted.
  - If concerned for PHACES syndrome, workup includes magnetic resonance imaging/magnetic resonance angiography of brain and neck, echocardiogram, and ophthalmology evaluation. Patients should be referred to a physician familiar with vascular lesions.
  - For multifocal hemangiomas (>5), obtain ultrasound of liver.
  - For IH on the chin or neck (beard distribution), ENT evaluation is recommended to evaluate for airway involvement.

## 15.5. TREATMENT

- For most uncomplicated hemangiomas, active nonintervention is the best management option. If large, ulcerated, or disfiguring, the treatment of choice is topical and/or oral beta-blockers.[10] Other options include intralesional/oral steroids, pulsed-dye laser, and surgical removal.

# 16. Nevus Simplex

## 16.1. CLINICAL PRESENTATION

- Pink macular patches (Fig. 14-13), generally on the eyelids, glabella, or nape of neck.
- Lesions on the eyelids usually improve at 1 year and fade by 3 years.
  - Those on the nape of the neck tend to persist.
  - No treatment is needed.

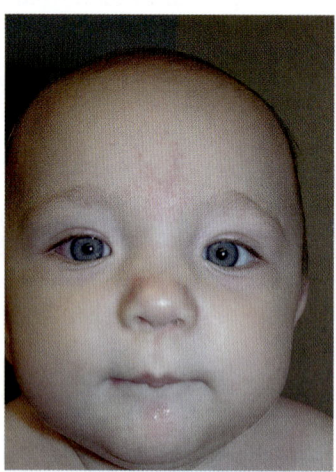

**Figure 14-13.** Nevus simplex (angel's kiss). (Reprinted with permission from White AJ. *The Washington Manual of Pediatrics*. 3rd ed. Wolters Kluwer; 2022:283-304. Figure 15-11.)

## Dermatitis

## 17. Atopic Dermatitis

### 17.1. CLINICAL PRESENTATION

- Characterized by pruritic, erythematous scaly patches, papules, and plaques.
- Secondary changes include lichenification, postinflammatory hyperpigmentation, or hypopigmentation.

### 17.2. EPIDEMIOLOGY

- There is a strong association with personal or family history of asthma and allergic rhinitis.
- Most eczema improves by 10 years of age, but severe atopic dermatitis can persist into adulthood.
- Severe, recalcitrant eczematous dermatitis may be associated with immunodeficiencies, including hyper-IgE syndrome, Wiskott-Aldrich syndrome, and severe combined immunodeficiency syndrome.
- Often associated with mutations in the *filaggrin* gene.[11]
- Children with eczema are prone to viral superinfection (eg, herpes simplex virus [HSV], molluscum contagiosum, coxsackie) and colonization with *Staphylococcus aureus*.[12]

### 17.3. SUBTYPES

- Infantile
  - From 2 months to 2 years
  - Commonly involves cheeks (Fig. 14-14A), scalp, trunk, and extensor surfaces of the extremities
- Childhood
  - From 2 years to adolescence
  - Commonly involves flexural surfaces, including antecubital, popliteal fossae, neck, wrists, and feet (Fig. 14-14B and C)
- Adolescent/adult
  - Flexural surfaces may be limited to hands and/or face.
- Nummular
  - Coin-shaped erythematous, oozing plaques that may have papules or vesicles at the periphery
  - Often occur on hands, arms, or legs (Fig. 14-14D)
- Dyshidrotic
  - Bilateral hand and/or foot dermatitis
  - Intensely pruritic with small vesicles along sides of fingers and toes

### 17.4. TREATMENT

- General skin care
  - Limit bathing to once daily in lukewarm water. Plain water is best. Use mild soaps (eg, Dove, Aveeno) only in small amounts and in the area necessary.
  - Apply moisturizers immediately after bathing. Ointments (eg, petroleum jelly [Vaseline] or Aquaphor) are more effective than are lotions.

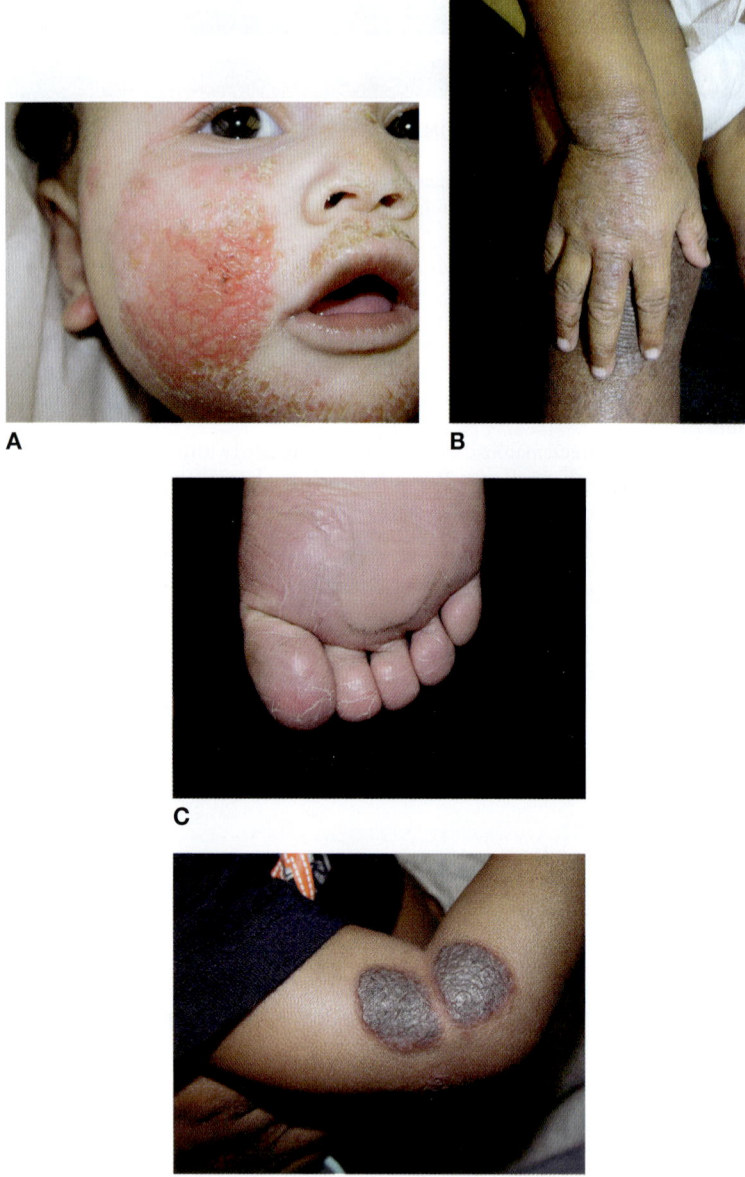

**Figure 14-14.** Atopic dermatitis. **A.** Infantile eczema with oozing plaques on the cheeks. **B.** Childhood eczema-lichenified plaques with excoriations. **C.** Juvenile plantar dermatosis (foot eczema). **D.** Nummular eczema. (Reprinted with permission from White AJ. *The Washington Manual of Pediatrics.* 3rd ed. Wolters Kluwer; 2022:283-304. Figure 15-14.)

- Education of patients, including emphasizing the chronicity of disease and the need for consistent application of prescribed treatment, can improve compliance and outcomes.
- Topical steroids[13]
  - Classification.
  - Low strength (eg, hydrocortisone 1% or 2.5% ointment) can be used for mild to moderate disease.
  - Mid strength (eg, triamcinolone 0.1% ointment) can be used for limited amounts of time on more severe, localized areas of disease. These agents can cause atrophy if used chronically.
  - High strength (eg, fluocinonide or clobetasol ointment) for palmar and plantar dermatitis or lichenified plaques.
  - Avoid using topical steroids on the face and intertriginous areas. Risks of topical steroids include skin atrophy, striae, and hypopigmentation.
- Immunomodulators
  - Topical tacrolimus (0.03% or 0.1%) or topical pimecrolimus (1%) may be useful in limited areas such as the face, where topical steroids may cause undesirable side effects with prolonged use.
  - These agents are recommended in children over age 2 years.
- Antihistamines
  - Oral diphenhydramine, hydroxyzine, or cetirizine may cause sedation, restricting their use to nighttime, to help with sleeping.
- Systemic steroids
  - Rarely used in short bursts for severe exacerbations.
  - Regular or long-term use is not recommended.
- Antibiotics
  - *S aureus* is the most common cause of bacterial superinfection. Dilute bleach baths can decrease colonization (1/4 cup for tub of water). Oral antibiotics may be necessary depending on the severity of infection. Methicillin-resistant *S aureus* is becoming more prevalent. Cultures to determine antibiotic susceptibility may be helpful.
- If eczema is still refractory, systemic therapy may be considered. Systemic immunosuppressants used to treat eczema include cyclosporine and methotrexate.[14] Biologic drug agents such as dupilumab (IL-4 and IL-13 inhibitor), tralokinumab-ldrm (IL-13 inhibitor), and Janus kinase inhibitors have recently been approved to treat atopic dermatitis in pediatric patients.[15]

## 18. Contact Dermatitis (Allergic)

### 18.1. CLINICAL PRESENTATION

- Erythematous papules and vesicles with oozing and crusting. Pruritus may be intense. This is a type IV (delayed/cell-mediated) hypersensitivity reaction.
- Common causes include poison ivy/oak, nickel, cosmetics and fragrances, topical medications, chemicals in diaper wipes, tape, or adhesives (Fig. 14-15A and B). The distribution often gives clues to the causative agent (eg, exposed areas for poison ivy, umbilicus for nickel, eyelids and face for nail polish or other cosmetics, buttocks and posterior thigh for toilet seat).
- May be accompanied by eczematous dermatitis at sites far from initial exposure (hypersensitivity reaction).

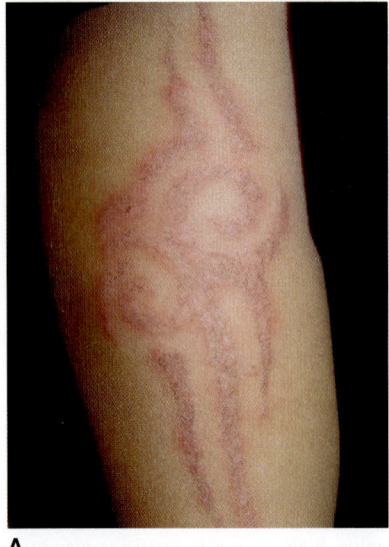

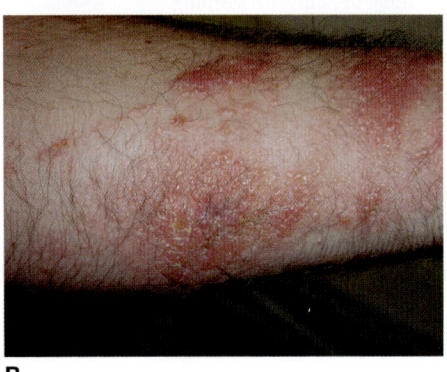

**Figure 14-15.** Contact dermatitis. **A.** Henna tattoo allergy. **B.** Poison ivy. (Reprinted with permission from White AJ. *The Washington Manual of Pediatrics*. 3rd ed. Wolters Kluwer; 2022:283-304. Figure 15-16.)

## 18.2. EVALUATION

- If condition is recurrent and no causative agent can be identified, skin patch testing may be indicated.

## 18.3. TREATMENT

- Contact with the offending allergen should be avoided. Topical mid-potency and high-potency steroids decrease inflammation. In severe eruptions, systemic steroids may be needed (2- to 3-week taper).

## 19. Diaper Dermatitis

- Many potential causes of diaper dermatitis, with the most common being irritant. Other causes: seborrheic dermatitis, candidiasis, psoriasis, zinc deficiency, and Langerhans cell histiocytosis.

### 19.1. CLINICAL PRESENTATION

- Irritant dermatitis: erythematous patches with maceration occur in diaper area, sparing the creases due to the moist environment. In more severe cases, papules, erosions, and ulcerations may be present.

### 19.2. EVALUATION

- Diagnosis is straightforward and uncomplicated. However, if the dermatitis is refractory to treatment, widespread, or unusual, additional studies (such as measurement of zinc levels or biopsy) may be warranted.

### 19.3. TREATMENT

- Treatment includes frequent diaper changes, avoidance of diaper wipes, liberal use of barrier creams, and low-strength topical steroids and/or topical antifungals.

## 20. Seborrheic Dermatitis

### 20.1. CLINICAL PRESENTATION

- Characterized by erythematous patches covered by thick, yellow scale on the vertex of the head and intertriginous areas.
- "Cradle cap" occurs on the scalp of infants (Fig. 14-16). Other commonly affected sites in babies include diaper area, axillae, and other creases. Dermatitis may be complicated by Candida or bacteria, with postinflammatory hypopigmentation.
  - It is most common at 2 to 10 weeks and may last for 8 to 12 months.

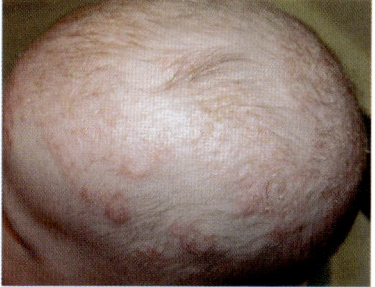

**Figure 14-16.** Seborrheic dermatitis. (Reprinted with permission from White AJ. *The Washington Manual of Pediatrics*. 3rd ed. Wolters Kluwer; 2022:283-304. Figure 15-15.)

## 20.2. TREATMENT

- Treatment in infants is hydrocortisone 0.5% to 1% cream or ointment.
- Scale may be removed with a soft brush while shampooing. Salicylic acid preparations should be avoided as they cause salicylism through absorption.
- Avoid "medicated shampoos" as this will aggravate eczema if this is a complicating factor.

# Infectious Diseases

# 21. Tinea

- Fungal infections in children commonly occur on the scalp (tinea capitis) (Fig. 14-17A and B), face (tinea faciei), and body (tinea corporis) (Fig. 14-18).
- Most often caused by *Microsporum* and *Trichophyton* species.
- Transmitted by contact with affected individuals, cats, or dogs.

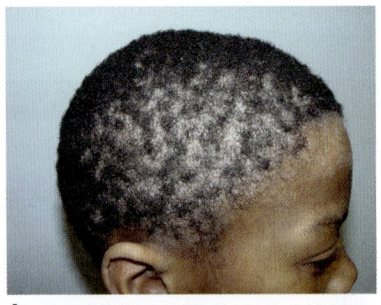

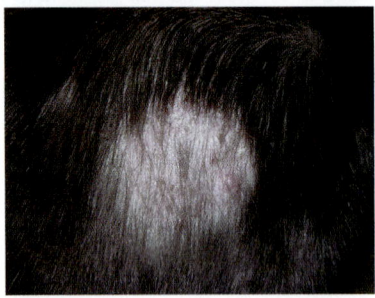

**Figure 14-17. A, B.** Tinea capitis. (Reprinted with permission from White AJ. *The Washington Manual of Pediatrics.* 3rd ed. Wolters Kluwer; 2022:283-304. Figure 15-17.)

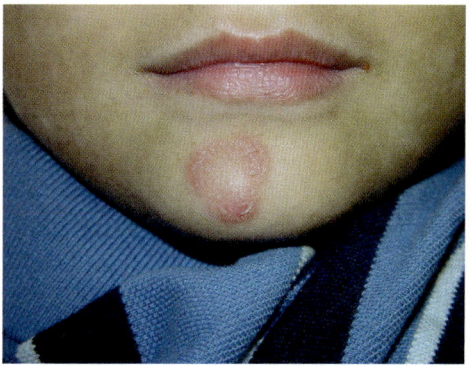

**Figure 14-18.** Tinea corporis. (Reprinted with permission from White AJ. *The Washington Manual of Pediatrics*. 3rd ed. Wolters Kluwer; 2022:283-304. Figure 15-18.)

### 21.1. CLINICAL PRESENTATION

- Scalp infections are characterized by scaling and patchy hair loss. They may be confused with seborrheic dermatitis if there is minimal hair loss and inflammation. A kerion is a sharply demarcated, tender, inflammatory pustular plaque.
- Tinea corporis is characterized by annular, scaly plaques or plaque with central clearing and erythematous scaly border.

### 21.2. EVALUATION

- Diagnosis may be made by clinical appearance, potassium hydroxide (KOH) slide "prep" showing branching hyphae, or fungal culture.

### 21.3. TREATMENT

- Scalp infections: topical antifungals are ineffective when used alone; requires systemic antifungal treatment (griseofulvin for 6-8 weeks minimum or terbinafine for 2 to 4 weeks, depending on fungal species), plus antifungal shampoo (selenium sulfide 2.5% or ketoconazole 1%-2%), 2 to 3 times per week
- Skin infections: topical antifungals (eg, miconazole, clotrimazole, terbinafine) BID for 3 to 4 weeks or until scaling clears

## 22. Verrucae

- Verrucae are caused by human papillomavirus infection of skin keratinocytes.

### 22.1. CLINICAL PRESENTATION

- Verruca vulgaris
  - Round papules with an irregular, papillomatous surface that disrupts skin lines (Fig. 14-19A)
    - Common on the hands but may occur anywhere

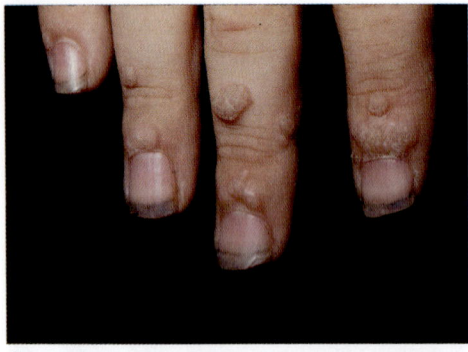

**A**

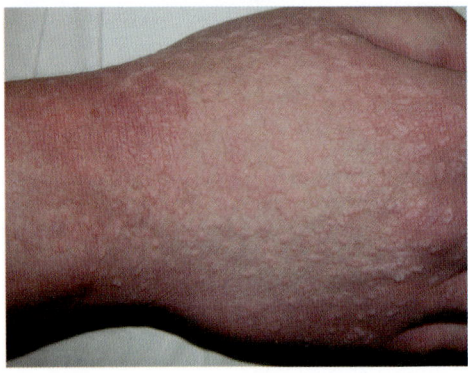

**B**

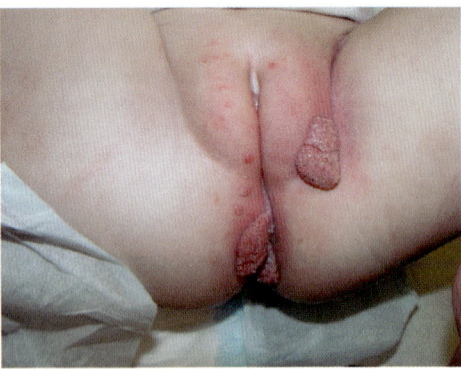

**C**

**Figure 14-19.** Warts. **A.** Verrucae vulgaris. **B.** Flat warts. **C.** Genital warts (condylomata acuminata). (Reprinted with permission from White AJ. *The Washington Manual of Pediatrics*. 3rd ed. Wolters Kluwer; 2022:283-304. Figure 15-19.)

- Verruca plantaris
  - Flat hyperkeratotic papules on plantar feet. Thrombosed capillaries may appear as black dots.
  - Painful with pressure of walking.
- Verruca plana
  - Skin-colored slightly raised, flat-topped papules (Fig. 14-19B).
  - They often occur in groups on the legs and face.

### 22.2. TREATMENT

- Most warts resolve spontaneously within 2 years. Therapeutic methods include:
  - Topical keratolytics (eg, salicylic acid) or cryotherapy available over the counter; however, they may be slow to work.
  - Liquid nitrogen cryotherapy performed every 2 to 4 weeks in office.
- Flat warts on legs: patients should avoid shaving because microtrauma can lead to new lesions.
- Refractory lesions: more intensive intervention, including pairing, Candida antigen injections, topical immunotherapy, laser therapy, or surgical removal, may be considered.
- Anogenital warts (Fig. 14-19C): use imiquimod. Therapy is usually 6 to 12 months, applied 2 to 3 times per week. May be caused by autoinoculation of common warts or vertical transmission during childbirth. Screening for sexual abuse in a child ages 2 to 14 years if warranted.

## 23. Molluscum Contagiosum

- Caused by a poxvirus; transmitted by swimming, bathing, or other close contact with an infected person

### 23.1. CLINICAL PRESENTATION

- Skin-colored pearly papules with central umbilication. If inflamed, they may become red, tender, pustular, and increase in size (Fig. 14-20).

### 23.2. TREATMENT

- Generally self-limited, and the condition often resolves in 12 months.
- For extensive or persistent lesions, curettage or topical cantharidin (blistering agent) may be effective. Imiquimod is not effective.

## Miscellaneous

## 24. Acne Vulgaris

- The etiology of acne is multifactorial. Causes include follicular plugging, increased sebum production, *Propionibacterium acnes* overgrowth, and inflammation.

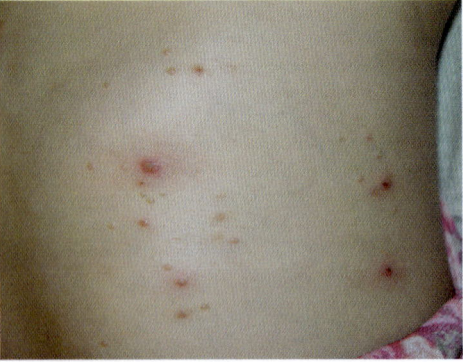

**Figure 14-20.** Molluscum contagiosum. (Reprinted with permission from White AJ. *The Washington Manual of Pediatrics.* 3rd ed. Wolters Kluwer; 2022:283-304. Figure 15-20.)

## 24.1. CLINICAL PRESENTATION (TYPES)

- Comedonal: open comedones (blackheads) and closed comedones (whiteheads) (Fig. 14-21A)
- Inflammatory: erythematous, inflammatory papules and pustules in addition to comedones
- Cystic: nodules and cysts on face, chest, and back (Fig. 14-21B)

## 24.2. TREATMENT

- General skin care: washing of face with soap or acne wash 2 times per day. Avoid scrubbing and excessive washing.
- Comedonal acne[16]
  - Benzoyl peroxide 2.5%, 5%, and 10% preparations. Benzoyl peroxide products should not be used at the same time as a topical retinoid.
  - Topical retinoids come in a variety of strengths: adapalene 0.1% (least potent) and 0.3%; tretinoin 0.025%, 0.05%, and 0.1% creams and gels; and tazarotene 0.05% and 0.1% cream (most potent). Start with the least potent for patients with dry or sensitive skin and work up as tolerated.
  - Benzoyl peroxide and retinoids can be irritating. Advise patients to use only a pea-sized amount on the face. Use every other day initially if redness/drying occurs, and then increase to daily as tolerance develops.
  - Products combining a topical antibiotic (clindamycin 1%, erythromycin) and benzoyl peroxide OR topical antibiotic and retinoid are available to simplify regimens.
- Inflammatory acne[9]
  - Add oral antibiotic (doxycycline, minocycline, tetracycline) to topical regimen for inflammatory acne. Per guidelines, oral antibiotics should be continued for 3 to 6 months to assess efficacy.
  - Advise patients to avoid excessive sun exposure and to use sunscreen to avoid photosensitivity, and to take antibiotics with food a large glass of water to minimize esophagitis.

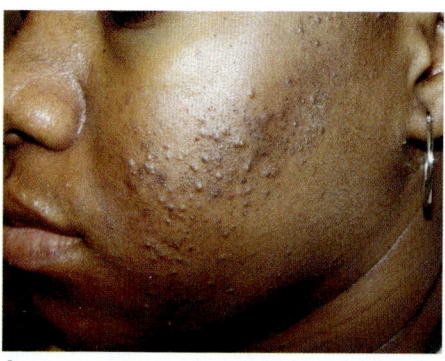

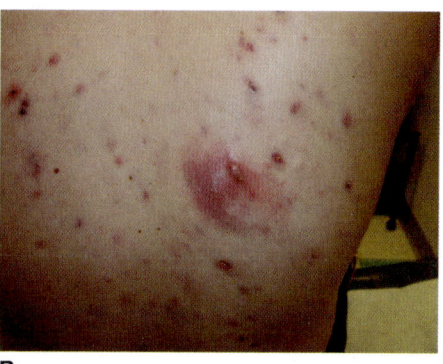

**Figure 14-21.** Acne vulgaris. **A.** Comedonal acne. **B.** Cystic acne. (Reprinted with permission from White AJ. *The Washington Manual of Pediatrics*. 3rd ed. Wolters Kluwer; 2022:283-304. Figure 15-13.)

- Cystic/nodular or scarring acne
  - Systemic retinoid therapy (isotretinoin).
  - Lab monitoring of lipids and liver function should be done at baseline and then repeated at peak dose.
- Strict contraception is required in females because the agent is teratogenic.
- For females, consider an endocrine workup if there are virilizing signs or irregular menses to look for androgen excess disorder (polycystic ovary syndrome).

## 25. Erythema Multiforme

### 25.1. CLINICAL PRESENTATION

- Characterized by erythematous papules or plaques that evolve into target lesions with dusky centers. Oral lesions may be present (Fig. 14-22).
- Most common precipitants are HSV infection, drug, or mycoplasma.

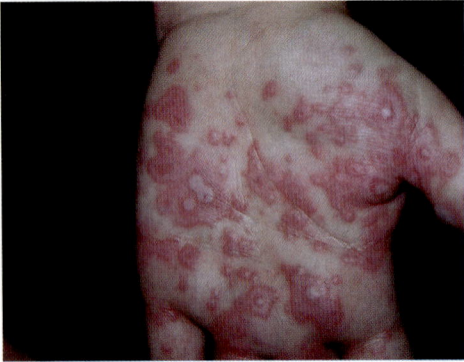

**Figure 14-22.** Erythema multiforme with typical target lesions. (Reprinted with permission from White AJ. *The Washington Manual of Pediatrics*. 3rd ed. Wolters Kluwer; 2022:283-304. Figure 15-21.)

## 25.2. TREATMENT

- Oral systemic steroids may be helpful if given early, for 7 to 10 days.
- Prophylactic acyclovir may be useful to prevent recurrent HSV-related disease.
- Antihistamines provide symptomatic relief.
- *See Chapter 5 for additional discussion of reactive viral exanthems.*

# REFERENCES

1. Groesser L, Herschberger E, Ruetten A, et al. Postzygotic HRAS and KRAS mutations cause nevus sebaceous and Schimmelpenning syndrome. *Nat Genet*. 2012;44(7):783-787.
2. Idriss MH, Elston DM. Secondary neoplasms associated with nevus sebaceous of Jadassohn: a study of 707 cases. *J Am Acad Dermatol*. 2014;70(2):332-337.
3. Siegel LH, Fraile Alonso C, Tuazon CFR, et al. Subcutaneous fat necrosis of the newborn: a retrospective study of 32 infants and care algorithm. *Pediatr Dermatol*. 2023;40(3):413-421.
4. Jahnke MN, O'Haver J, Gupta D, et al. Care of congenital melanocytic nevi in newborns and infants: review and management recommendations. *Pediatrics*. 2021;148(6):e2021051536.
5. Shirley MD, Tang H, Gallione CJ, et al. Sturge-Weber syndrome and port-wine stains caused by somatic mutation in GNAQ. *N Engl J Med*. 2013;368(21):1971-1979.
6. Cottrell CE, Bender NR, Zimmermann MT, et al. Somatic PIK3R1 variation as a cause of vascular malformations and overgrowth. *Genet Med*. 2021;23(10):1882-1888.
7. Keppler-Noreuil KM, Sapp JC, Lindhurst MJ, et al. Clinical delineation and natural history of the PIK3CA-related overgrowth spectrum. *Am J Med Genet A*. 2014;164A(7):1713-1733.
8. Dutkiewicz AS, Ezzedine K, Mazereeuw-Hautier J, et al. A prospective study of risk for Sturge-Weber syndrome in children with upper facial port-wine stain. *J Am Acad Dermatol*. 2015;72(3):473-480.
9. Valdebran M, Lee LW. Hemangioma-related syndromes. *Curr Opin Pediatr*. 2020;32(4):498-505.
10. Léauté-Labrèze C, Dumas de la Roque E, Hubiche T, Boralevi F, Thambo JB, Taïeb A. Propranolol for severe hemangiomas of infancy. *N Engl J Med*. 2008;358(24):2649-2651.
11. Palmer CN, Irvine AD, Terron-Kwiatkowski A, et al. Common loss-of-function variants of the epidermal barrier protein filaggrin are a major predisposing factor for atopic dermatitis. *Nat Genet*. 2006;38(4):441-446.
12. Eichenfield LF, Tom WL, Chamlin SL, et al. Guidelines of care for the management of atopic dermatitis: section 1. Diagnosis and assessment of atopic dermatitis. *J Am Acad Dermatol*. 2014;70(2):338-351.
13. Eichenfield LF, Tom WL, Berger TG, et al. Guidelines of care for the management of atopic dermatitis: section 2. Management and treatment of atopic dermatitis with topical therapies. *J Am Acad Dermatol*. 2014;71(1):116-132.

14. Sidbury R, Davis DM, Cohen DE, et al. Guidelines of care for the management of atopic dermatitis: section 3. Management and treatment with phototherapy and systemic agents. *J Am Acad Dermatol.* 2014;71(2):327-349.
15. Wollenberg A, Werfel T, Ring J, Ott H, Gieler U, Weidinger S. Atopic dermatitis in children and adults—diagnosis and treatment. *Dtsch Arztebl Int.* 2023;120(13):224-234.
16. Eichenfield LF, Krakowski AC, Piggot C, et al. Evidence-based recommendations for the diagnosis and treatment of pediatric acne. *Pediatrics.* 2013;131(suppl 3):S163-S186.

# 15 Geriatric Dermatology
Spencer Ng, MD, PhD

Diseases of older adults are becoming increasingly important as life expectancy increases worldwide. To promote healthy aging, it is important to understand and recognize the skin changes that occur over one's lifetime. Structural and physiologic skin changes, coupled with years of environmental insults, make the older adults especially susceptible to dermatologic disorders.[1]

As the skin ages, cellular turnover slows, with progressive loss of cells in the epidermis, dermis, and extracellular matrix.[2,3] Histologically, the rete pegs, which help to hold the epidermis to the dermis, are retracted,[4] leading to skin that is wrinkled, lax, and friable.[5,6] Years of sun exposure predispose the older adults to benign skin conditions (**solar lentigines**, **rosacea**) as well as premalignant and malignant skin conditions (**actinic keratoses**, **basal cell carcinoma**, **squamous cell carcinoma**, **lentigo maligna**, **malignant melanoma**).

Reduced stratum corneum lipid biosynthesis impairs permeability barrier function,[7] increasing the likelihood of **xerosis, pruritus, and seborrheic dermatitis**. There is decreased cutaneous blood flow and remodeling of microvasculature,[8,9] increasing the risk for vascular abnormalities such as **actinic (solar) purpura**, **stasis dermatitis**, **chronic leg ulcers**, and **pressure ulcers** (Fig. 15-1). Thermoregulation is also weakened due to fewer sweat glands and diminished subcutaneous fat,[5] increasing the older adult's sensitivity to moisture, heat, and cold (**skin maceration**, **intertrigo**, **erythema ab igne**).

A parallel blunting of normal immune function in the older adults produces higher levels of autoimmune skin disorders such as **bullous pemphigoid** and **pemphigus vulgaris**. Immunologic senescence also increases the potential for reactivation of latent viruses such as **herpes zoster (shingles)**. Despite immune senescence, inflammatory disorders of the skin, such as atopic dermatitis, may be underrecognized as a common etiology for xerosis and pruritus with a reported prevalence of 2% to 3% in those ages 65 and up. Functional decline of the skin barrier and skewing of adaptive immunity toward T-helper 2 responses may result in recurrence of prior atopic dermatitis (ie, from childhood/adolescence) or result in new-onset atopic dermatitis.[10]

With age comes skin growths that are often unwanted and unsightly, such as the exceedingly common **seborrheic keratosis**. Endearingly termed "wisdom spots," these benign skin thickenings are hereditary and increase proportionally with age. They are often confused by patients with skin cancer and as such are a frequent cause for referral to the outpatient dermatology clinic.

The etiology of allergic responses in the older adults can be challenging to diagnose. Patients often present with itchy, inflamed skin. The prevalence of polypharmacy in the older adults increases their risk for drug reactions and **urticaria**. Although elderly individuals have increased cumulative exposures to allergens,[11] normal immune senescence leads to diminished clinical manifestations, making diagnosis more difficult. Overall, it seems that the incidence of **allergic contact dermatitis** decreases with age; however, some allergens such as fragrance demonstrate increased

---

*The authors would like to acknowledge the first edition authors* Kathleen Nemer and David Sheinbein.

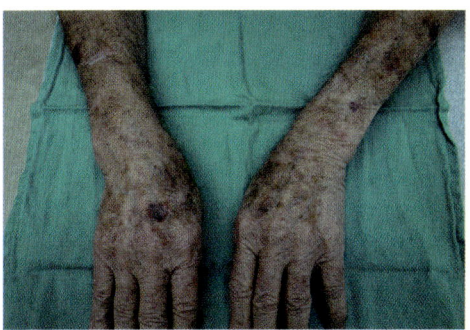

**Figure 15-1.** Purpuric, irregular macules of actinic (solar) purpura with prominent veins, skin wrinkling, and hemosiderin staining.

sensitization rates in the older adults.[12] The presence of ulcerated skin also increases sensitization rates, for example, in patients with chronic leg ulcers.[13]

When treating the elderly patient, the physician must take into consideration the patient's physical ability to comply with the recommended therapy as well as socioeconomic factors that impact compliance. Older patients often present with multiple comorbidities and the potential for cognitive dysfunction and/or impaired vision, hearing, and/or mobility. One medical problem can lead to a cascade of others. For example, a diabetic elderly patient is at risk for sensory, motor, and autonomic neuropathy, leading to limited sensation, decreased mobility of the lower extremities, and foot trauma. Immunosuppression in diabetics places them at higher risk for chronic fungal infection (**tinea pedis**, **onychomycosis**). Incidental foot trauma, coupled with fungal pathogens, creates a portal of entry for bacterial invasion of subcutaneous tissues (**cellulitis**).[14]

When treating elderly patients, it is important to consider extrinsic factors necessary for compliance. Some patients may not have adequate housing, nutrition, or the financial resources necessary for adequate compliance. For those who do have housing in long-term care facilities, there is increased risk for transmission of contagious infestations such as **scabies**. Scabies can cause a generalized eruption resembling erythroderma (generalized scaling and erythema over an extensive part of the body) in the older adults, the institutionalized, and those with immunosuppression or neurologic dysfunction. The inability to scratch in these patients can lead to **crusted or Norwegian scabies**, a more severe form of scabies with a higher mite burden.

Polypharmacy in the older adults increases the risk for medication confusion, while skin fragility increases safety concerns with overuse of topical medications prescribed. Given these factors, simple regimens for the shortest course possible are preferable in elderly patients. Extra effort may be necessary on the clinician's part to write down medication instructions for patients and caregivers so that they are accurately followed.

Many of the dermatologic conditions afflicting the older adults are seen in a wide range of ages. These entities are listed by chapter in Table 15-1 with a short clinical description of "*what to look for*" when distinguishing between them. Further details can be found within the appropriate chapter. The remaining common skin ailments in the older adults are discussed, with an emphasis on general skin care for dry, itchy skin, as these are intertwined as two of the most common skin complaints seen in the outpatient elderly patient.

| TABLE 15-1 | Common Elderly Dermatoses | |
|---|---|---|
| **Disorder** | ***Look For...*** | **Page** |
| **Inflammatory disorders** | | |
| Rosacea | Facial flushing, localized erythema, telangiectasias, erythematous papules and pustules on the nose, cheeks, brow, and chin; rhinophyma is more common in men. | |
| Allergic contact dermatitis | Red, itchy, burning rash in the distribution of allergen exposure. Look for well-demarcated borders and geometric shapes. Eyelid edema is seen when the allergen is innocently transferred from finger to lid. In nursing home patients, consider rubber catheters and body lotions as potential culprits. Patch testing may be necessary to identify the offending allergen. | |
| Seborrheic dermatitis | Loose, branlike, or greasy white scales often with background erythema. Characteristic sites: scalp (dandruff), eyebrows, eyelids, nasolabial folds, within and behind ears, sternum, umbilicus, groin (scrotum, labia minora), and perianal area. This is a common, chronic entity in the older adults and can be quite severe in HIV and Parkinson disease. | |
| **Infections and infestations** | | |
| Tinea pedis | Pruritic plaques on the dorsum of the foot; advancing edge with prominent erythema and scale. Plantar surface with powdery, white scale in a "moccasin" distribution. Interdigital web space scaling and white maceration (fourth web space most common). | |
| Intertrigo | Erythema or erosions of opposing skin surfaces: axillae, groin, perineum, inframammary creases, and abdominal folds. Patients are often obese and/or diabetic. In obese patients, look for inflammation in neck creases, popliteal or antecubital fossae, thigh and groin folds, and under pendulous breasts. Satellite papules suggest *Candida*. | |
| Herpes zoster (shingles) | 1-3 d prodrome of burning pain/paresthesias followed by an eruption of grouped papules and vesicles on an erythematous base. Usually confined to a distinct dermatome and not crossing midline. Postherpetic neuralgia can be quite painful and is more common in those over 70 years old. | |

| TABLE 15-1 | Common Elderly Dermatoses (*continued*) | |
|---|---|---|
| **Disorder** | ***Look For...*** | **Page** |
| Cellulitis | Rapidly progressive areas of skin edema, redness, warmth, tenderness, and lymphangitic streaking. Fever, malaise, and chills are common in immunosuppressed individuals. Tinea pedis and diabetes are risk factors. | |
| Scabies | Look for burrows: fine, threadlike, serpiginous lines with a terminal tiny black speck (the mite) with surrounding small erythematous papules and vesicles in the interdigital web spaces of the hands, flexor wrists, elbows, areolae, axillae, umbilicus, genitals, and buttocks. Spares the head and neck. Pruritus is intense, especially at night. Pruritic lesions on the areola in women and penis and scrotum in men are highly suggestive of scabies. Scabies is very contagious. Inquire about symptoms in family members and caretakers. | |
| Crusted/ Norwegian scabies | Thick, crusted plaques may be localized but are more often generalized involving the scalp, face, trunk, extremities, and periungual areas. Patients may present with generalized erythema and scaling. Typical burrows may be absent. The diagnosis is frequently missed, and transmission continues to those in physical contact with the individual. Always consider this diagnosis in any older adults, institutionalized, or immunocompromised patient with pruritus. | |
| **Reactive disorders and drug eruptions** | | |
| Stasis dermatitis | Bilateral erythema, hyperpigmentation, and scaling on the ankle and distal lower legs. Often, there is edema, varicosities, and atrophic patches indicative of venous insufficiency. Advanced disease may have a woody induration due to chronic adipose tissue ischemia (lipodermatosclerosis), characterized by an "inverted champagne bottle" due to fibrosis in the distal leg and edema in the proximal leg. Stasis dermatitis is often confused with cellulitis. Unlike cellulitis, stasis dermatitis is usually *scaly* and *bilateral*. | |
| Urticaria (hives) | Well-circumscribed, erythematous, edematous papules, patches, or plaques, often with a pale center. No single lesion lasts >24 h. May occur anywhere on the body but most often on the trunk. | |

(*continued*)

| TABLE 15-1 | Common Elderly Dermatoses (*continued*) | |
| --- | --- | --- |
| Disorder | Look For... | Page |
| Morbilliform drug eruption | Blanchable red macules and papules arising on the trunk and spreading symmetrically to the proximal extremities. Areas of pressure may be more severely affected. Pruritus is common. Superficial desquamation (scaling) occurs as the rash resolves. Onset is usually within 7-14 d of initiating a medication. | |
| **Benign skin lesions** | | |
| Seborrheic keratoses | Tan, brown, black, waxy, "stuck-on" appearing papules with a well-defined border. Pigmentation may vary within a single lesion. They occur anywhere except the palms, soles, and mucous membranes. **No malignant potential** but can be itchy and annoying; irritated by clothing (bra straps, underwear elastic) and jewelry (necklaces). Patients often scratch them off only to have them grow back. | |
| Solar lentigo | Tan to dark brown irregular macules on areas of sun exposure including the face, upper chest, shoulders, dorsal arms, and hands. Caused by chronic sun exposure. Present in 90% of Caucasians over 60 years old. A solar lentigo that looks different from the others or is enlarging or darkening should be biopsied to rule out lentigo maligna. | |
| **Malignant skin lesions** | | |
| Basal cell carcinoma | Nonhealing, pearly papule with a rolled border and telangiectasias on sun-exposed skin (face, trunk). Can bleed and ulcerate. Increased risk in fair-skinned patients. | |
| Actinic keratosis | Erythematous, raised, rough papules with associated scale; their "gritty" texture makes them easier felt than seen. | |
| Squamous cell carcinoma | Nonhealing, red papule, plaque, or nodule on sun-exposed skin (face, scalp, trunk, extremities). Over time, the tumor often develops a depressed center. Increased risk in fair-skinned and solid organ transplant patients. | |
| Lentigo maligna | Irregularly bordered, hyperpigmented (tan-brown) flat patch usually on the face of an elderly person. Predilection for the nose and cheeks. Looks like a "stain" on the skin of a fair-skinned person with a history of significant sun exposure. | |

| TABLE 15-1 | Common Elderly Dermatoses (*continued*) | |
|---|---|---|
| Disorder | Look For... | Page |
| Malignant melanoma | **Asymmetry:** draw a line through the lesion and the two sides do not match.<br>**Border:** irregular, notched, or scalloped borders.<br>**Color:** different shades of brown, tan, black, red, or white.<br>**Diameter:** >6 mm is concerning (size of a #2 pencil eraser).<br>**Evolution:** changing in size, shape, or color; pain, pruritus, or bleeding.<br>Caucasian men: most common location is the back.<br>Caucasian women: most common location is the back and legs. | |
| **Disorders of the hair and nails** | | |
| Onychomycosis | Thickened, yellowed fingernails or toenails (latter more common). Associated subungual debris and onycholysis (lifting of the nail plate from the nail bed at its distal end, resembling a half-moon). Commonly associated with concurrent tinea pedis. | |
| Brittle nail syndrome (Fragilitas unguium) | Look for excessive longitudinal ridging, roughness, and brittleness of the nail plate (trachyonychia/onychorrhexis) and horizontal lamellar splitting at the distal nail plate (onychoschizia). | |
| **Cutaneous manifestations of systemic disease** | | |
| Bullous pemphigoid | Large, tense bullae on an erythematous base filled with serous or blood-tinged fluid. Most often seen on the forearms, lower abdomen, and thighs of elderly individuals over 60 years old. Pruritus is very common and may precede bullae. Bullae are *tense* compared to the flaccid bullae of pemphigus vulgaris and are rarely seen on the mucosa. | |
| Pemphigus vulgaris | Flaccid bullae that break easily, leaving denuded erosions and risk for bacterial infection; frequently begins with oral lesions; blister spreads apart with application of pressure; first onset is in individuals 50-60 years old. | |
| Lichen sclerosus et atrophicus | Flat, ivory white, shiny scarlike plaques with a violaceous border. Most commonly found on the vulva and perianal skin in women and glans and prepuce of the penis in men but can be extragenital. Severely pruritic. Squamous cell carcinoma can arise in genital lesions. Complications related to genital scarring include dyspareunia, urinary obstruction, ulceration, painful erection, and phimosis. When on the genitals, the lesions may have purpura, and elderly abuse must be ruled out. | |

(*continued*)

| TABLE 15-1 | Common Elderly Dermatoses (*continued*) | |
|---|---|---|
| Disorder | Look For... | Page |
| **Geriatric dermatology** | | |
| Actinic purpura | See below. | |
| Erythema ab igne | See below. | |
| Leg ulcers | See below. | |
| Skin maceration | See below. | |
| Xerosis/Pruritus | See below. | |
| **The Washington Manual of Outpatient Internal Medicine**[15] | | |
| Pressure ulcers | Erythema, shallow erosion, or ulceration over a bony prominence or pressure point (sacrum, heels, occiput, elbows). More prevalent in patients who are bed or wheelchair bound. | pp. 771-775 |

# 1. Actinic Purpura

## 1.1. BACKGROUND

- Actinic purpura, also known as solar or senile purpura, is a benign form of purpura found almost exclusively in the older adults. Years of ultraviolet radiation induces atrophy of the dermis, rendering dermal blood vessels vulnerable to minor trauma. While the trauma itself often goes unrecognized, it causes noticeable leakage of red blood cells into the dermis.

## 1.2. CLINICAL PRESENTATION (FIG. 15-2)

- Asymptomatic violaceous macules and patches with irregular borders and sharp margins on the dorsal hands and extensor forearms. Ecchymoses may vary in deepness of color depending on their age and can persist for several weeks. They are most pronounced in fair-skinned individuals. Other signs of actinic damage are often present.

## 1.3. EVALUATION

- This is a clinical diagnosis. Of note, patients usually do not give a history of trauma and are often taking medications that exacerbate the condition (warfarin, clopidogrel, aspirin).

## 1.4. TREATMENT

- Minimize trauma to the skin.
- Protect the forearms from the sun with sunscreen and from trauma with a double layer of clothing. Long athletic socks with the feet cut off at the ankle can provide a protective layer for the arms when around the house/long-term care facility.

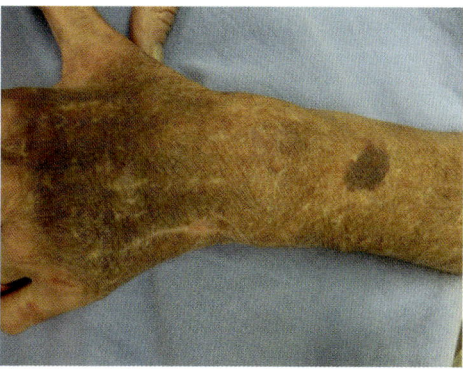

**Figure 15-2.** Hemosiderin deposition with a sharp demarcation between normal and abnormal skin. The linear white scars suggest dermal atrophy.

## 2. Erythema Ab Igne

### 2.1. BACKGROUND

- Erythema ab igne, derived from Latin for "redness from fire," is characterized by hyperpigmentation caused by long-term exposure to heat. The older adults are especially susceptible given prolonged exposure to hot water bottles, heating pads, or electric blankets. Sitting near a wood stove or fireplace as well as using a laptop computer on the lap are also risk factors. The disorder is seen more commonly in women.

### 2.2. CLINICAL PRESENTATION

- Reticular (netlike) or mottled patches of pink, purple, red, and eventually brown (from melanin deposition) in areas of heat exposure. Telangiectasia and other poikilodermatous changes (hypopigmentation, hyperpigmentation, or atrophy) can appear in long-standing cases. Burns do not occur, but pruritus or mild burning paresthesias can be present. The resultant pigmentation changes can be permanent.

### 2.3. EVALUATION

- This is a clinical diagnosis. When erythema ab igne is suspected, ask the patient specific questions regarding direct heat exposure (eg, heating pad, hot water bottle, exposure to radiant heat from a radiator, stove, or fireplace). Do not confuse with livedo reticularis and cutis marmorata, which are more erythematous and vascular appearing, have no associated hyperpigmentation, and are not related to heat exposure (more likely to be related to cold exposure).

### 2.4. TREATMENT

- Eliminate the source of the chronic heat exposure. In mild cases, the hyperpigmentation may remit. Elderly individuals, especially those with dementia, warrant an environmental safety assessment.

## 3. Leg Ulcers

### 3.1. BACKGROUND

- 90% of leg ulcers result from venous insufficiency, 5% result from arterial disease, and 5% are due to miscellaneous causes including diabetic microangiopathy, pyoderma gangrenosum, malignancies, vasculitis, and infections.[15]
- Venous ulcers are caused by incompetent one-way venous valves, leading to insufficient venous blood return, leg venous hypertension, aberrant tissue perfusion, and ischemia. Risk increases with age, a history of thrombosis, phlebitis, obesity, or leg injury such as fracture.
- Arterial ulcers are caused by inadequate blood supply to the skin from progressive atherosclerosis (peripheral vascular disease) or arterial embolization. Risk increases with diabetes mellitus, smoking, hyperlipidemia, obesity, rheumatoid arthritis, coronary artery disease, hypertension, hyperhomocysteinemia, male sex, and a sedentary lifestyle.

### 3.2. CLINICAL PRESENTATION

- Venous ulcers
  - Shallow, irregular borders; yellow, fibrinous exudate.
  - Most common on the medial malleolus in areas of preceding stasis dermatitis. May become circumferential over time.
  - Associated features include leg and ankle edema, varicose veins, yellow-brown pigmentation secondary to hemosiderin deposition, eczematous changes with scaling and crusting (stasis dermatitis), and lymphedema.
  - Pulses are normal.
  - Ulcers are not painful.
- Arterial ulcers
  - Sharply defined, punched out ulcer with a pale base over bony prominences with surrounding smooth, shiny skin.
  - Most common on the lateral malleolus, tips of the toes, and heel.
  - Associated features include cyanosis, pallor, cool extremities, and loss of hair.
  - Pulses are diminished and capillary refill is delayed (more than 3-4 seconds).
  - Ulcers are painful and patients often give a history of claudication. Pain is relieved by dependency of the extremity (eg, dangling the affected limb off the edge of the bed).

### 3.3. EVALUATION

- Ulcers presenting with the distinct characteristics of either venous or arterial disease can be diagnosed clinically. Skin biopsy is often useful in the diagnosis of enigmatic ulcers; however, consideration must be given to the long healing time of biopsy sites on the lower leg, where ulcers are most common.
- In cases of doubt, the best tests to distinguish between arterial and venous disease are ankle-brachial index (ABI) to evaluate for arterial disease and duplex ultrasound to evaluate for venous insufficiency. The correct diagnosis is significant because the management differs for each. For example, compression stockings are a mainstay of treatment for venous disease but worsen arterial disease.

- ABI values:
  - Normal ABI: 1.0 to 1.3
  - Noncompressible calcified vessel: greater than 1.3
  - Positive peripheral arterial disease: less than 0.9
- A vascular surgeon should evaluate any patient with a decrease in ABI.

## 3.4. TREATMENT[16,17]

- Venous ulcers
  - Treatment aims to improve venous return with **leg elevation** and **compression stockings**. Compression stockings should be tailored to fit the patient and the degree of venous insufficiency. Recommended pressure gradients are as follows:
    - **15 to 20 mm Hg**: mild varicose veins and minor leg swelling
    - **20 to 30 mm Hg**: moderate edema and moderate to severe varicosities
    - **30 to 40 mm Hg**: chronic venous insufficiency, severe edema, deep vein thrombosis and postthrombotic syndrome, venous ulceration, lymphedema, and orthostatic hypotension
  - Wet-to-dry dressings provide excellent mechanical débridement for 2 to 3 days, but longer use can interfere with wound healing. Keep wounds clean, covered, and moist with occlusive dressings. Cleanse with saline. Unna wraps are effective in severe cases.
  - Choice of wound dressing should be based on the amount of exudate, the depth of the ulceration, and the presence of slough.
  - Flat, shallow wounds with a low to medium amount of exudate do well with the following:
    - **Semipermeable films** (Tegaderm, OpSite Plus)
    - **Hydrocolloids** (DuoDERM, Tegasorb)
    - **Hydrogels** (IntraSite, Nu-Gel)
    - **Foam** (Allevyn brands)
  - Cavities and undermining wounds with a high amount of exudate do well with the following:
    - **Alginates** (Tegagen, Sorbsan, AlgiSite)
  - Ulcers with extensive necrotic tissue should be débrided. Treat secondarily infected wounds with systemic antibiotics and antimicrobial dressings:
    - **Iodosorb**
    - **Silver-impregnated dressings** (Acticoat, Aquacel Ag, Arglaes)
  - Associated stasis dermatitis may benefit from mid- to high-potency topical corticosteroids applied twice daily. Protect the ulcer with Vaseline petroleum jelly prior to application of corticosteroid.
  - Use of pentoxifylline 400 mg two to three times daily has been shown to be an effective adjunctive therapy in addition to compression therapy for the healing of venous ulcers.[18]
  - Ulcers recalcitrant to medical treatment may need surgical intervention including punch grafts, split-thickness grafts, epidermal or dermal engineered grafts, and ablation of the superficial venous system (VNUS procedure).
- Arterial ulcers
  - Treatment aims to improve arterial blood flow with wound care, revascularization, and risk factor modification.
  - Arterial ulcers can be treated similarly to venous ulcers (above) with the exception of compression stockings, which *worsen* ischemic ulcers. Arterial ulcers tend to

have slough but less exudate; thus, hydrogel dressings (IntraSite, Nu-Gel, Curasol) that rehydrate wounds and promote autolytic débridement are most efficacious.
- Risk factor modifications:
  - Strict blood sugar control and meticulous foot care in diabetics
  - Tobacco cessation
  - Antiplatelet therapy with aspirin or clopidogrel
  - Antihypertensive therapy
  - Lipid-lowering therapy: goal LDL cholesterol less than 100 mg/dL and in very high-risk patients less than 70 mg/dL
  - Encourage exercise as tolerated
- Amputation can be avoided with revascularization procedures: angioplasty, stenting, catheter-based plaque excision, or open lower extremity bypass.
- Nonhealing ulcerations, gangrene, rest pain, and worsening claudication are indications for surgical consideration.

# 4. Skin Maceration

## 4.1. BACKGROUND

- Maceration is defined as the softening and breaking down of skin resulting from prolonged exposure to moisture.[17] Excess moisture may be secondary to urinary or fecal incontinence, excessive sweating, occlusive dressings, or produced by a wound bed. In obese individuals, lesions may occur between skin folds. Macerated, moist skin can lead to pressure ulcers. For a detailed discussion of pressure ulcers, see *The Washington Manual of Outpatient Internal Medicine,* pp. 716-718.[18]

## 4.2. CLINICAL PRESENTATION

- Erythematous, abraded, or excoriated skin; there can be blisters and white or silver patches. Can affect any area constantly in contact with moisture.

## 4.3. EVALUATION

- Older adults who are bedbound or incontinent of urine/feces are at risk of developing lesions on the buttocks or sacrum. These areas should be checked regularly by caregivers for both skin maceration and pressure ulcers.

## 4.4. TREATMENT[19]

- Eliminate the cause of moisture:
  - Toileting program for incontinence
  - Condom catheter
  - Indwelling catheter (if condom catheter not adequate)
  - Fecal incontinence collector
- Protect the skin from moisture:
  - Clean gently with a mild, nondrying soap (Dove, Oil of Olay, or Cetaphil) after each incontinent episode.
  - Apply a moisture barrier (Vaseline, Proshield, Smooth and Cool, Calmoseptine, or zinc oxide).

- For irritated perianal skin, it is useful to apply an over-the-counter low-potency steroid (1% hydrocortisone cream) mixed with a low-potency antifungal (clotrimazole cream [Canesten or Lotrimin]).
- Use disposable briefs that wick moisture from the skin; use linen incontinence pads when disposable briefs worsen perineal dermatitis.

# 5. Xerosis/Pruritus

## 5.1. BACKGROUND

- Dry, itchy skin is a frequent ailment in the older adults. Skin thinning, coupled with decreased permeability barrier function, leads to persistently dry skin.[7] Dryness (xerosis) is the number one cause of itchy skin (pruritus). Other causes of pruritus in the older adults are listed in Table 15-2. When a common cause of pruritus cannot be identified, other avenues must be explored. Pruritus without a rash may be caused by several disparate underlying systemic diseases, listed in Table 15-3. A thorough workup should be undertaken if any such disease is suspected.
- Medication-induced pruritus should be entertained in those individuals with intractable itching after the more usual causes have been excluded. Common drugs associated with pruritus in the older adults include the following[20-22]:
  - **Narcotics** (opioids)
  - **Antihypertensives** (calcium channel blockers, beta adrenergic blockers, angiotensin-converting enzyme inhibitors, angiotensin II antagonists [sartans])
  - **Statins**
  - **Antidiabetic drugs** (biguanides, sulfonylurea derivatives)
  - **Antibiotics**
  - **Antiepileptics**
  - **Antimalarials** (hydroxychloroquine)
  - **Psychotropic drugs** (tricyclic antidepressants, selective serotonin reuptake inhibitors, neuroleptics)
  - **Chemotherapeutics**
  - **Nonsteroidal anti-inflammatory drugs**
  - **Corticosteroids**
  - **Sex hormones**
  - **Antithyroid agents**
  - **B vitamins** (cyanocobalamin, niacin, thiamine)

## 5.2. CLINICAL PRESENTATION

- Dull, rough, flaky, dry, cracked skin. There can be fine branlike scales that flake off easily. Can present as large patches of dryness or smaller, nummular lesions. Repeated scratching can result in lichenification (thickened skin), excoriations, infection, and traumatic purpura.
- Xerosis usually worsens in the wintertime, exacerbated by low humidity, frequent bathing, and harsh soaps. Severe xerosis may present as asteatotic eczema, also known as *eczema craquelé* or *winter itch*. The skin is rough and dry with fine scale and interconnected fissures resembling cracked porcelain. Asteatotic eczema classically involves the lower legs but may involve the upper arms, anterior thighs, and lower back.[23]

## TABLE 15-2 Pruritus in the Older Adults

**Autoimmune blistering diseases**

Acquired epidermolysis bullosa
Bullous pemphigoid
Dermatitis herpetiformis
Pemphigus vulgaris

**Autoimmune connective tissue diseases**

Dermatomyositis
Sjögren syndrome
Systemic sclerosis

**Cutaneous lymphomas**

Mycosis fungoides and its variants
Sézary syndrome

**Erythematous papulosquamous diseases**

Darier disease
Grover disease
Hailey-Hailey disease
Lichen planus
Palmoplantar pustulosis
Pityriasis rubra pilaris
Polymorphic light eruption
Psoriasis

**Inflammatory diseases**

Allergic contact dermatitis
Atopic dermatitis (eczema)
Dyshidrotic eczema
Urticaria

**Other benign skin conditions**

Lichen sclerosus et atrophicus
Seborrheic dermatitis
Seborrheic keratosis

**Skin infections and infestations**

Cutaneous larva migrans
Folliculitis
Herpes simplex
Herpes zoster
Insect bites and arthropod reactions
Intertrigo
Lice (pediculosis)
Scabies
Tinea

**Xerosis (dry skin)**

## TABLE 15-3  Systemic Diseases With Associated Pruritus

**Endocrine diseases**

Hyperthyroidism
Hypothyroidism
Hyperparathyroidism
Diabetes

**Hematologic diseases**

Polycythemia vera (pruritus follows contact with heat, especially hot water)
Hodgkin lymphoma
Non-Hodgkin lymphoma
Leukemias
Myeloma multiplex
Iron deficiency
Systemic mastocytosis
Hypereosinophilic syndrome
Myelodysplastic syndromes

**Infectious diseases**

HIV infection/AIDS
Infestations (see above)

**Kidney disease**

Chronic kidney disease

**Liver diseases (look for jaundice)**

Primary biliary cirrhosis
Primary sclerosing cholangitis
Extrahepatic cholestasis
Hepatitis B and C

**Malnutrition**

Vitamin deficiencies (iron, vitamin A, vitamin D, zinc, B vitamins)

**Neurologic diseases**

Postherpetic itch
Notalgia paresthetica
Brain injury/tumor (frequently unilateral pruritus)
Sclerosis multiplex
Small fiber neuropathy

**Other malignancies**

Solid tumors (paraneoplastic pruritus)
Carcinoid syndrome
Cutaneous lymphomas (mycosis fungoides, Sézary syndrome)

**Psychogenic diseases**

Obsessive-compulsive disorder (OCD)
Anxiety
Neurotic excoriations
Delusions of parasitosis

## 5.3. EVALUATION

- The physical examination should include a search for any other skin manifestations. While pruritus is most often related to xerosis, care should be taken to palpate for thyroid, liver, or lymph node abnormalities, especially if systemic disease is suspected.
- Suggested baseline evaluations for pruritus of unknown etiology are listed in Table 15-4.

## 5.4. TREATMENT

- Xerosis and pruritus in the older adults can create substantial suffering and often prove difficult to treat. Treatment focuses on general skin care with avoidance of provocative factors and frequent topical moisturization.
- Bathing
  - Take short baths or showers (<5 minutes).
  - Avoid hot water (use tepid water), especially in the wintertime.
  - Avoid bath oils, which can lead to falls from slippery feet.
  - Apply an emollient (ointment is best) within 3 minutes of bathing for maximal effect.
  - Invest in a humidifier.
- Soaps
  - Use mild, nondrying soaps such as Dove, Oil of Olay, Cetaphil, Tone, or Purpose.
  - Use of washcloths and loofahs is discouraged as they can harbor bacteria.
  - Limit soap to axilla and groin.
- After bathing
  - Pat dry and apply thick moisturizers while the skin is still wet.
  - Ointments such as Vaseline and Aquaphor are the most lubricating and occlusive, making them the most potent. The downside is that they can be greasy and thus more difficult to apply.
  - Creams are less lubricating than ointments but more lubricating than gels, lotions, and solutions. They also are more likely to have additives that may irritate the skin (lanolin, aloe vera, and parabens). Thus, if a patient complains of burning or stinging with a cream, try switching to the comparable ointment. Recommended creams include Aveeno, Eucerin, CeraVe, Curél, Cetaphil, Vanicream, or Lubriderm.
  - Apply ointments/creams multiple times daily.
  - Occlusion with plastic wrap or gloves after application of emollients increases their potency.

| TABLE 15-4 | Suggested Evaluations for Pruritus of Unknown Etiology |
|---|---|
| Complete blood count with differential | |
| Basic metabolic panel | |
| Iron studies (iron, ferritin) | |
| Thyroid-stimulating hormone | |
| Liver function tests | |
| Human immunodeficiency virus test | |
| Chest radiograph | |
| Vitamin levels | |

- Antipruritics
  - Camphor 1% to 3% and menthol (Sarna) provide a cooling sensation and should be stored in the refrigerator for maximal effect.
  - Topical anesthetics (benzocaine), antihistamines (diphenhydramine), and neomycin are best avoided because of the high rate of contact dermatitis.
  - Systemic antihistamines (H1-receptor antagonists) are helpful for sedative effect (cetirizine, loratadine, hydroxyzine, doxepin).
  - In recalcitrant cases, low-dose mirtazapine (7.5 mg qhs) or gabapentin (300 mg qhs) can be used for pruritus and carefully titrated up if tolerated and effective.
- Corticosteroids
  - Mild to mid-potency topical steroids may be used on inflamed pruritic skin.
  - As with emollients, occlusion increases potency. Given the potential for skin thinning, steroid occlusion should be reserved for severe, resistant lesions and for a limited amount of time (such as in the evening while watching television).
  - Mid-potency topical corticosteroids (classes 3-4):
    - Triamcinolone cream or ointment: apply twice daily
    - Mometasone cream or ointment: apply twice daily
    - Fluocinolone cream or ointment: apply twice daily
  - Low-potency topical corticosteroids for thinner skin (eg, face, groin) (classes 6-7):
    - Desonide cream, lotion, or ointment: apply twice daily
    - Hydrocortisone 1% (over the counter) or 2.5% cream or ointment: apply twice daily
- In sum:
  - Patients can minimize the effect of xerosis by increasing the ambient humidity in their living environment, modifying their bathing technique, and using emollients multiple times daily to replace the lipid components of their skin.
  - A word about the use of systemic agents to treat inflammatory skin disease in geriatric patients:
    - Although not Food and Drug Administration–approved for the treatment of xerosis/pruritus specifically, use of biologics targeting the T-helper 2 immune axis (ie, IL-4/IL-13 receptor antagonists, IL-13 antagonists) have demonstrated efficacy in treating these symptoms in patients with underlying atopic dermatitis and prurigo nodularis.[24]
    - Initial clinical trials for the use of IL-4/IL-13 receptor antagonists, such as dupilumab, included patients from the ages of 18 to 65, excluding more elderly patients. However, more recent studies specifically in geriatric patients have shown it is just as efficacious in treating atopic dermatitis and safe as in younger patients.[25]
    - Use of small molecule inhibitors of the Janus kinase (JAK) or related family of proteins to treat atopic dermatitis and psoriasis have recently been Food and Drug Administration approved and have demonstrated efficacy in elderly patients.[26] However, increased rates of treatment cessation secondary to adverse effects have been reported in this particular demographic.[27]
    - More traditional immunosuppressive medications such as prednisone or cyclosporine should be used with caution in the elderly population due to frequent comorbidities such as diabetes and kidney disease, which may be worsened with the use of such medications.[28]

# REFERENCES

1. Farage MA, Miller KW, Berardesca E, Maibach HI. Clinical implications of aging skin: cutaneous disorders in the elderly. *Am J Clin Dermatol.* 2009;10(2):73-86.
2. Kligman AM. Perspectives and problems in cutaneous gerontology. *J Invest Dermatol.* 1979;73(1):39-46.
3. Branchet MC, Boisnic S, Frances C, Robert AM. Skin thickness changes in normal aging skin. *Gerontology.* 1990;36(1):28-35.
4. Waller JM, Maibach HI. Age and skin structure and function, a quantitative approach (I): blood flow, pH, thickness, and ultrasound echogenicity. *Skin Res Technol.* 2005;11(4):221-235.
5. Gilchrest BA. Skin aging and photoaging: an overview. *J Am Acad Dermatol.* 1989;21(3 Pt 2):610-613.
6. Tindall JP, Smith JG. Skin Lesions of the aged and their association with internal changes. *JAMA.* 1963;186:1039-1042.
7. Elias PM, Ghadially R. The aged epidermal permeability barrier: basis for functional abnormalities. *Clin Geriatr Med.* 2002;18(1):103-120. vii.
8. Chang E, Yang J, Nagavarapu U, Herron GS. Aging and survival of cutaneous microvasculature. *J Invest Dermatol.* 2002;118(5):752-758.
9. Tsuchida Y. The effect of aging and arteriosclerosis on human skin blood flow. *J Dermatol Sci.* 1993;5(3):175-181.
10. Jull AB, Arrol B, Parag V, Waters J. Pentoxifylline for treating venous leg ulcers. *Cochrane Database Sys Review.* 2012;12(12):CD001733.
11. Na CR, Wang S, Kirsner RS, Federman DG. Elderly adults and skin disorders: common problems for nondermatologists. *South Med J.* 2012;105(11):600-606.
12. Buckley DA, Rycroft RJ, White IR, McFadden JP. The frequency of fragrance allergy in patch-tested patients increases with their age. *Br J Dermatol.* 2003;149(5):986-989.
13. Saap L, Fahim S, Arsenault E, et al. Contact sensitivity in patients with leg ulcerations: a North American study. *Arch Dermatol.* 2004;140(10):1241-1246.
14. Al Hasan M, Fitzgerald SM, Saoudian M, Krishnaswamy G. Dermatology for the practicing allergist: *Tinea pedis* and its complications. *Clin Mol Allergy.* 2004;2(1):5.
15. Rosman I, Lloyd B, Jassim O. Dermatology. In: De Fer TM, Brisco MA, Muller RS, eds. *The Washington Manual of Outpatient Internal Medicine.* 1st ed. Lippincott Williams & Wilkins; 2010:831-861.
16. Hafner A, Sprecher E. Ulcers. In: Bolognia JL, Jorizzo JL, Schaffer JV, eds. *Dermatology.* 3rd ed. Elsevier Saunders; 2012:1729-1746.
17. Menaker GM, Mehlis SL, Kasprowicz S. Dressings. In: Bolognia JL, Jorizzo JL, Schaffer JV, eds. *Dermatology.* 3rd ed. Elsevier Saunders; 2012:2365-2379.
18. Anderson KN. *Mosby's Medical Nursing and Allied Health Dictionary.* Mosby-Year Book; 1998.
19. Reuben DB, Herr KA, Pacala JT, Pollock BG, Potter JF, Semla TP. *Geriatrics at your fingertips.* 13th ed. American Geriatrics Society; 2011.
20. Reich A, Ständer S, Szepietowski JC. Drug-induced pruritus: a review. *Acta Derm Venereol.* 2009;89(3):236-244.
21. Reich A, Ständer S, Szepietowski JC. Pruritus in the elderly. *Clin Dermatol.* 2011;29(1):15-23.
22. Tripathi S, Kim B. The Science of Chronic Itch: a current review of the pathophysiology & clinical presentations of chronic pruritus to help you manage your itchy patients. *Rheumatologist.* 2014;8(12):32-42.
23. Piérard GE, Quatresooz P. What do you mean by eczema craquelé? *Dermatology.* 2007;215(1):3-4.
24. Silverberg JI, Lynde CW, Abuabara K. Efficacy and safety of dupilumab maintained in adults ≥ 60 years of age with moderate-to-severe atopic dermatitis: analysis of pooled data from four randomized clinical trials. *Am J Clin Derm.* 2023;24(3):469-483.
25. Zhou X, Yang G, Chen X. Efficacy and safety of dupilumab in older patients (aged 80 years and above) with atopic dermatitis: a prospective study. *Drugs Aging.* 2023;40(10):933-940.
26. Hren HG, Khattri S. Use of systemic Janus kinase inhibitors for dermatologic indications in the elderly: a retrospective study of 67 cases. *J Am Acad Derm.* 2024;90(4):816-819.
27. Rajasimhan S, Pamuk O, Katz JD. Safety of Janus kinase inhibitors in older patients: a focus on the thromboembolic risk. *Drugs Aging.* 2020;37(8):551-558.
28. Endo JO, Wong JW, Norman RA. Geriatric dermatology: part I. Geriatric pharmacology for the dermatologist. *J Am Acad Derm.* 2013;68(4):521.e1-521.e10.
29. Khalid S, Carr DB. Geriatrics. In: De Fer TM, Brisco MA, Muller RS, eds. *The Washington Manual of Outpatient Internal Medicine.* 1st ed. Lippincott Williams & Wilkins; 2010:699-722.

# 16 Sun Safety

M. Laurin Council, MD, MBA

Exposure to ultraviolet (UV) light is the most important modifiable risk factor for skin cancer. Regular use of broad-spectrum sunscreen can reduce the risk of sunburn, prevent skin cancer, and decrease skin aging. Clothing provides some protection from UV radiation; the amount of protection depends on the weave of the fabric, dye color, fabric material, and dryness. Tanning bed use has been associated with a substantial increased risk for both melanoma and nonmelanoma skin cancer. All patients should be counseled to avoid excessive UV exposure, including indoor tanning.

## 1. Sunscreens

- A primer on UV radiation
  - UV light is the portion of the electromagnetic spectrum that encompasses the wavelengths 100 to 400 nm. The UV spectrum is divided into three bands: UVC (100-280 nm), UVB (280-320 nm), and UVA (320-400 nm). The ozone layer blocks all UVC and 90% of UVB rays produced by the sun; subsequently, the vast majority of the UV radiation that reaches the earth's surface is UVA.[1,2]
  - UV penetration into the skin varies with wavelength, with longer wavelengths penetrating deeper into the skin. UVB causes cross-linking of deoxyribonucleic acid (DNA), leading to pyrimidine dimer formation and pyrimidine-pyrimidone 6,4-photoproducts. UVA induces generation of reactive oxygen species leading to DNA strand breaks.[1]
  - Short-term effects of UV radiation on the skin include sunburn and tanning. UVB induces an inflammatory response that generates the prototypical erythema and blistering of a sunburn. Immediate tanning occurs secondary to UVA-induced oxidation and redistribution of the existing melanin. Delayed tanning peaks 3 days after UV exposure and is due to increased melanin synthesis and increased numbers of melanocytes.[1]
  - Long-term effects of chronic sun exposure include photoaging and photocarcinogenesis. The chronic inflammation induced by repetitive exposure to excessive UV radiation results in skin wrinkling, irregular skin pigmentation, and thickening of the skin that leads to a leathery appearance. The DNA damage induced by UV radiation is known to be important in the pathogenesis of skin cancer.[1,2]
- The UV index
  - The UV radiation level varies with latitude, altitude, time of day, and time of year. UV levels are higher at lower latitudes (closer to the equator), higher altitudes, during midday, and during summer months. Only a small fraction of UV light is filtered by clouds.[2]
  - The UV index was developed as a tool to provide the public with an objective measure of UV radiation levels and raise awareness for the need to use sun protection (Table 16-1).[3]

---

*The authors would like to acknowledge the first edition authors Rachel Braden and Kim Brady.*

### TABLE 16-1  The UV Index

| | UV Index | Associated Risk |
|---|---|---|
| Low | 0-2 | No danger to the average person |
| Moderate | 3-5 | Little risk of harm from unprotected sun exposure |
| High | 6-7 | High risk of harm from unprotected sun exposure |
| Very high | 8-10 | Very high risk of harm from unprotected sun exposure |
| Extreme | 11-14 | Extreme risk of harm from unprotected sun exposure |

The index is color coded to ease public recognition and facilitate inclusion of the index in weather forecasts.

- Rationale for use
  - UV radiation is a known carcinogen.[4] However, complete sun avoidance is neither always possible nor practical.
  - The development of both melanoma and nonmelanoma skin cancers is clearly associated with exposure to UV radiation from the sun.[1-6] Sunburn at any age increases an individual's risk for skin cancer.[1,5]
  - Broad-spectrum sunscreens with at least sun protection factor (SPF) 15 have been proven to decrease the risk of actinic keratoses and squamous cell cancers.[1,3,7] There is limited evidence to support efficacy for prevention of basal cell carcinoma and melanoma. Regular sunscreen use also can prevent photoaging.[1,7]
- Mechanism of action
  - The active agents in sunscreen form a protective coating on the surface of the stratum corneum that attenuates UV radiation in one of two ways: reflection or absorption.
  - **Physical blockers** or "inorganic" sunscreens, such as zinc oxide or titanium dioxide, form a film of inert metal particles on the skin that reflect both UVA and UVB. Advances in nanotechnology have allowed for the development of micronized inorganic sunscreens, which are less opaque and more cosmetically acceptable.[1]
  - **Chemical absorbers** or "organic" sunscreens function as UV filters, which absorb the energy in UVA, UVB, or both; this energy is converted to a negligible amount of heat. The specific absorption spectrum of each chemical varies, and most sunscreens contain a combination of multiple chemical agents to provide broad-spectrum protection and act as stabilizing agents (Table 16-2).[1,7] Aminobenzoates, cinnamates, salicylates, octocrylene, and ensulizole provide protection against UVB, while benzophenones, avobenzone, ecamsule, and meradimate provide UVA protection.
- Sun protection factor
  - The **sun protection factor (SPF)** is a commonly used measure of efficacy for sunscreens. The SPF is the ratio of the minimal erythema dose of sunscreen-protected skin to the minimal erythema dose of unprotected skin.[1] It is expressed as a factor reflecting the relative amount of time skin can be exposed to sunlight without developing erythema, such that an SPF of 10 would allow 10 times as much time in the sun with the same resultant erythema as would unprotected skin. This assumes perfect use with a thick application of at least 2 mg/cm$^2$. In reality, most people do not apply sunscreen according to this recommendation.[3,5]

### TABLE 16-2  The Absorption Spectrum of Ingredients Commonly Used in Chemical and Physical Sunscreens

|  | Absorption Spectrum | |
|---|---|---|
| **Chemical Absorbers** | UVB | UVA |
| Benzophenones | | |
|   Dioxybenzone | × | |
|   Oxybenzone | × | × |
|   Sulisobenzone | | × |
| Cinnamates | | |
|   Cinoxate | × | |
|   Octinoxate | × | |
| Salicylates | | |
|   Homosalate | × | |
|   Octisalate | × | |
|   Trolamine salicylate | × | |
| PABA derivatives | | |
|   PABA (*para*-aminobenzoic acid) | × | |
|   Padimate O | × | |
| Miscellaneous | | |
|   Avobenzone | | × |
|   Ecamsule | | × |
|   Ensulizole | × | |
|   Meradimate | | × |
|   Octocrylene | × | |
| **Physical blockers** | | |
|   Titanium dioxide | × | × |
|   Zinc oxide | × | × |
|   Iron oxide | × | × |

- The SPF is related to the percentage of blocked erythemal radiation (Fig. 16-1). This relationship is nonlinear, such that a sunscreen with SPF 20 blocks 95% of erythemal radiation, while a sunscreen with SPF 40 blocks 97.5%.[1] Sunscreens with a higher SPF do not remain effective longer than do those with a lower SPF and still must be reapplied frequently.[3,6]
- Because UVB radiation is responsible for the erythema produced during a sunburn, **SPF only measures efficacy against UVB**. There is no standard to measure protection against UVA light, but there are in vitro assays utilizing spectrophotometry to calculate the percentage of UVA rays absorbed by a given chemical, as well as in vivo assays measuring either immediate or delayed skin pigment darkening.
- Safety
  - The first commercial sunscreen was developed in 1928. Sunscreens have been widely used since the 1970s and have an excellent safety profile.

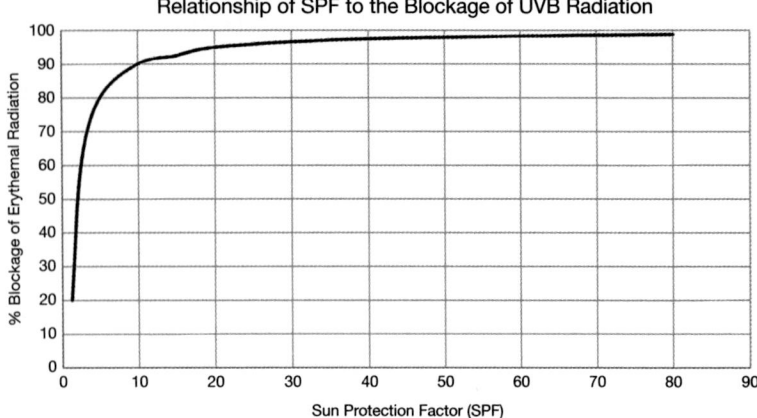

**Figure 16-1.** The relationship of SPF to the blockage of UVB radiation. This is a nonlinear relationship, and as SPF increases beyond 30, there is minimal added protection.

- The main risks associated with sunscreen use are **minor skin irritation**, which is common, and **allergic contact dermatitis**, which is rare.[1] The most common agents implicated in allergic contact dermatitis include the chemical absorbers oxybenzone, padimate O, and avobenzone. Sunscreens containing only physical blockers are available for patients who develop allergic reactions to one of these agents or for those who have sensitive skin that is prone to irritation.
- UV exposure stimulates vitamin D production in the skin. Casual sun exposure (5-15 min/d, 2 to 3 times per week) can provide enough vitamin D for most people. **Adequate vitamin D can safely be obtained via dietary sources** without exposure to the risks of UV radiation, and there is no clear evidence that regular sunscreen use causes vitamin D deficiency.[8]
- Regulation
  - Sunscreens are regulated by the Food and Drug Administration (FDA) as over-the-counter medications. In 2012, the FDA updated labeling requirements for sunscreens. Any sunscreen marketed as **"broad spectrum"** has to pass tests proving efficacy against **both UVA and UVB**.[7] In 2019, the FDA released further revisions in its proposed rule for sunscreen drug products for over-the-counter human use.[9]
  - Products that are not broad spectrum or that have SPF less than 15 are labeled with a warning to caution that they only prevent sunburn and should not be used for the prevention of skin cancer or early skin aging.
  - Sunscreens can no longer be labeled as "waterproof" or "sweatproof." Sunscreens labeled as **"water resistant" and "very water resistant"** must pass a standardized test to assure they retain their protective effects after prolonged immersion of the skin in water for 40 or 80 minutes, respectively.[7]
  - There is a labeling cap of SPF 60+ on sunscreens in the United States, as sunscreens greater than SPF 50 have not been proven to provide increased protection.
  - In the 2019 proposed rule, the FDA classified two commonly used sunscreen ingredients, zinc oxide and titanium dioxide, as GRASE (Generally Recognized As Safe and Effective) in concentrations up to 25%. For the remainder of sunscreen ingredients studied, the FDA declared insufficient data to permit final classification.[10]

- Application
  - Patients, especially those with lighter skin types, should be counseled to use sunscreen on a daily basis.
  - Sunscreen used for daily sun protection should be **broad spectrum and have an SPF of at least 15**. All areas of exposed skin should be covered with an adequate layer of sunscreen, including the face.
  - **During outdoor activities with exposure to sunlight**, sunscreen should be used that has an **SPF of at least 30**. Sunscreen should be **reapplied every 2 hours**, and more frequently if skin is exposed to water (sweat, swimming). Sunscreen use should not be used with the aim of increasing the duration of sun exposure.

## 1.1. SUN PROTECTIVE CLOTHING

- The UV protection factor
  - UV protection claims for clothing are rated according to the "**Ultraviolet Protection Factor (UPF)**," which is analogous to the SPF rating system for sunscreens. A UPF of 25 means that only 1/25th of UV radiation will pass through the fabric. While SPF only measures a sunscreen's efficacy against UVB radiation, UPF measures efficacy against both UVA and UVB rays.[3,6]
- Rationale for use
  - The UPF of clothing varies depending on several factors, and more protection is provided by tighter weaves, darker dyes, synthetic fabrics, and dry fabrics. Many clothing manufacturers have begun specifically developing and marketing UV-protective clothing. These fabrics have enhanced protection from UV light by virtue of either construction with a dense weave or dyeing with chemicals that function as UV filters.
  - While UV-protective clothing has undergone various standardized tests analyzing UV transmission through fabrics, it is important to remember that unlabeled clothing also provides protection from UV light.[3]
  - Hats should have a brim wide enough to shade the entire face (typically >2 in). The eyes are also vulnerable to UV-induced damage. Sunglasses should be chosen that provide broad-spectrum UV protection.[5]

## 1.2. TANNING BED USE

- Risks associated with indoor tanning:
  - Indoor tanning increases the risk for developing both melanoma and nonmelanoma skin cancers. Risks appear to be dose and age dependent, with the youngest and most frequent users at highest risk.[11,12]
  - Any change in skin pigmentation is a sign of overexposure to UV light and resulting DNA damage. A "base tan" from indoor tanning correlates to only an SPF of 1 to 2, and a tan from outdoor tanning correlates to an SPF of 2 to 3.1.
  - The U.S. Centers for Disease Control and Prevention (CDC) estimates that one in three Caucasian young adult women, the population at highest risk for future skin cancers, engage in indoor tanning each year.[13]
  - The average intensity of UV radiation from indoor tanning devices correlates to a UV index of 13 or 14 (extreme), which is up to five times the amount of UV exposure of natural light. The amount and type of UV radiation emitted varies widely between devices and often exceeds FDA-recommended limits.[5]
  - In addition to increasing skin cancer risk, tanning beds carry additional risks including sunburns, damage to the eyes, and skin infections caused by exposure to improperly sanitized devices.

- Regulations
  - In 2009, the World Health Organization (WHO) classified indoor tanning beds as class 1 human carcinogens.[4,13] Many countries, including France, Spain, Germany, Italy, Norway, and the United Kingdom, have subsequently banned the use of tanning beds for those under age 18. Australia and Brazil recently instituted total bans on indoor tanning for cosmetic purposes.
  - In the United States, tanning bed restrictions have thus far been legislated on a state by state basis. Several states have banned use of tanning beds by minors, and others require parental consent. Some states have instituted limits on tanning bed frequency or tanning time limits.
  - The FDA recently reclassified tanning bed devices from class I (low-risk) to class II (moderate-risk) devices.[14] Tanning beds must now carry a visible black box warning explicitly stating that the device should not be used by persons under 18 years of age.
- Alternatives to tanning bed use
  - **Sunless tanning lotions** contain dihydroxyacetone (DHA), a color additive that binds to the stratum corneum and colors the skin to produce a darkened appearance, which does not provide any additional protection against UV radiation. These lotions are **only FDA approved for external application**.
  - **Spray tanning** involves the use of DHA as a misting spray. There are insufficient safety data regarding DHA exposure to mucous membranes, periorbital surfaces, or inhalational exposure; therefore, use of DHA in this fashion is not FDA approved.
  - Pills containing large doses of canthaxanthin or other food color additives have been illegally marketed as "tanning pills" in the United States. The dyes deposit in the skin, imparting a darker color. The dyes also deposit in other organs of the body, including the eyes, and retinopathy is a known side effect.
  - Injectable analogs of melanocyte-stimulating hormone, which increase melanogenesis, have been developed and illegally marketed in the last decade. Patients should be counseled that commercially marketed injections claiming to induce melanogenesis are unapproved and may be hazardous to their health.
- Counseling
  - All patients should be counseled regarding the dangers of excessive UV radiation and the importance of sun safety including sun avoidance, sunscreen, and the use of protective clothing.[1,3,5] The U.S. Preventive Services Task Force has specifically recommended that primary care physicians conduct a brief behavioral counseling intervention warning of the dangers of indoor tanning for those at highest risk: patients with fair skin aged 6 months to 24 years.[15]
  - Some studies have suggested that counseling focused on the appearance-related side effects of sun exposure is more successful than are cancer prevention–focused messages.

# REFERENCES

1. Bolognia JL, Jorizzo JL, Schaffer JV. *Dermatology*. 3rd ed. Elsevier Saunders; 2012.
2. Lucas R, McMichael M, Smith W, et al; World Health Organization. *Solar Ultraviolet Radiation: Global Burden of Disease from Solar Ultraviolet Radiation*. World Health Organization Public Health and the Environment; 2006.
3. U.S. Environmental Protection Agency, Office of Air and Radiation. *SunWise Program*. Accessed December 18, 2014. http://www2.epa.gov/sunwise

4. International Agency for Research on Cancer Working Group on the Evaluation of Carcinogenic Risks to Humans; World Health Organization. Radiation. *IARC Monogr Eval Carcinog Risks Hum.* 2012;100:7-303.
5. U.S. Department of Health and Human Services. *The Surgeon General's Call to Action to Prevent Skin Cancer.* U.S. Department of Health and Human Services, Office of the Surgeon General; 2014.
6. Centers for Disease Control and Prevention. *Skin Cancer: Sun Safety.* Accessed December 18, 2014. http://www.cdc.gov/cancer/skin/basic_info/sun-safety.htm
7. U.S. Food and Drug Administration; U.S. Department of Health and Human Services. Labeling and effectiveness testing; sunscreen drug products for over-the-counter human use. Final rule. *Fed Regist.* 2011;76:35620-35665.
8. Ross AC, Taylor CL, Yaktine AL, et al; Institute of Medicine (US). *Dietary Reference Intakes for Calcium and Vitamin D.* National Academies Press (US); 2011.
9. The Federal Register. 2019. https://www.federalregister.gov/documents/2019/02/26/2019-03019/sunscreen-drug-products-for-over-the-counter-human-use
10. CPT. *An Overview of the FDA Changes to Sunscreen Regulation in 2019.* https://cptclabs.com/wp-content/uploads/CPT-Overview-FDA-Sunscreen-Regulation-2019.pdf
11. Wehner MR, Shive ML, Chren MM, Han J, Qureshi AA, Linos E. Indoor tanning and non-melanoma skin cancer: systematic review and meta-analysis. *BMJ.* 2012;345:5909.
12. Colantonio S, Bracken MB, Beecker J. The association of indoor tanning and melanoma in adults: systematic review and meta-analysis. *J Am Acad Dermatol.* 2014;70:847-857.
13. Centers for Disease Control and Prevention (CDC). Use of indoor tanning devices by adults—United States, 2010. *MMWR Morb Mortal Wkly Rep.* 2012;61:323-326.
14. Ernst A, Grimm A, Lim HW. Tanning lamps: health effects and reclassification by the Food and Drug Administration. *J Am Acad Dermatol.* 2015;72:175-180.
15. US Preventive Services Task Force. Behavioral counseling to prevent skin cancer: US Preventive Services Task Force recommendation statement. *JAMA.* 2018;319(11):1134-1142.

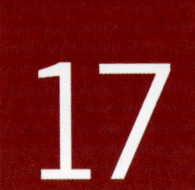

# Dermatologic Therapies

Emily Cole, MD, MPH

Commonly encountered skin diseases encompass a broad etiologic spectrum including infectious, neoplastic, and autoimmune/inflammatory. Accordingly, a wide variety of classes of therapeutic agents are used in treating dermatologic disease. Given space limitations, only selected therapies that are commonly used, particularly notable, and/or likely to be less familiar to the generalist practitioner will be discussed here. In particular, the reader should refer to outside sources for complete information on pharmacokinetics, contraindications, side effects, cautions in pregnant or breastfeeding patients, monitoring guidelines, and drug-drug interactions as these are beyond the scope of this chapter.[1-4] The reader is also referred to the sections of this manual on specific disease entities for additional therapeutic information.

The skin forms the body's interface with the external environment, which also makes it easily accessible for treatment with topical or intralesional therapies, modes of drug administration that are somewhat unique to dermatology. Sunscreens are a special category of topically applied compounds and are discussed in Chapter 16. Some disorders can also be treated with light-based therapies including photodynamic therapy, lasers, or phototherapy (see Section 4 of this chapter). These modalities provide a concentrated, local therapeutic effect at the site of pathology without significant systemic absorption. Therefore, they often have a favorable side effect profile. Finally, some dermatoses do require systemically acting agents, which are administered via standard oral or parenteral routes.

## 1. Topical Therapy Overview

- Drugs formulated for transdermal administration can target localized skin disease via direct diffusion or the systemic circulation via dermal capillaries. The latter requires that the compound be of low molecular weight and lipophilic and exhibit efficacy at relatively low doses and/or serum concentrations. Because of these constraints, relatively few systemic agents are administered transdermally. Examples include clonidine, testosterone, estrogen, and fentanyl.
- As discussed in Chapter 2, the skin's barrier function is performed by the outermost layer of the epidermis, termed the cornified layer or stratum corneum. It forms a relatively impermeable barrier that prevents water and nutrient loss while effectively blocking entry of most external substances, including pharmaceuticals. The barrier is arranged in a "bricks and mortar" configuration comprising a protein-rich cellular component (keratinocytes or corneocytes) and a lipid-laden extracellular matrix. Topical delivery of drugs is accomplished by small amounts of diffusion through the stratum corneum. Therefore, compounds with the greatest bioavailability will be of low molecular weight and lipophilic.
- Most of a topically applied drug remains on the skin surface because of poor absorption. This remaining drug is subject to loss from factors such as exfoliation,

---

*The authors would like to acknowledge the first edition authors* Kyle Eash and Ian Hornstra.

sweating, washing, rubbing, degradation, etc. Clinicians should be cognizant of this fact when determining dosing interval and, in the case of superpotent glucocorticoids or topical chemotherapeutics, counseling about the potential for exposure of others (especially neonates) in the home environment.
- The rate of percutaneous absorption of a drug is proportional to the soluble concentration in the vehicle (C) and the partitioning coefficient (k). This partitioning coefficient k describes the ability of the drug to move out of the vehicle and into the stratum corneum. Both variables C and k are highly dependent on the vehicle in which the drug is delivered.

## 1.1. VEHICLES

- Formulations include creams, ointments, lotions, gels, solutions, foams, and patches.
- Many specific components in vehicles enhance absorption via positive effects on solubility and/or partitioning. Examples of enhancers include ethanol and propylene glycol. Often, components that increase absorption come at a cost of increased risk of irritant or allergic side effects.
- The properties of the vehicle can have a marked effect on drug potency. Thus, a given pharmaceutical compound can have a wide range of potencies depending on its formulation. This is exemplified in the classification of glucocorticoids wherein the same drug can fall into several different potency classes depending on its concentration and vehicle, for example, cream versus ointment versus gel (Table 17-1).[5,6]
- In practice, ointments are generally more potent than are creams or lotions. Although nominally equipotent alternative formulations have been developed, the occlusion, hydration, and augmented barrier function provided by ointments makes them more clinically effective in most cases.
- Solutions or gels can be used on hair-bearing skin or for a drying effect, while creams, lotions, or foams rub in to the skin easily and may be preferred to greasy ointments by some patients.
- Alcohol-containing formulations should be avoided on fissured or eroded skin because they will cause stinging and pain in these instances.

## 1.2. CLINICAL FACTORS AFFECTING DRUG ABSORPTION

- The thickness and composition of the stratum corneum and thus drug absorption varies by body site and must be considered when administering topical therapy. A rough guideline in order from most to least permeable is scrotum/genital region, face/scalp/axillae, trunk/extremities, palms/soles, and nails.
- Hydration of the skin via soaking or prolonged occlusion increases barrier permeability and, thus, drug delivery. Occlusion with impermeable or semipermeable material (plastic wrap, medical tape, cloth dressing, or old clothing) is a reliable and easy way to increase drug delivery and therefore efficacy. Aside from increased hydration, occlusion also prevents loss of yet-to-be absorbed drug from the skin surface.
- Skin folds (inguinal, gluteal, inframammary, and axillary regions) are naturally hydrated and occluded regions, and care should be taken to avoid potent formulations with the potential for overdosage and side effects in these areas (eg, ointments, superpotent topical glucocorticoids).
- Drug absorption is increased in skin disorders that are characterized by impaired skin barrier function. A classic example is atopic dermatitis. In most cases, this

### TABLE 17-1 Potency Classification of Selected Topical Glucocorticosteroid Products

| Name | Trade Name(s) | Vehicle(s) | Concentration (%) |
|---|---|---|---|
| **Class 1 (superpotent)** | | | |
| Betamethasone dipropionate, augmented | Diprolene | O, L, G | 0.05 |
| Clobetasol | Temovate, Clobex, Olux | O, C, L, G, F, Sh, Sol, Sp | 0.05 |
| Halobetasol | Ultravate | O, C | 0.05 |
| Fluocinonide | Vanos | C | 0.1 |
| Flurandrenolide | Cordran | Tape | 4 µg/cm$^2$ |
| Diflorasone diacetate | Psorcon | O | 0.05 |
| **Class 2 (potent)** | | | |
| Betamethasone dipropionate | Diprolene AF, Diprosone | C, O | 0.05 |
| Halcinonide | Halog | O, C, Sol | 0.1 |
| Fluocinonide | Lidex | O, C, G, Sol | 0.05 |
| Desoximetasone | Topicort | O, C | 0.25 |
| Desoximetasone | Topicort | G | 0.05 |
| **Class 3 (upper midstrength)** | | | |
| Betamethasone dipropionate | Diprosone | C, L | 0.05 |
| Betamethasone valerate | Luxiq | F | 0.12 |
| Desoximetasone | Topicort LP | C | 0.05 |
| Diflorasone diacetate | Psorcon, Florone | C | 0.05 |
| Fluticasone propionate | Cutivate | O | 0.005 |
| Fluocinonide | Lidex-E | C | 0.05 |
| Mometasone furoate | Elocon | O | 0.1 |
| Triamcinolone acetonide | Kenalog, Aristocort, Triderm | O, C | 0.5 |
| **Class 4 (midstrength)** | | | |
| Clocortolone pivalate | Cloderm | C | 0.1 |
| Desoximetasone | Topicort E | C | 0.25 |
| Fluocinolone acetonide | Synalar | O | 0.025 |
| Flurandrenolide | Cordran | O | 0.05 |
| Hydrocortisone valerate | Westcort | O | 0.2 |
| Mometasone furoate | Elocon | C, L, Sol | 0.1 |
| Triamcinolone acetonide | Kenalog | O, C, Sp | 0.1 |

| TABLE 17-1 | Potency Classification of Selected Topical Glucocorticosteroid Products (*continued*) | | |
|---|---|---|---|
| Name | Trade Name(s) | Vehicle(s) | Concentration (%) |
| **Class 5 (lower midstrength)** | | | |
| Betamethasone dipropionate | Diprosone | L | 0.05 |
| Betamethasone valerate | Beta-Val, Betatrex, Valisone | C | 0.05 |
| Desonide | DesOwen, Desonate | O, G | 0.05 |
| Fluocinolone acetonide | Synalar | C | 0.025 |
| Flurandrenolide | Cordran | C, L | 0.05 |
| Hydrocortisone butyrate | Locoid | O, C, L, Sol, Sp | 0.1 |
| Hydrocortisone valerate | Westcort | C | 0.2 |
| Prednicarbate | Dermatop | O, C | 0.1 |
| Triamcinolone acetonide | Kenalog | L, O | 0.1, 0.025 |
| **Class 6 (mild)** | | | |
| Alclometasone dipropionate | Aclovate | O, C | 0.05 |
| Betamethasone valerate | Beta-Val, Valisone | L | 0.1 |
| Desonide | DesOwen, LoKara, Verdeso | C, L, F | 0.05 |
| Fluocinolone acetonide | Synalar, Capex, Derma-Smoothe | C, Sol, Sh, Oil | 0.01 |
| Triamcinolone acetonide | Kenalog, Aristocort | C, L | 0.025 |
| **Class 7 (least potent)** | | | |
| Hydrocortisone | Hytone, Cortaid, Cortizone | O, C, L, Sol, Sp | 2.5-0.5 |
| Hydrocortisone acetate | Pramosone | O, C, L, F | 2.5-1.0 |

O, ointment; C, cream; L, lotion; G, gel; F, foam; Sp, spray; Sol, solution, Sh, shampoo.
Data from Jacob SE, Steele T. Corticosteroid classes: a quick reference guide including patch test substances and cross-reactivity. *J Am Acad Dermatol*. 2006;54(4):723-727; Tadicherla S, Ross K, Shenefelt PD, Fenske NA. Topical corticosteroids in dermatology. *J Drugs Dermatol*. 2009;8(12):1093-1105.

is therapeutically advantageous. However, in disorders characterized by severe epidermal dysfunction (eg, toxic epidermal necrolysis, congenital ichthyosis) or with the increased skin permeability of preterm infants, caution must be taken as uptake will be dramatically increased, possibly resulting in significant serum levels of drug.

## 1.3. QUANTITY OF APPLICATION

The volume of medication is an important consideration, with respect to both the total volume to be dispensed to the patient for a given treatment area and duration and the amount used per application by the patient or caregiver. Although some formulas are discussed below as rough guidelines, in clinical practice, the actual amounts required can be quite variable.

- Medication should be applied in a thin layer not to exceed 0.1 mm in thickness.
- One "fingertip unit" is the amount of ointment dispensed in a line from the distal crease to the tip of the index finger, is equivalent to 0.5 g, and can cover the area of two flat hands.
- Practically speaking then, a single application to one hand would require 0.5 g of medication, the face and neck 1.25 g, one arm 1.75 g, one leg 3 g, and either the front or back of the trunk 3 g. Therefore, once-daily application for 10-day duration requires approximately a 15-g tube for the arm, hand, or face, but at least a 50-g tube for the leg or trunk.
- Total body application can vary from 20 to 100 g depending on patient characteristics, thickness of application, and preparation.
- Several studies have objectively quantified these parameters and provide a useful guide for dispensing and application of topical medications (Table 17-2).[7,8]

| TABLE 17-2 | Dosing Estimates for Topical Therapy in Adults | | | |
|---|---|---|---|---|
| Area/Region | FTU | Flat Hand Areas | Single Application (Grams) | BID Application × 1 Week (g) |
| 25 × 25 cm, 625 cm² | 2 | 4 | 1 | 14 |
| Face and neck | 2.5 | 5 | 1.25 | 17.5 |
| Single arm, excluding hand | 3.5 | 7 | 1.75 | 24.5 |
| One hand, both sides | 1.5 | 3 | 0.75 | 10.5 |
| Trunk, one side (chest and abdomen or back) | 6 | 12 | 3 | 42 |
| Buttocks/groin | 2 | 4 | 1 | 14 |
| Single leg and thigh, excluding foot | 6 | 12 | 3 | 42 |
| One foot | 2 | 4 | 1 | 14 |
| **Total body** | **42.5** | **85** | **~21** | **~300** |

FTU, fingertip unit; BID, twice daily.
Data from Long CC, Finlay AY. The finger-tip unit—a new practical measure. *Clin Exp Dermatol.* 1991;16(6):444-447; Long CC, Mills CM, Finlay AY. A practical guide to topical therapy in children. *Br J Dermatol.* 1998;138(2):293-296.

# 2. Glucocorticosteroids

These are the most commonly prescribed anti-inflammatory medications in dermatology and medicine at large. They have efficacy in many inflammatory dermatoses but can have significant side effects, especially with long-term (>4 weeks) therapy. Accordingly, they come in a wide variety of formulations and routes of administration.

## 2.1. MECHANISM OF ACTION

These drugs are various modifications of the four-ring cholesterol-based structure of the endogenous hormone cortisol. They bind to the glucocorticoid receptor, a cytosolic hormone receptor, which then translocates to the nucleus and modifies the transcription of a wide variety of genes involved in inflammation. They also interact with other key inflammatory transcription factors. Glucocorticosteroids (CS) can also exert direct effects without receptor binding. The end result is decreased levels of proinflammatory molecules including cytokines and prostaglandins and decreased activation, cell number, and localization of most inflammatory cells including neutrophils, eosinophils, and lymphocytes.

## 2.2. HYPOTHALAMIC-PITUITARY-ADRENAL (HPA) AXIS

The HPA axis controls the production of cortisol by the adrenal glands. Peak secretion of cortisol occurs in the morning. CS suppress the adrenal production of cortisol via negative feedback. Generally, morning dosing is used to minimize HPA suppression. Split (twice daily) dosing can be used to increase efficacy at a cost of increased side effects. A dose of 5 mg/d of prednisone approximates physiologic levels of cortisol. Three weeks or less treatment duration is considered short-term therapy; in these cases, adrenal function is usually sufficiently preserved so that tapering is not required from an adrenal recovery standpoint.

## 2.3. PHARMACOLOGY

CS are readily orally bioavailable, with peak plasma levels 30 to 90 minutes after administration and wide tissue distribution. They are bound to serum proteins, so free levels are increased in the setting of low serum proteins as can be seen in liver or kidney disease. Additionally, some CS (hydrocortisone and prednisolone) require functioning hepatic enzymes for conversion to their active metabolites. Because they are hormonally and transcriptionally mediated, the effects of CS persist for some time after the drug has been metabolized.

## 2.4. TOPICAL AND INTRALESIONAL THERAPY

Principles of topical therapy are discussed in Section 1 of this chapter.
- **Indications/use.** Include but are not limited to psoriasis, various forms of dermatitis including contact, atopic, stasis, and seborrheic (Chapter 3); prurigo nodularis, urticaria, and drug eruptions (Chapter 5); vitiligo (Chapter 6); alopecia areata (Chapter 9); and autoimmune/connective tissue disease including discoid lupus (Chapter 10).[9]

- **Dosing.** Topical CS (TCS) are divided into seven potency classes based on topical vasoconstrictor assays and objective clinical activity (Table 17-1).[5,6]
  - The clinician should choose the potency based on type, severity, extent, and location. Preparations are applied up to twice daily, although daily application may be sufficient.
  - The least potent agent that is expected to achieve a response should be chosen, and the potency and/or frequency of application should be tapered as rapidly as possible while still maintaining a response.
  - ***Intralesional* triamcinolone acetonide** in concentrations ranging from 2 to 40 mg/mL diluted in saline can be administered via 30-gauge needle directly into the dermis, thus bypassing the need for cutaneous absorption and delivering a higher concentration of CS directly to the site of pathology. This therapy is generally administered by a dermatologist and reserved for deeper, thicker, and/or more severe disease processes.
- **Therapeutic considerations**
  - Agents of potency class 3 or greater should generally be avoided in pediatric patients.
  - TCS are very safe in general; serious or important adverse effects are rare and typically involve exceedingly long-term use or gross misapplication of the medication.
  - High-potency formulations should be avoided when treating large areas, as some systemic absorption can occur.
  - Common side effects with *short-term* use include mild itching, burning, redness, and stinging that are usually transient. More rarely, true urticaria, irritant contact dermatitis, or allergic contact dermatitis can develop (Chapters 3 and 5). Allergy can develop to vehicle components or the CS molecule itself.
  - **Desoximetasone (Topicort)** is in a distinct structural class from other topical steroids. It is sometimes used in cases where TCS allergy is suspected based on the theory that there is a decreased chance of allergic cross-reactivity.
  - The most common and important side effect with prolonged (more than 2-3 weeks) therapy is **cutaneous atrophy** (Fig. 17-1). Clinically, atrophy is characterized by thin, lax, shiny, wrinkled skin, often with easy bruising (purpura), lightening or

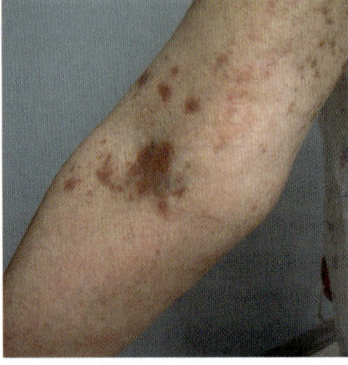

**Figure 17-1.** Cutaneous atrophy due to topical corticosteroid use. Close-up of the right antecubital fossa shows decreased pigmentation; thin, translucent skin; and prominent blood vessels. (Courtesy Milan J. Anadkat, MD.)

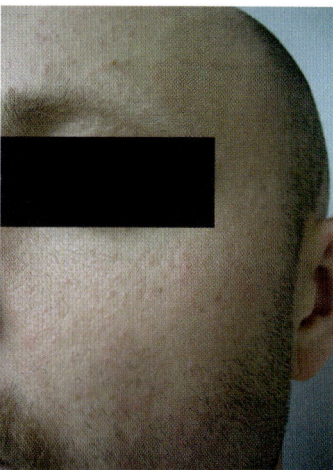

**Figure 17-2.** Perioral dermatitis. This disorder occurs on the face in the setting of topical steroid use and is characterized by redness, acnelike papules, and eczemalike scaling and flaking. (Courtesy Milan J. Anadkat, MD.)

darkening of the skin (pigmentary changes/dyspigmentation), prominently visible small blood vessels (telangiectasias), and, in severe cases, ulceration.
- Rebound upon discontinuation of TCS and loss of efficacy to ongoing treatment (tachyphylaxis) are known to occur. A related disorder known as **perioral dermatitis** (Fig. 17-2) occurs on the face after prolonged or potent TCS exposure. Its clinical appearance can have features of acne rosacea and/or atopic dermatitis (Chapter 3). The treatment for perioral dermatitis is discontinuation of TCS and use of a topical calcineurin inhibitor and/or tetracycline class antibiotics if needed.
- An infectious etiology, particularly superficial fungal species such as **candida** or **tinea** (Chapter 4), should be considered in eruptions that worsen or recur with TCS therapy.

## 2.5. SYSTEMIC THERAPY

- **Indications/use.** Severe dermatitis (Chapter 3), urticaria, drug eruptions (Chapter 5), and a number of systemic diseases with skin manifestations including vasculitis, sarcoidosis, lupus erythematosus, dermatomyositis, scleroderma, and bullous diseases (Chapter 10).
- **Dosing.** Prednisone is readily available and can be easily titrated and tapered. A relatively standard dose would be 40 to 60 mg/d (0.5-1 mg/kg) tapered over a 2- to 4-week period, initially in intervals of 20 mg and then in 10 mg, 5 mg, or even lower amounts as the dose is lowered (see HPA above). Generally, cutaneous inflammatory disease does not respond satisfactorily to lower doses or shorter courses of CS, and some diagnoses require prolonged or chronic therapy in the case of bullous or autoimmune disease, respectively.
- **Therapeutic considerations**
  - Short-term therapy for acute dermatoses such as contact dermatitis, drug eruptions, or urticarial is generally safe and well tolerated.

- Adverse effects with even short-term therapy include mood changes, insomnia, increased appetite and weight gain, fluid retention, hypertension, insulin resistance, and poor wound healing.
- Systemic fungal infection is a contraindication to therapy. Risk of infection of all types is increased in patients on systemic CS.
- With prolonged therapy, patients are at risk for a number of serious adverse events that can affect multiple body systems. These side effects are a major limitation on the use of CS and include osteoporosis, osteonecrosis, growth retardation, myopathy, cataracts, glaucoma, peptic ulcer disease, intestinal perforation, hyperglycemia, obesity, hypertension, atherosclerosis, adrenal suppression including adrenal crisis, mood changes, and psychosis.
- Cutaneous findings in patients on CS therapy are distinctive and include atrophy, purpura, striae, hirsutism, and acne.
- Vitamin D and calcium supplementation at standard doses (1.5 g and 800-1,000 U, respectively) is easy to implement and should be recommended to all patients on systemic CS.
- For patients expected to be on greater than 3-month duration of therapy, an assessment of osteoporotic fracture risk should be performed including baseline bone mineral densitometry via dual-energy x-ray absorptiometry scan. Since the greatest bone loss occurs in the first 6 months of therapy, bisphosphonate therapy should be initiated promptly.

## 3. Retinoids

These compounds are structural and functional analogues of vitamin A. Endogenous retinoids (vitamin A and its derivatives) function in embryonic development and in proliferation, differentiation, and maintenance of various epithelial surfaces. They have a key role in the epidermis and its various appendages; thus, synthetic retinoids, with the exception of ATRA (all *trans* retinoic acid) for a rare subtype of leukemia, are almost exclusively utilized for a number of dermatologic disorders.

### 3.1. MECHANISM OF ACTION

Both endogenous and synthetic retinoid compounds exert a diverse set of effects on epithelial and immune cells in the skin including decreased inflammation, promotion of apoptosis, decreased tumor formation, decreased keratinization, alterations in the extracellular matrix, and decreased sebum production. A complete understanding of the cellular and molecular basis of these effects is lacking, but it is known that retinoids bind RAR and/or RXR nuclear hormone receptors, which then induce a complex transcriptional program that is then responsible, at least in part, for the observed effects.

### 3.2. PHARMACOLOGY AND TERATOGENICITY

- Retinoids are lipophilic compounds. They are orally bioavailable on the order of 25% to 60%, and, although not required, absorption is increased by administration with a fat-containing meal. Topical retinoids have minimal systemic absorption. Systemic retinoids are metabolized in the liver and excreted via biliary and renal routes.
- Retinoids are extremely potent teratogens. There is no known minimal safe level of retinoid compounds during pregnancy. Exposure, especially during the first trimester when organogenesis occurs, may lead to craniofacial, cardiovascular, central nervous system, and limb anomalies that result in abortion, preterm birth, or perinatal death.

- These drugs are therefore absolutely contraindicated in pregnancy, lactation, and patients attempting to conceive. Topical retinoids range from pregnancy categories C to X, while all systemic retinoids are category X. Patients of childbearing potential should be counseled about these risks, and appropriate contraceptive measures and serial serum pregnancy tests are required before, during, and after therapy. Contraception methods and documentation of negative pregnancy status is performed for 1 month prior to initiation of therapy, monthly during therapy, and for at least 1 month after therapy for all patients of childbearing potential.
- The elimination half-life of retinoids is variable, from 1 hour to 120 days. Prolonged elimination is due to the lipophilic nature of the compound and resulting depot storage in adipose tissue. Because of this property, patients on acitretin (but not other retinoids) must undergo contraception for 2 to 3 years after cessation of therapy.
- Although the theoretical systemic exposure and therefore teratogenic risk is much lower, topical retinoids are also avoided during pregnancy and lactation. Similarly, retinoid therapy in the partner of a patient of childbearing potential who is pregnant or attempting to become pregnant should be avoided.

## 3.3. TOPICAL RETINOID COMPOUNDS

Topical retinoid compounds in common dermatologic use include **tretinoin (Retin-A)**, **adapalene (Differin)**, and **tazarotene (Tazorac)**. They all act via binding the RAR receptor. They are all available in gel and cream formulations, with some also available in lotion or solution format.
- **Indications/use.** The most common indication for the use of a topical retinoid is inflammatory or comedonal acne vulgaris (Chapter 3). They are first-line treatment for this common disorder. The other indication the general practitioner should be aware of is the use of topical retinoids (including low-potency, over-the-counter, vitamin A cosmeceutical products) for cosmetic benefit in the treatment of photoaging.
- **Dosing.** A small amount of medication should be applied in a thin layer to dry skin nightly or every other night. Maximal efficacy is not evident until 1 to 2 months of therapy.
- **Therapeutic considerations.** Aside from the risk of teratogenicity discussed above, the major side effect of topical retinoids is skin irritation, also known as retinoid dermatitis. Moisturizing lotions and sunscreens can decrease the irritation. Patients should be encouraged to continue treatment through mild irritation because after approximately 1 month, it generally improves as the skin develops tolerance to the medication. For severe irritation, decreased concentration, frequency, and/or duration of application may be necessary.
- **Bexarotene** gel acts via the RXR receptor and is used topically to treat early-stage CTCL (cutaneous T-cell lymphoma; see Chapter 8).

## 3.4. SYSTEMIC RETINOID DRUGS

Systemic retinoid drugs include isotretinoin, acitretin, and bexarotene. Isotretinoin binds the RAR receptor, while acitretin only weakly interacts with retinoid receptors, yet exerts significant activation of these receptors and their pathways.
- **Isotretinoin (Accutane)** is the mainstay of treatment for severe, scarring, or recalcitrant acne vulgaris. It is the only agent known to induce long-term remission in the disease. This may be related to the fact that it is the only retinoid that decreases sebum production.
  - **Dosing.** Generally 0.5 to 1.0 mg/kg/d. Both disease flares and the most severe cutaneous side effects are often seen in the first month of therapy; therefore,

half-strength doses are often used initially. In practice, patients are usually started at between 20 and 40 mg daily and titrated to a maximal dose of 40 to 80 mg. A total dose of 120 mg/kg is recommended to achieve sustained remission, corresponding to a typical duration of treatment of 4 to 6 months.
- **Therapeutic considerations.** Isotretinoin is regulated by the government-mandated iPLEDGE program, primarily because of the combination of its teratogenicity and frequent use in young females of childbearing age. Patients, providers, and pharmacies must be enrolled before the medication can be dispensed. The program and its website (www.ipledgeprogram.com) formalize and document the functions of obtaining consent, monitoring pregnancy avoidance measures, and confirming nonpregnant status via human chorionic gonadotropin testing. In addition to its teratogenicity and dermatitis side effects, the other common and important side effects of isotretinoin therapy are myalgias and arthralgias and elevations in lipid levels and liver enzymes. All are generally self-limited with discontinuation or dose reduction; chronic hepatitis, liver failure, and pancreatitis are exceedingly rare complications. The laboratory parameters (aspartate aminotransferase, alanine transaminase, total cholesterol, triglycerides) should be monitored at the initiation of and at regular intervals during therapy.
- **Acitretin (Soriatane)** is a treatment option for psoriasis. An additional indication is severe hand eczema. It is particularly effective in the erythrodermic or pustular variants (as opposed to plaque type) of psoriasis. Effective doses are between 25 and 75 mg (~0.5-1.0 mg/kg) daily, although patients are often started at 10 mg daily to minimize the initial worsening of disease that often occurs. Side effects and their management are as noted above.
- **Bexarotene (Targretin)** at initial doses of 150 mg/m$^2$ titrated to 300 mg/m$^2$ daily is Food and Drug Administration approved for the treatment of CTCL, but doses as low as 75 mg can be effective. Additional side effects not previously noted above include hypothyroidism, leukopenia, and agranulocytosis. Patients on therapy require thyroid hormone replacement and lipid-lowering treatment.

## 4. Phototherapy

A number of dermatologic disorders have been known for years to respond to ultraviolet (UV) radiation. More recent advances have moved from using broad-spectrum light to highly specific wavelengths of the UV spectrum. The UV spectrum is between 200 and 400 nm and can be divided, from shortest to longest wavelength, into UVC (200-290 nm), UVB (290-320 nm), UVA2 (320-340 nm), and UVA1 (340-400 nm). Two common and important types of light-based therapies in dermatology are narrow-band UVB (NBUVB), which uses high-intensity UV radiation limited to 311 to 313 nm, and photochemotherapy with psoralens plus UVA (PUVA).

### 4.1. DETERMINING RESPONSE TO UV RADIATION

In the phototherapy setting and general clinical practice, dermatologists often determine a given patient's intrinsic photosensitivity, reflecting not only pigmentation levels but also other genetic factors. This can be done with Fitzpatrick skin phototyping, which utilizes a clinical scale based on pigmentation and response to sunlight ranging from one to six (Table 17-3). A more objective assessment can be obtained with phototesting, where small areas of normally covered skin are exposed to a range

**TABLE 17-3** Skin Phototypes (Fitzpatrick Scale)

| Skin Type | Unexposed Skin Color | Burn | Tan | Associated Features |
|---|---|---|---|---|
| I | White | Always | Never | Blue or green eyes, red or blond hair, freckles |
| II | White | Easily/usually | Minimal/difficult | Variable |
| III | White to beige | Sometimes/mild | Average/gradually | Variable |
| IV | Beige to light brown | Rarely | Easily | Variable |
| V | Dark brown | Extremely rare | Very easy/dark | Variable |
| VI | Black | Never | Very easy/dark | Dark brown eyes, dark brown or black hair |

Data from Fitzpatrick TB. The validity and practicality of sun-reactive skin types I through VI. *Arch Dermatol.* 1988;124(6):869-871.

of UV doses to determine a minimal erythema dose. Erythema is assessed at its peak, 24 hours after UVB exposure. In general, light-based dermatologic therapies are contraindicated in patients with known history of a photosensitizing disorder or genetic susceptibility to UV-induced carcinogenesis.

### 4.2. NBUVB

- **Mechanism of action.** UV light is absorbed by DNA, forming DNA photoproducts (primarily pyrimidine dimers). This induces p53 and causes cell cycle arrest or apoptosis, thus decreasing epidermal or immune cell proliferation. UVB also alters cytokine expression patterns (in both DNA damage–dependent and DNA damage–independent mechanisms) and causes associated immunosuppressive and anti-inflammatory effects.
- **Indications/use.** NBUVB is used to treat psoriasis, atopic dermatitis (Chapter 3), pruritus, vitiligo (Chapter 6), and CTCL (Chapter 8).
- **Dosing.** Patients are typically treated 3 times per week initially until remission or maximal improvement is achieved. Dose (ranging from 200-1,200 mJ/cm$^2$) is initially determined based on phototesting or phototyping and then increased in standard increments until persistent asymptomatic erythema is obtained. Treatment is paused and resumed at lower doses if painful erythema develops. After maximal response is achieved, maintenance therapy of twice and then once weekly treatments is continued for several months.
- **Therapeutic considerations.** Maximal response may not be evident until after 6 to 8 weeks of therapy (18-24 treatments). The major adverse effect is phototoxicity. Treatment compliance and/or availability is primarily hampered by the need for frequent office visits. UV carcinogenesis (Chapters 8 and 14) is a concern, but the risk appears to be quite low for NBUVB as opposed to sunlight exposure, tanning beds, broadband UVB, or PUVA.[10]

## 4.3. PUVA

In this treatment, patients are given a photosensitizing agent (psoralens), which absorbs light at 330 to 335 nm. The skin is then exposed to UVA radiation with peak emission at 352 nm. This combination produces a therapeutically beneficial phototoxic effect. Psoralens are a family of plant-derived compounds, several of which have been used for PUVA therapy.

- **Mechanism of action.** When activated by UV radiation, psoralens cross-link DNA, leading to cell cycle arrest and decreased cellular proliferation. It also forms reactive oxygen species. Via these and other as yet undetermined pathways, keratinocyte and lymphocyte apoptosis occurs with resulting normalization of keratinocyte differentiation and decreased inflammation.
- **Indications/use.** Psoriasis (Chapter 3) and CTCL (Chapter 8). With the advent of new systemic therapies, the use of PUVA in psoriasis has greatly decreased because of equivalent efficacy and a better side effect profile.
- **Dosing.** 8-methoxypsoralens 0.6 to 0.8 mg/kg is administered 1 to 3 hours prior to UVA exposure ranging from 0.5 to 5 J/cm$^2$ as determined by phototyping. Psoralens are also available via bath or topical applications. Treatments are 2 to 4 times per week during the initial clearing phase followed by maintenance treatments at decreased frequency. In contrast to NBUVB, erythema from PUVA peaks at 72 hours after treatment. Thus, dose increases are never more frequent than every 3 days.
- **Therapeutic considerations.** PUVA is carcinogenic, and patients are at an increased risk of cutaneous squamous cell carcinoma. Otherwise, the major side effects are nausea with oral psoralens, phototoxicity during treatment, and cumulative photodamage. PUVA induces melanogenesis and a distinctive increase in skin pigmentation (Fig. 17-3) to a greater degree than do other sources of UV light.

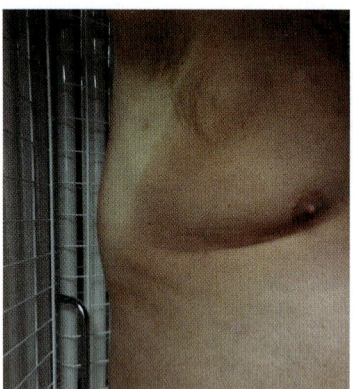

**Figure 17-3.** Psoralens plus ultra violet A (PUVA)-induced hyperpigmentation. A patient on chronic therapy for cutaneous T-cell lymphoma demonstrates the characteristic dark, orange-hued pigmentation of a "PUVA tan." Once the pigmentation develops, the skin disease becomes less responsive (hardened) to equivalent doses of light. (Caroline Mann, MD and Pat Cashel-Lee, LPN.)

# 5. Selected Antimicrobials

The skin is a common site of a wide variety of infections and infestations (Chapter 4). The reader is referred to more detailed dermatologic or infectious disease texts for details of treatment,[1,4] although general principles of treatment should be already familiar to most generalist practitioners. However, several unique situations where antimicrobials are utilized in dermatology merit comment here.

## 5.1. SUPERFICIAL SKIN INFECTIONS

Folliculitis, minor wounds, paronychia, and impetigo (Chapter 4) may be amenable to topical treatment only. Clindamycin, erythromycin, gentamicin, mupirocin, and polymyxin B/neomycin/bacitracin are readily available in topical formulations. They can be applied to the affected areas of skin 2 to 4 times per day and are generally well tolerated without side effects. Gentamicin has activity where psuedomonal or other gram-negative species may be a concern. Mupirocin has good activity against methicillin-resistant *Staphylococcus aureus*.

## 5.2. ACNE

The pathogenesis of acne (Chapter 3) is complex, with aseptic inflammation, sebum production, hormonal influences, and *Propionibacterium acnes* and other commensal bacteria all playing a role.
- Several topical and oral antibiotics are efficacious in the treatment of both acne vulgaris and acne rosacea because of their anti-inflammatory and antibacterial properties.
- Topical formulations of azelaic acid, benzoyl peroxide, clindamycin, and dapsone are effective in treating mild to moderate inflammatory acne. Of note, benzoyl peroxide–containing washes and gels do not require a prescription and have at least partial efficacy for most types and severity of acne. The major limitation to use of benzoyl peroxide is irritation and the fact that the compound will bleach clothing.
- Topical metronidazole and sodium sulfacetamide are first-line treatments for acne rosacea.
- For more severe inflammatory acne, oral tetracycline antibiotics are used. Doxycycline and minocycline at doses from 50 to 200 mg/d are both very effective at controlling acne. In contrast to isotretinoin, they unfortunately do not alter the natural history of the disease.
- Despite causing more gastrointestinal upset, doxycycline is preferred in most cases because of the risk of cutaneous hyperpigmentation and rare reports of severe drug reactions with minocycline therapy.

## 5.3. ATOPIC DERMATITIS

Some dermatologic disorders are characterized by the propensity for chronic or periodic superinfection or overgrowth with *S aureus* bacteria naturally present on the skin.
- Atopic dermatitis (Chapter 3) is the prototype for this phenomenon, but any clinical state with altered epidermal barrier function is susceptible. A more novel but growing population of these susceptible patients are those treated with targeted EGFRi (epidermal growth factor receptor inhibitor) chemotherapy for epithelial-derived malignancies.

- *S aureus* overgrowth contributes to worsening of atopic dermatitis, and often, patients will require prolonged (1 month or more), repeated, or chronic antistaphylococcal antibiotic therapy. Skin swab culture to confirm infection and facilitate identification of susceptibility profile should always be performed prior to initiating therapy.
- Cephalosporins such as cephalexin 500 mg 2 to 3 times per day are used for methicillin-sensitive strains, while resistant strains are typically treated with trimethoprim/sulfamethoxazole 800/160 mg once or twice daily. Clindamycin and tetracycline are other orally available antistaphylococcal antibiotics.
- In this patient population, decontamination methods such as dilute bleach baths, mupirocin to nares and fingernails, or antibiotic washes such as chlorhexidine can also be helpful.

## 6. Topical Immunomodulators and Chemotherapeutics

### 6.1. TOPICAL CALCINEURIN INHIBITORS

These drugs are nonsteroidal anti-inflammatory agents. They are a "steroid-sparing" option for treating steroid-responsive dermatoses such as atopic dermatitis and other inflammatory skin disorders. Calcineurin inhibitors avoid the main side effect of TCS, cutaneous atrophy. Thus, they are particularly useful around the eyes, on the face, or on the genital and intertriginous areas.

- **Mechanism of action.** These drugs bind to FK506-binding protein, interacting with calcineurin and preventing the dephosphorylation of the transcription factor NFAT and transcription of inflammatory cytokines.
- **Indications/use.** Atopic dermatitis, eyelid dermatitis, seborrheic dermatitis, perioral dermatitis, psoriasis, vitiligo (Chapters 3 and 6).
- **Dosing. Pimecrolimus (Elidel)** is supplied as a 1% cream, and **tacrolimus (Protopic)** is available as a 0.1% or 0.03% ointment. Both can be applied 1 to 2 times per day.
- **Therapeutic considerations.** The most common side effect that leads some patients to discontinue use is burning and stinging at the application site. Caution is advised in the setting of herpes simplex virus (HSV or varicella-zoster virus) infection.

### 6.2. TOPICAL JANUS KINASE INHIBITORS (JAKi)

These drugs are also steroid-sparing anti-inflammatory agents that are currently approved for the treatment of atopic dermatitis (Chapter 3) and vitiligo (Chapter 6).

- **Mechanism of action**. Ruxolitinib (Opzelura) blocks the activation of JAK1 and JAK2 enzymes, resulting in decreased production of inflammatory cytokines and growth factors.
- **Indications/use**. Atopic dermatitis, vitiligo.
- **Dosing**. Ruxolitinib (Opzelura) is supplied as a 1.5% cream. It is applied topically twice daily to affected body areas, up to 20% of total body surface area.
- **Therapeutic considerations**. The most common side effects are acne or itching at the injection site and nasopharyngitis. Caution should be taken in patients at high risk for serious/opportunistic infections or sepsis.

### 6.3. TAPINAROF (VTAMA)

- This drug is a topical steroid-sparing anti-inflammatory agent approved for use in plaque psoriasis and atopic dermatitis and functions as an agonist of aryl hydrocarbon receptors. It is supplied as a 1% cream and is applied topically once daily to affected areas of skin. The most common adverse reactions include folliculitis, nasopharyngitis, and contact dermatitis.

## 6.4. PHOSPHODIESTERASE-4 (PDE-4) INHIBITORS

Several topical PDE-4 inhibitors are available for use in dermatology. These medications work via inhibition of phosphodiesterase-4, resulting in increased intracellular cyclic adenosine monophosphate levels.
- **Crisaborole (Eucrisa)** is approved for mild to moderate atopic dermatitis. It is supplied as a 2% topical ointment and is applied to affected areas of skin twice daily. The most common adverse reaction is stinging or burning at the application site.
- **Roflumilast (Zoryve)** is approved for use in plaque psoriasis and atopic dermatitis. It is supplied as 0.15% and 0.3% creams and should be applied to affected areas of skin once daily. The most common side effects included headache, diarrhea, and injection site pain.

## 6.5. CALCIPOTRIENE (DOVONEX)

This is a synthetic vitamin $D_3$ derivative that is currently approved for the treatment of plaque psoriasis but has been used off-label for other conditions including actinic keratosis (AK), atopic dermatitis, lichen planus, and alopecia areata, particularly in combination with other topical therapies. It works through regulation of the production and growth of keratinocytes and is available as a cream, ointment, solution, or foam as well as numerous combination formations, primarily with topical corticosteroids.

## 6.6. IMIQUIMOD (ALDARA)

This drug is a topical immune activating agent used in the treatment of viral (Chapter 4) or neoplastic (Chapter 8) lesions.
- **Mechanism of action.** Imiquimod stimulates antiviral and antitumor immune responses via activation of toll-like receptor 7 (TLR7), resulting in increased cytokines and cell-mediated immunity.
- **Indications/use.** It is first-line therapy for anogenital human papillomavirus infection (genital warts). It is also an effective option for treating superficial cutaneous malignancies, namely AK, superficial basal cell carcinoma (sBCC), and squamous cell carcinoma in situ (SCCIS), should these lesions not be good candidates for destructive or excisional therapies (Chapters 8 and 11).
- **Dosing.** Imiquimod is supplied as a 5% or 3.75% cream. Warts and AK are treated with thrice weekly application for up to 16 weeks, while malignancies (sBCC or SCCIS) are treated 5 times per week for 6 weeks or more as tolerated.
- **Therapeutic considerations.** Patients should be counseled that irritation and inflammation is expected and desired at the treatment site (Fig. 17-4). Therapy can be discontinued or interrupted prior to the prescribed time period if excessive inflammation develops. In these cases, it is likely that the tumor or infection has cleared and the patient only needs to be observed at regular intervals for any sign of clinical persistence or recurrence after the inflammation has subsided.

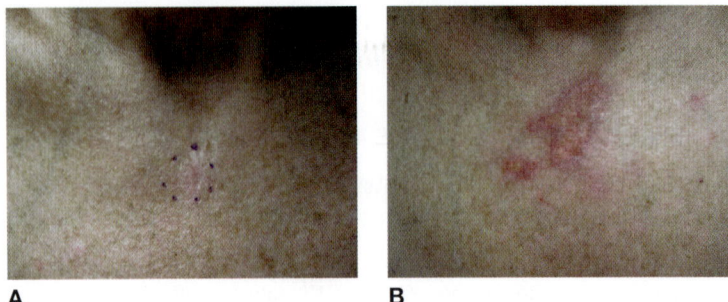

**Figure 17-4.** Inflammatory response in an superficial basal cell carcinoma treated with imiquimod. Before **(A)** and after **(B)** 7 weeks of treatment. (Courtesy Milan J. Anadkat, MD.)

### 6.7. 5-FLUOROURACIL (5-FU, EFUDEX)

This drug is a topical chemotherapeutic agent useful in the treatment of viral, premalignant, or malignant skin lesions (Fig. 17-5).
- **Mechanism of action.** 5-FU is a pyrimidine analog that blocks DNA synthesis and causes DNA breakage, leading to selective apoptosis of rapidly dividing and/or malignant cells.
- **Indications/use.** This therapy is extremely useful for "field treatment" of patients with numerous actinic keratoses and areas of extensively UV-damaged skin where actinic keratoses are likely to arise but are not yet clinically evident. It is an alternative to the destructive or physical methods (cryotherapy or photodynamic therapy) discussed in Chapter 11. Like imiquimod, 5-FU is a topical treatment option for cutaneous or genital warts, sBCC, and SCCIS as well (Chapters 4 and 8).
- **Dosing.** The drug is supplied in a cream or solution at several concentrations. Typical dosing is the 5% cream applied twice daily for 2 weeks for the treatment of AK and up to 6 weeks for the treatment of basal cell carcinoma or SCCIS.
- **Therapeutic considerations.** Similar to imiquimod, 5-FU typically induces a marked inflammatory response characterized by variable degrees of erythema, pain, swelling, and crusting followed by eventual re-epithelialization (Fig. 17-6). The inflammation is related to the degree of actinic damage and underlying keratinocyte dysplasia and

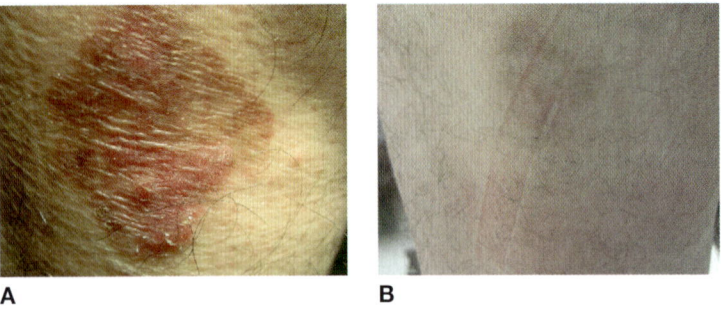

**Figure 17-5.** Clearance of squamous cell carcinoma in situ after treatment with 5-fluorouracil. Before **(A)** and after **(B)** 6 weeks of treatment. (Courtesy Milan J. Anadkat, MD.).

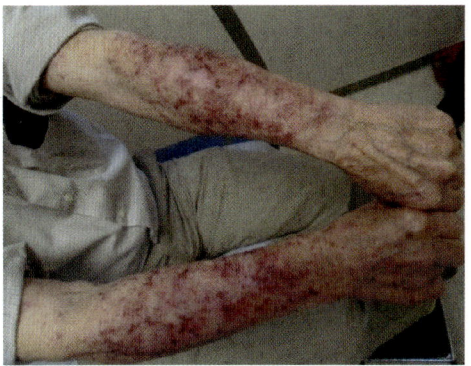

**Figure 17-6.** Inflammatory response to 2 weeks of 5-fluorouracil treatment of actinic keratosis of the arms.

is a marker of therapeutic efficacy. Early cessation of therapy because of pronounced inflammation is acceptable and likely still results in significantly effective treatment. Patients should be assessed for persistent or recurrent lesions once the treated area has normalized. Topical 5-FU is pregnancy category X.

## 7. Systemic Immunosuppressive and Immunomodulatory Agents

Many inflammatory and/or autoimmune skin disorders require systemic treatments. Prototypical examples include psoriasis (Chapter 3) and cutaneous lupus (Chapter 10), respectively, but there are a great many additional diseases and therapies of interest to the dermatologic specialist that are beyond the scope of this manual. Commonly used therapies for this broad group of disorders include hydroxychloroquine, cyclosporine, azathioprine, mycophenolate mofetil, dapsone, methotrexate, and biologics. This last category refers to a wide variety of biomolecules including proteins, receptors, or antibodies that specifically target specific immune and/or cell signaling pathways. The development of biologics has only been possible because of recent technologic advances in molecular biology. These agents represent a profound leap forward in therapy for a wide variety of dermatologic and nondermatologic systemic autoimmune, inflammatory, and neoplastic diseases. Drugs in common use in dermatology and their targets include rituximab (Rituxan, CD20, B cells), omalizumab (Xolair, IgE, mast cells), anakinra (Kineret, IL-1), and dupilumab (Dupixent, IL-4/IL-13). Common antipsoriatic agents include ustekinumab (Stelara, IL-12/IL-23, T cells), IL-17 inhibitors (secukinumab [Cosentyx], ixekizumab [Taltz], and brodalumab [Siliq]), IL-23 inhibitors (risankizumab [Skyrizi], guselkumab [Tremfya], and tildrakizumab [Ilumya]), apremilast (Otezla, phosphodiesterase-4, cyclic adenosine monophosphate), and the anti-tumor necrosis factor-α (anti-TNF-α) agents etanercept, adalimumab, and infliximab that target dendritic cells, neutrophils, and IL-17–secreting T cells. Common first-line systemic treatments for plaque psoriasis will be discussed here; the reader is referred to additional resources for complete information.[1,2]

## 7.1. METHOTREXATE

- **Mechanism of action.** The drug exerts its anti-inflammatory effect by decreasing immune cell proliferation. It blocks key enzymes required for nucleotide synthesis and thus inhibits DNA replication and cell division.
- **Indications/use.** Methotrexate is a steroid-sparing immunosuppressive agent Food and Drug Administration approved for the treatment of severe, debilitating, or recalcitrant psoriasis (Chapter 3). Additional indications include CTCL (Chapter 8), dermatomyositis, systemic sclerosis, and other glucocorticoid-responsive dermatoses (Chapter 10).
- **Dosing.** Supplied in 2.5-mg tablets, methotrexate is given orally once weekly and titrated to clinical response. Standard doses are between 10 and 25 mg. To decrease toxicity, the authors generally prescribe all patients 1-mg folic acid tablets to be taken daily except on the day of methotrexate administration. It is also available in parenteral (intramuscular or intravenous) formulations.
- **Therapeutic considerations.** A number of adverse effects are possible with methotrexate therapy; thus, patients should be selected, counseled, and monitored appropriately.
  - Gastrointestinal toxicity (oral ulcers, nausea, vomiting) is common and reduced with folate supplementation and/or parenteral administration.
  - Serious hematologic toxicity in the form of pancytopenia can occur even early in the course of therapy and at low doses. This can be potentiated by other drugs that inhibit folate metabolism; common examples are dapsone or trimethoprim/sulfamethoxazole.
  - There is a risk of hepatotoxicity in the form of cirrhosis and fibrosis; it is increased with cumulative dose and duration of therapy and/or additional hepatic insults such as chronic hepatitis, current or former alcohol use, or other preexisting liver disease. Patients should be tested for hepatitis virus infection prior to initiating therapy.
  - The need for screening liver biopsy is no longer absolutely recommended; it can be determined by patient risk factors and consultation with a hepatologist.
  - Methotrexate is renally cleared, and drug levels may be elevated in patients with chronic kidney disease.
  - Complete blood count and assessment of hepatic and renal function (CMP) should be performed at regular intervals (no less frequent that monthly with changes in dose and every 3-4 months when on a stable dose).
  - Methotrexate is an abortifacient and teratogen. Its use is contraindicated in pregnant or lactating patients. Reliable contraception and serum pregnancy testing are required.
  - The risk of infection is increased with therapy, and caution should be exercised in patients with active infection or additional underlying immunosuppressive conditions. Consideration should be given to HIV testing prior to initiating therapy.

## 7.2. ANTI-TNF AGENTS

- **Mechanism of action.** These drugs bind to soluble or membrane-bound TNF-α, thus blocking signaling and inducing apoptosis with resulting decrease in downstream inflammatory cytokines (IL-17, IL-22, and IL-23) and cell types (dendritic cells, macrophages, neutrophils, Th17, and Th22 T cells).[11]

- **Indications/use.** Severe psoriasis or psoriatic arthritis (Chapter 3). Also approved for rheumatoid arthritis, juvenile idiopathic arthritis, and inflammatory bowel disease (adalimumab and infliximab). A number of off-label dermatologic uses have been reported, including cutaneous lupus, dermatomyositis, and sarcoidosis (Chapter 10).
- **Dosing. Etanercept (Enbrel)** is a fusion protein of the TNF receptor and IgG. It is available in 25-mg or 50-mg syringes for subcutaneous administration. Standard dosing is 50 mg twice weekly for the first 3 months and then once weekly thereafter, but 25 mg twice weekly or an initial dose of only 50 mg weekly can also be used. **Adalimumab (Humira)** is a fully human monoclonal antibody directed against TNF. Standard maintenance dosing is 40 mg subcutaneous every 2 weeks. Frequency can be increased to weekly for recalcitrant disease, and at the initiation of therapy, higher and more frequent doses are given (ie, first dose of 80 mg followed by 40 mg 1 week later). **Infliximab (Remicade)** is a mouse-human chimeric anti-TNF antibody. It is administered intravenously at 5 mg/kg, initially at weeks 0, 2, and 6 and then every 8 weeks, although the dose frequency and level can be adjusted up to 10 mg/kg to achieve a satisfactory response.
- **Therapeutic considerations.** Given their efficacy, TNF inhibitors have a favorable side effect profile compared to traditional, nonbiologic immunosuppressives. Serious infections are the most important adverse effect.
  - Patients are particularly susceptible to tuberculosis (TB) infection. Therefore, baseline and annual monitoring of TB infection status is required for all patients on therapy and can be accomplished via testing of the skin (PPD test), serum (Quantiferon or T-SPOT interferon-γ release assays), or lungs (chest radiograph).
  - Other reported adverse effects are the development of malignancy including melanoma and other skin cancers or lymphoma, heart failure, multiple sclerosis, or lupuslike autoimmune disease.
  - Hepatitis B reactivation has occurred, but patients with hepatitis C can often be successfully treated.
  - Infusion reactions and/or hypersensitivity can occur. In the case of infliximab, these can be managed with slow infusion rates and premedication.
  - Development of antidrug antibodies with concomitant loss of efficacy, particularly with infliximab, can be managed with concurrent low-dose immunosuppression with corticosteroids, azathioprine, or methotrexate.
  - Anti-TNF agents are category B, so they can be used if necessary in pregnant patients.
  - Baseline assessment of blood counts, electrolytes, kidney function, liver function, hepatitis serology, and TB status should be obtained prior to starting therapy. HIV status should also be assessed in at-risk individuals.

## 7.3. JANUS KINASE INHIBITORS (JAKi)

JAK inhibitors are a new class of drugs that are also steroid-sparing anti-inflammatory agents approved for atopic dermatitis, alopecia areata, and psoriatic arthritis.
- **Mechanism of action**. These medications block the activation of JAK enzymes, including JAK1, JAK2, JAK3, and TYK2, resulting in decreased production of inflammatory cytokines and growth factors.
- **Indications/use**. Atopic dermatitis, alopecia areata (deuruxolitinib/Leqselvi, ritlecitinib/Litfulo).

- **Dosing**. **Upadacitinib (Rinvoq)** is JAK1/JAK2 inhibitor approved for the treatment of atopic dermatitis and psoriatic arthritis. It is available in 15-, 30-, and 45-mg tablets and 1 mg/mL oral solution. Standard dosing is 15 mg once daily in psoriatic arthritis and 15 to 30 mg once daily in atopic dermatitis. **Tofacitinib (Xeljanz)** is a nonselective inhibitor of JAK proteins with the highest inhibitory activity against JAK3. It is approved for the treatment of psoriatic arthritis, and standard dosing is 5 mg twice daily or 11 mg once daily of the extended-release tablet. **Deucravacitinib (Sotyktu)** is a selective TYK2 inhibitor approved for the treatment of moderate to severe plaque psoriasis. It is available in 6-mg tablets, and standard dosing is 6 mg once daily. **Abrocitinib (Cibinqo)** is a JAK1 inhibitor approved for the treatment of atopic dermatitis. It is available in 50-, 100-, and 200-mg tablets. Standard dosing is 100 mg once daily, but 200 mg once daily can be prescribed if adequate response is not achieved on the lower dose. **Baricitinib (Olumiant)** is a JAK1/JAK2 inhibitor approved for the treatment of severe alopecia areata. It is available in 1-, 2-, and 4-mg tablet, and standard dosing is 2 mg once daily, but dose can be doubled to 4 mg once daily if adequate results are not achieved on the lower dose. **Deuruxolitinib (Leqselvi)** is a JAK1/JAK2 inhibitor approved for moderate to severe alopecia areata. It is supplied as 8-mg tablets, and typical dosing is 8 mg twice daily. **Ritlecitinib (Litfulo)** is a JAK3 inhibitor approved for the treatment of severe alopecia areata. It is supplied as 50-mg capsules, and standard dosing is 50 mg once daily.
- **Therapeutic considerations**. One of the most significant recent changes to the therapeutic armamentarium in dermatology has been the addition of JAK inhibitors. However, these medications carry serious risks that require careful consideration from prescribing physicians.
  - The most common side effects of JAK inhibitors are mild and include nasopharyngitis, bronchitis, urinary tract infections, headache, and nausea.
  - Patients have an increased risk of serious infections including TB. All patients should be screened for latent TB prior to initiation of therapy, via skin testing (a PPD test), serum (Quantiferon or T-SPOT interferon-γ release assays), or lungs (chest radiograph). Patients should be regularly monitored for serious infections while on and following completion of therapy, including bacterial, viral, invasive fungal, and other opportunistic infections.
  - Other serious adverse events including major cardiovascular events (myocardial infarction, stroke, or cardiovascular death), thrombosis (deep vein thrombosis, pulmonary embolism, or arterial thrombosis), lymphoma, other malignancies, and increased all-cause mortality. Caution should be taken in those patients at increased risk for major cardiovascular events or thrombosis including smokers or those with hypertension or dyslipidemia. Therapy should be discontinued in patients who have experienced a major cardiovascular or thrombotic event.
  - Currently, the effects of JAK inhibitor use in pregnancy is unknown. However, animal studies have shown an increased risk for birth defects, and use in pregnant patients should be avoided.

## 7.4. VACCINATION

If feasible, clinicians should attempt to have patients up-to-date on vaccinations prior to initiating immunosuppressive therapy.[12] Live vaccines should be given at least 6 weeks prior to therapy, while inactivated vaccines are given up to 2 weeks prior to treatment. Inactivated vaccines can be given while on therapy, but the immunologic response and resulting immunity may be suboptimal. Live vaccines are contraindicated in immunosuppressed patients including those on TNF inhibitors. Common live vaccines to avoid include varicella, herpes zoster, intranasal flu, and MMR. Other live vaccines sometimes given to select populations include BCG, smallpox, and yellow fever.

# REFERENCES

1. Bolognia JL, Jorizzo J, Schaffer JV, eds. *Dermatology*. 3rd ed. Elsevier/Saunders; 2012.
2. Wolverton SE, ed. *Comprehensive Dermatologic Drug Therapy*. 3rd ed. Saunders/Elsevier; 2013.
3. Mann MW, Berk DR, Popkin DL, Bayliss SJ. *Handbook of Dermatology: A Practical Manual*. Wiley; 2009.
4. Saag MS, Eliopoulos GM, Chambers HF, Gilbert GN, eds. *Sanford Guide to Antimicrobial Therapy 2014*. 44th ed. Antimicrobial Therapy Inc.; 2014.
5. Jacob SE, Steele T. Corticosteroid classes: a quick reference guide including patch test substances and cross-reactivity. *J Am Acad Dermatol*. 2006;54(4):723-727.
6. Tadicherla S, Ross K, Shenefelt PD, Fenske NA. Topical corticosteroids in dermatology. *J Drugs Dermatol*. 2009;8(12):1093-1105.
7. Long CC, Finlay AY. The finger-tip unit—a new practical measure. *Clin Exp Dermatol*. 1991;16(6):444-447.
8. Long CC, Mills CM, Finlay AY. A practical guide to topical therapy in children. *Br J Dermatol*. 1998;138(2):293-296.
9. Drake LA, Dinehart SM, Farmer ER, et al. Guidelines of care for the use of topical glucocorticosteroids. American Academy of Dermatology. *J Am Acad Dermatol*. 1996;35(4):615-619.
10. Hearn RMR, Kerr AC, Rahim KF, Ferguson J, Dawe RS. Incidence of skin cancers in 3867 patients treated with narrow-band ultraviolet B phototherapy. *Br J Dermatol*. 2008;159(4):931-935.
11. Lynde CW, Poulin Y, Vender R, Bourcier M, Khalil S. Interleukin 17A: toward a new understanding of psoriasis pathogenesis. *J Am Acad Dermatol*. 2014;71(1):141-150.
12. Chirch LM, Cataline PR, Dieckhaus KD, Grant-Kels JM. Proactive infectious disease approach to dermatologic patients who are taking tumor necrosis factor-alfa antagonists: Part II. Screening for patients on tumor necrosis factor-alfa antagonists. *J Am Acad Dermatol*. 2014;71(1):11.e1-11.e7. quiz 18-20.

# Index

Note: Italicized *f* and *t* refer to figures and tables

## A
ABCDEs of melanoma, 2, 166
Abrocitinib, 21, 360
Abscesses, 74, 74*f*
Accutane, 349. *See also* Isotretinoin
Acetaminophen, 115
Acitretin, 50, 192*t*, 350
Acne, 24–29
  antimicrobials, 353–354
  bacterium, 24
  clinical presentation
    comedonal acne, 24
    conglobata, 26
    drug-induced acne, 26
    fulminans, 26
    inflammatory acne, 24
    nodulocystic acne, 25*f*
    postadolescent acne, 26
    truncal, 25*f*
  comedone formation, 24
  evaluation, 26
  fulminans, 26
  genetics, 24
  hormonal influences, 24
  neonatal, 291, 292*f*
  sebum production, 24
  treatment, 26–29
  vulgaris, 14, 311–313
Acne keloidalis nuchae (AKN), 273*f*
  folliculitis keloidalis nuchae, 252*t*
  management, 272
  men of African descent, 272
  treatments, 272
    community intervention, 274*t*
    intralesional energy-based devices, 274*t*
    oral, 274*t*
    surgery/procedures, 274*t*
    topicals, 274*t*
Acne postinflammatory hyperpigmentation, 252*t*
Acne scarring, 259*t*–260*t*
Acne vulgaris, 260–261
Acroangiodermatitis, 96
Acrochordons, 149–150, 149*f*
Actinic keratosis, 15, 161, 316, 318*t*–322*t*
Actinic purpura, 318*t*–322*t*, 322–323
Acute cutaneous lupus erythematosus (ACLE), 201
Acute generalized exanthematous pustulosis (AGEP), 116, 118, 119*f*
Acyclovir, 71, 115
Adalimumab (Humira), 20, 266*t*, 359

Adapalene, 27
Adaptive immunity, 19
Adipocytes, 18
Adrenergic urticaria, 104
Adult and pediatric dermatology, SOC
  acne keloidalis nuchae, 272, 273*f*
  acne vulgaris, 258*f*, 260–261
  allergic contact dermatitis, 261–262, 263*f*
  atopic dermatitis, 261
  central centrifugal cicatricial alopecia, 272–276, 275*f*
  cutaneous sarcoidosis, 269–270, 271*f*
  cutaneous T-cell lymphoma, 267, 268*f*
  discoid lupus erythematosus, 267–269, 269*f*
  folliculitis keloidalis nuchae, 272, 273*f*
  hidradenitis suppurativa, 263–267, 265*f*
  pseudofolliculitis barbae, 270–272, 272*f*
  scarring alopecia, 272
  seborrheic dermatitis, 262–263, 264*f*
  traction alopecia, 276, 277*f*
*Aeromonas hydrophila* infections, 76
Aesthetic dermatology, 233–250
  chemical peels, 241–243
    caustic agents, 241
    evaluation, 242
    postoperative care, 243
    primary objective, 241
    treatment, 242–243
    types, 241–242
  cosmetic peel techniques, 241
  hair restoration, 247–248
    clinical presentation, 247
    evaluation, 247
    hair loss/alopecia, 247
    treatment, 247–248
  laser and energy-based devices, 243–246
    chromophores, 243–244
    clinical presentation, 244
    components, 243–244
    evaluation, 244–245
    laser devices and associated indications, 245*t*
    lasers, 244
    treatment, 245–246
  microneedling, 248–249
    clinical presentation, 248
    devices, 248
    evaluation, 248–249
    treatment, 249
  neurotoxins, 233–237
    applications, 233–234
    BoNT, 233
    botulinum toxin formulations, 235*t*

Aesthetic dermatology (*Continued*)
  clinical presentation, 233–234
  evaluation, 234–236
  patient counseling, 236–237
  posttreatment care, 236–237
  treatment, 236
 sclerotherapy, 246
  evaluation, 246
  reticular and varicose veins, 246
  treatment, 246
 soft tissue fillers, 233
  aseptic techniques, 240
  clinical presentation, 239
  dermal fillers, 239
  evaluation, 239
  HA, 238
  precautions, 240
  treatment, 239–240
Aldara, 355–356, 356*f*
Alexandrite, 244
Alginates, 325
Allergic contact dermatitis (ACD), 261–262, 263*f*
Alopecia areata, 13, 185–186, 185*f*
*Amblyomma americanum,* 90
Amelanotic melanoma, 166*f*
American Joint Committee on Cancer (AJCC), 161–163, 167–168
American Society of Clinical Oncology, 216
Amyopathic dermatomyositis, 205
Anagen effluvium, 187
Androgenetic alopecia, 183–185, 184*f*
Androgenic alopecia, 12
Anesthesia, 216
Angiomas, 150–151, 150*f*
Angiosarcoma, 17
Anifrolumab, 203, 206
Ankle-brachial index (ABI), 324
Anticoagulant, 215–216
Antifungal agents, 53
Antihypertensive therapy, 326
Antimicrobial peptides (AMPs), 13
Antimicrobials
 acne, 353–354
 atopic dermatitis, 353–354
 superficial skin infections, 353
Antineutrophil cystoplasmic antibodies (ANCA), 17–18
Antipruritics, 331
Antiseptics, 217–218
Antisynthetase syndrome, 203
Anti-TNF agents, 358–359
Aplasia cutis congenita, 291–292, 292*f*
Apocrine gland carcinoma, 13
Apocrine sweat glands, 13
Aquagenic urticaria, 104
Arterial ulcer, 324–325
Atopic dermatitis (AD), 11, 15, 252*t*, 261, 303–305
 antimicrobials, 353–354
 childhood, 261
 clinical presentation, 303
  adolescent and adult, 33
  childhood, 33
  infantile, 33
  skin lesions, 32, 32*f*
  symptoms, 33
 epidemiology, 303
 evaluation, 33
 persistence, 252*t*
 physical and histological features, 262*t*
 pigmentary alterations, 261
 prevalence, 29
 pruritus (itching), 261
 seborrheic dermatitis, 41
 subtypes
  adolescent/adult, 303
  childhood, 293, 304*f*
  dyshidrotic, 303
  infantile, 303, 304*f*
  nummular, 303
 treatment, 299
  avoid triggers, 33
  cyclosporine, 50
  emollients, 33
  immunomodulatory agents, 36
  light therapy, 35
  topical calcineurin inhibitors, 35
  topical steroids, 34, 34*t*–35*t*
Atrophie blanche, 95
Autoeczematization, 97
Autoimmune blistering diseases, 328*t*
Autoimmune connective tissue diseases, 328*t*
Autoimmune drug reactions, 316–317
Autoimmune skin disorders, 316
Autosomal recessive inherited disorder, 14
Avelumab, 21
Azathioprine, 36, 129, 206
Azzalure/dysport, 235*t*

**B**

Bacterial endocarditis prophylaxis, 216
Balsam of Peru, 36–37
Baricitinib, 21, 360
Basal cell carcinoma (BCC), 157–160, 280, 282*f*, 316, 318*t*–322*t*
 biopsy, 158
 clinical features, 157–158, 159*f*
 follow-up and prevention, 160
 history, 158
 incidence, 161–163
 locally advanced\metastatic, 160
 MMS, 158
 pathogenesis, 157
 prognosis, 160
 risk factors, 157
Bazex-Dupre-Christol syndrome, 157
B cells, 20
Beau lines, 196*t*–199*t*

Benign skin lesions, 146–156
  acrochordons, 149–150, 149f
  angiomas, 150–151, 150f
  cysts, 154–155
  dermatofibroma, 151, 151f
  keloids, 153–154, 153f
  lentigines, 151–152, 152f
  lipomas, 155–156, 155f
  nevi, 146–148
  sebaceous hyperplasia, 152–153, 153f
  seborrheic keratoses, 148–149, 148f, 318t–322t
  solar lentigo, 318t–322t
Benzathine penicillin G, 84
Betamethasone, 131
Bevacizumab, 17
Bexarotene, 177, 349–350
Bimekizumab (Bimzelx), 20, 266t
Binimetinib, 21
Biopsy
  BCC, 158
  melanoma, 167
  punch biopsy technique, 3–4, 4f
  SCC, 161
  shave biopsy technique, 3–4, 4f
Bleeding, 228
Bleomycin, 138
Blue nevi, 146, 147f
Body lice, 79
Body odor, 13
Body surface area (BSA), 175
*Borrelia burgdorferi,* 87
Botox, 235t
Botulinum toxin (BoNT), 233
Brentuximab, 178
Breslow thickness, 167–169
Brodalumab, 20
Bulbous corpuscles, 14
Bullous disorders, 209–211
  bullous pemphigoid, 209, 210f
  clinical presentation, 209
  dermatitis herpetiformis, 209
  evaluation, 209–210
  pemphigus foliaceus, 209
  pemphigus vulgaris, 209
  treatment, 210–211
Bullous pemphigoid (BP), 15, 209, 210f, 211
Busulfan, 138

## C

Cafe au lait macules, 296–297
Calcinosis cutis, Raynaud phenomenon, esophageal dysmotility, sclerodactyly, telangiectasia (CREST), 21
Calcipotriene, 131
*Candida* infection, 65
Capillary malformation, 299–300, 300f
Carbapenem, 77
Carbon dioxide laser, 244
Ceftriaxone, 77

Cellulitis
  clinical features, 72, 73f
  diagnosis, 73f
  infections and infestations, 318t–322t
  pyogenic infection, 72
  treatment, 73
Cemiplimab, 21
Centers for Disease Control and Prevention (CDC), 337
Central centrifugal cicatricial alopecia (CCCA), 188–190, 189f, 252t, 272–276, 275f
Cephalexin, 354
Cephalic pustulosis, 291
Cephalosporins, 354
Chemical peels, 241–243
  caustic agents, 241
  evaluation, 242
  postoperative care, 243
  primary objective, 241
  treatment, 242–243
  types, 241–242
Cherry angiomas. *See* Angiomas
Childhood atopic dermatitis, 33
Chloramphenicol, 91
Cholinergic urticaria, 104
Chronic leg ulcers, 316
Chronic lupus erythematous, 12
Chronic urticaria (CU), 106
Ciclopirox olamine, 53
C-kit receptor tyrosine kinase, 16
Classic dermatomyositis, 203, 204f
Clobetasol propionate, 192t
*Clostridium botulinum,* 233
Clotrimazole, 64
Cobimetinib, 21
Colchicine, 101
Cold urticaria, 104
Collagen, 17
Comedonal acne
  clinical presentation, 39–40, 312, 313f
  topical retinoids, 48
Common warts, 58, 59f
Community acquired MRSA (CA-MRSA) infections, 75
Complete blood count (CBC), 28
Complexion-associated melanosis, 254
Compound nevi, 146, 147f
Condyloma acuminata, 58
Congenital dermal melanocytosis, 136, 297, 298f
Congenital melanocytic nevi (CMN), 297–299, 298f
Congenital syphilis, 82
Conglobata, acne, 26
Contact dermatitis
  allergic contact dermatitis
    clinical presentation, 39–40
    nickel allergic, 36
    poison ivy, 36
  Balsam of Peru, 37
  clinical presentation, 299, 306f

Contact dermatitis (*Continued*)
  differential diagnosis, 52
  evaluation, 299
  irritant contact dermatitis, 36, 40
  patch tested substances, 37t–39t
  patch testing, 41, 41f, 42t
  treatment, 299
    oral steroids, 42
    topical calcineurin inhibitors, 35
    topical steroids, 34
Contact urticaria, 104
Corticosteroids, 34, 34t–35t, 48, 331
Crabs, 13
Crisaborole, 355
Crusted scabies, 317, 318t–322t
Cryoglobulinemia, 18
Cryosurgery, 225
Cutaneous cysts. *See* Cysts
Cutaneous innervation, 14
Cutaneous sarcoidosis, 269–270, 271f
Cutaneous squamous cell carcinoma (cSCC), 280, 281f
Cutaneous T-cell lymphomas (CTCL), 174–178, 267, 268f
  histone deacetylase inhibitors, 178
  histopathology, 175
  immunophenotyping, 177
  light therapy, 177
  mycosis fungoides, 174, 176f
  physical examination, 175
  radiation therapy, 177
  retinoids, 178
  Sézary syndrome, 174, 176f
  T-cell receptor gene rearrangement studies, 177
  topical therapy, 177
Cutaneous T-cell lymphoma mortality, 252t
Cutaneous vasculitis
  cutaneous manifestations, 97
  definition, 97
  evaluation, 100–101
  histopathologic finding, 97
  laboratory testing, 97
  targeted history and physical exam assessment, 100
  treatment, 101
Cutis marmorata telangiectatica congenita, 300
Cyclophosphamide, 138
Cyclosporine, 107, 129
  atopic dermatitis, 35
  psoriasis, 50
Cystic acne, 312, 313f
Cysts, 154–155
  epidermal inclusion
    clinical presentation, 154
    treatment, 155
  evaluation, 155
  milia
    clinical presentation, 154
    treatment, 155
  pilar
    clinical presentation, 154
    treatment, 155

# D

Dabrafenib, 21
Dactinomycin, 138
Dapsone, 101, 203
Darier-Roussy sarcoid, 19
Daunorubicin, 138
Delayed pressure urticaria, 104
Dendritic cells (DCs), 16
DermaBlade, 216
Dermal cells, 17
Dermal melanocytosis, 136–138, 254, 256f
Dermatitis, 313f
  atopic dermatitis, 303–305, 304f
  contact dermatitis, 305–307
  diaper, 307
  seborrheic, 307–308, 307f
Dermatitis herpetiformis (DH), 209
Dermatofibroma, 151, 151f
Dermatofibrosarcoma protuberans, 252t, 281, 283f
Dermatographism, 103, 103f
Dermatologic inequities, 251
Dermatologic surgery, 215–232
  preoperative assessment, 215–219
    anesthesia, 218–219
    anesthetic concerns, 218–219
    anticoagulant use, 215–216
    antiseptics, 217–218
    implantable cardiac devices, 216
    infection precautions, 216–217
    informed consent, 217
    surgical preparation, 217
  procedural techniques, 219–227
    cryosurgery, 225
    deroofing, 226–227
    electrodesiccation and curettage, 226
    elliptical excision, 221–223, 222f–223f
    excision, 221–223
    Mohs micrographic surgery, 224–225
    punch biopsy, 220–221
    shave biopsy, 219–220
    snip removal, 221
    surgical repairs, 223–224
  surgical complications, 228–230
    bleeding, 228
    dehiscence, 230, 230f
    hematoma, 228, 229f
    infection, 229, 229f
  wound dressing, 227–228
  wound healing, 228
Dermatology, 251
Dermatomyositis (DM), 203–206
  autoimmune inflammatory myopathy, 203
  clinical presentation
    amyopathic dermatomyositis, 205
    antisynthetase syndrome, 203

classic dermatomyositis, 203, 204f
drug induced, 205
extracutaneous involvement, 205
and malignancy, 205
evaluation, 205
skin manifestations and pathogenic autoantibodies, 203
treatment, 205–206
Dermatosis papulosa nigra (DPN), 148, 259t–260t, 278–280, 280f
Dermis, 11–12, 11f
Desmosomes, 10, 15–16
Desoximetasone, 346
Deucravacitinib, 20, 360
Deuruxolitinib, 360
Dexamethasone, 131
Diaper dermatitis, 307
Dihydrotestosterone (DHT) stimulation, 12
Discoid lupus erythematosus (DLE), 13, 190, 191t, 201–202, 202f, 252t, 267–269, 269f
Disorders of pigmentation, 125–143
 dermal melanocytosis, 136–138
 drug-induced pigmentation, 138–140
 erythema dyschromicum perstans, 140–141
 idiopathic guttate hypomelanosis, 141
 melasma, 131–134
 oculocutaneous albinism, 134–136
 pityriasis alba, 141
 postinflammatory hyperpigmentation, 141–143
 postinflammatory hypopigmentation, 143
 vitiligo, 125–131
Dissecting cellulitis, 192–193
Doxorubicin, 138
Doxycycline, 91, 194
Drug eruptions, 116–122
 AGEP, 118, 119f, 121t, 122
 anaphylaxis, 116, 121t
 angioedema, 117
 anticoagulant-induced skin necrosis, 120
 DIHS, 116
 DRESS, 116, 118, 121t
 exanthematous eruption, 116, 121t
 fixed drug eruption, 117, 118f, 121t
 photosensitivity, 116–117
 reactions to chemotherapy, 116
 SJS, 116, 120, 121t
 stasis dermatitis, 316, 318t–322t
 TEN, 116, 120, 120f, 121t
 urticaria, 117, 121t, 316–317, 318t–322t
Drug-induced acne, 26
Drug-induced hypersensitivity syndrome (DIHS), 118
Drug-induced pigmentation, 138–140
Drug reaction with eosinophilia and systemic symptoms (DRESS), 116, 118, 121t
Dry skin. *See* Xerosis
Dupilumab, 20

**E**

Ecchymosis, 98
Eccrine hidradenoma, 14
Eccrine sweat glands, 13
Econazole, 64
Ectodermal dysplasia, 15–16
Eczema, 15
Efudex, 356–357, 356f
Ehlers-Danlos syndrome, 17
Elastin, 17
Elderly dermatoses. *See* Geriatric dermatology
Enbrel, 359
Encorafenib, 21
Endocrine diseases, 329t
Endogenous retinoids, 348
Endothelial cells, 17
Eosinophils, 19
Epidermal cells, 15
Epidermal inclusion cysts, 154
 clinical presentation, 154, 154f
 treatment, 155
Epidermis, 10
Epidermodysplasia verruciformis, 16
Epidermolysis bullosa disease, 15
Epidermolytic ichthyosis disease, 15
Epinephrine, 218
Eponychium, 15
Erbium-doped yttrium aluminum garnet (Er:YAG), 244
Erysipelas, 73–74
Erythema, 254–256, 257f
Erythema ab igne, 316, 323–324
Erythema dyschromicum perstans, 140–141
Erythema induratum of Bazin (EIB), 86
Erythema multiforme, 313–314, 314f
Erythema nodosum, 12
Erythema toxicum neonatorum, 292–293
 clinical presentation, 292, 293f
 evaluation, 293
 treatment, 293
Erythemal radiation, 335
Erythematous papulosquamous diseases, 328t
Erythroderma, 175, 177
Erythromelalgia, 14
Erythrotelangiectatic rosacea
 clinical presentation, 29, 30f
 treatment, 31
Etanercept, 20, 359
Excisional biopsy, 167
Exogenous inoculation, 85
External beam radiation therapy (EBRT), 177

**F**

Familial Mediterranean fever, 105
Fibrillin, 17
Fibroblasts, 17
Fibrofolliculoma, 13
Fibronectin, 17
Fine needle aspiration (FNA), 168
Finger and toenail skin, 15

Flat warts, 58
Fluocinonide, 192t
5-fluorouracil (5-FU), 158, 356–357, 356f–357f
Folliculitis decalvans, 193–194
Folliculitis keloidalis nuchae, 272, 273f
Food and drug administration (FDA), 336
Free nerve endings, 14
Fulminans, acne, 26
Fungal cultures, 2
Fungus, 13
Furuncles
- adolescents and young adults, 74
- clinical features, 74–75, 74f
- hair follicle, 74
- predisposing factors, 74
- purulent material, 74

## G

Geriatric dermatology, 316–332
- actinic purpura, 316, 322–323, 323f
- allergic contact dermatitis, 316–317, 318t–322t
- benign skin lesions, 318t–322t
- erythema ab igne, 316, 323–324
- hair and nails disorder, 318t–322t
- infections and infestations
  - cellulitis, 318t–322t
  - crusted/norwegian scabies, 318t–322t
  - herpes zoster (shingles), 316, 318t–322t
  - intertrigo, 316, 318t–322t
  - scabies, 318t–322t
  - tinea pedis, 317, 318t–322t
- leg ulcers, 316, 324–326
- maceration, 316, 326–327
- malignant skin lesions
  - actinic keratosis, 326–327
  - BCC, 318t–322t
  - lentigo maligna, 318t–322t
  - melanoma, 318t–322t
  - SCC, 318t–322t
- pruritus, 327–332
- reactive disorders and drug eruptions, 318t–322t
- rosacea, 316, 318t–322t
- seborrheic dermatitis, 316
- systemic disease, 318t–322t
- xerosis (see Xerosis)

Glucocorticosteroids, 345–348
- dosing, 342t–343t, 346
- hypothalamic pituitary axis, 345
- indications/use, 347
- intralesional therapy, 345–347
- mechanism of action, 345
- pharmacology, 345
- potency classification, 342t–343t
- systemic therapy, 347–348
- therapeutic considerations
  - allergy, 346
  - candida/tinea, 347
  - cutaneous atrophy, 346–347, 346f
  - desoximetasone, 346
  - perioral dermatitis, 347
  - topical therapy, 345–347

Green nail syndrome, 196t–199t
Griseofulvin, 64
Guselkumab, 20
Guttate psoriasis, 45

## H

Hair bulb, 12
Hair disorders, 183–200
- alopecia areata, 184f, 185–186, 186t
- anagen effluvium, 187
- androgenetic alopecia, 183–185, 184f, 185t
- central centrifugal cicatricial alopecia, 188–190, 189f
- discoid lupus erythematosus, 190, 191t
- dissecting cellulitis, 192–193, 193f
- folliculitis decalvans, 193–194
- hirsutism, 194–196, 195t
- hypertrichosis, 194, 195t
- lichen planopilaris, 190–192, 191f, 192t
- onychomycosis, 196t–199t
- secondary scarring alopecias, 194
- telogen effluvium, 186–187, 187t
- trichotillomania, 187–188, 188f

Hair follicle malformation syndromes, 15–16
Hair functions, 12
Hair restoration
- clinical presentation, 247
- evaluation, 247
- hair loss/alopecia, 247
- treatment, 247

Halo nevi, 146
$H_2$ antihistamines, 107
$H_1$ antihistamines, 107
Head lice, 79
Hematogenous dissemination, 86
Hematologic diseases, 329t
Hematoma, 228, 229f
Hemidesmosomes, 10, 15
Herald patch, 43
Hereditary nonpolyposis colorectal carcinoma (HNPCC) syndrome, 14
Herpes simplex virus type 1 (HSV-1), 67
Herpes simplex virus type 2 (HSV-2), 67
Herpes zoster, 69, 70f, 316, 318t–322t
Hidradenitis suppurativa (HS), 252t, 259t–260t, 263–267, 265f
- FDA-approved biologic treatments, 266t
- treatments, 266t

Hirsutism, 194–196, 195t
Histone deacetylase inhibitors, 178
Hives. See Urticaria
Hormone-induced cystic acne, 26–27
HSV infection, 11
Human papillomavirus, 16
Humira, 359
Hyaluronic acid (HA), 17, 233, 239–240

Hydrocolloids, 325
Hydrogels, 325
Hydroxychloroquine, 192*t*
Hyperhidrosis, 13
Hyperpigmentation, macular, 95
Hyperthermia, 13
Hypertrichosis, 194–196, 195*t*
Hypertrophic scars, 17, 153
Hypocalemia, 45
Hyponychium, 15

## I

Ichthyosis vulgaris, 15
Idiopathic guttate hypomelanosis, 141
Imatinib, 138
Imiquimod, 355–356
Immunology
    adaptive immunity, 19
    innate immunity, 18
Immunophenotyping, 177
Immunosuppressants, 266*t*
Impetigo, 70*f*, 71
Implantable cardiac devices, 216
Incisional biopsy, 167
Indoor tanning, 337
Infantile atopic dermatitis, 33
Infantile hemangioma, 17, 300–302
Infections, skin
    cellulitis, 318*t*–322*t*
    herpes zoster, 316, 318*t*–322*t*
    intertrigo, 316, 318*t*–322*t*
    pruritus, 318*t*–322*t*
    scabies, 318*t*–322*t*
Infestations
    pruritus, 318*t*–322*t*
    tinea pedis, 317, 318*t*–322*t*
Inflammatory acne, 312
    clinical presentation, 24
    treatment
        benzoyl peroxide, 27
        clindamycin, 27
        isotretinoin, 28
        oral antibiotics, 28
        sodium sulfacetamide, 27
Infliximab, 20, 359
Infundibulum, 12
Innate immunity, 18
Innate lymphoid cells (ILCs), 18
Intense pulsed light (IPL), 244–245
Intercellular adhesion molecule 1 (ICAM-1), 17
Intradermal nevi, 146, 147*f*
Intralesional steroids, 154
Intralesional triamcinolone acetonide, 346
Inverse psoriasis, 46
Iodosorb, 325
Ipilimumab, 20–21
Irritant contact dermatitis, 36
Isotretinoin, 28, 31, 349
Isthmus, 12
Itchy skin. *See* Pruritus

Ivermectin, 80
Ixekizumab, 20

## J

Janus kinase inhibitors (JAKi), 21
Jeuveau, 235*t*
Junctional nevi, 146, 147*f*

## K

Kaposi sarcoma, 17
Keloids, 17, 153*f*, 252*t*, 259*t*–260*t*, 278, 279*f*
Keratin, 15
Keratinocytes, 15
Keratohyalin granules, 15
Ketoconazole, 53, 64, 291
Kidney disease, 329*t*
Koebner phenome, 45

## L

Lactate dehydrogenase (LDH), 169
Lamellar corpuscles, 14
Laminin, 17
Langerhans cells, 10, 16, 19
Laser and energy-based devices, 243–246
    chromophores, 243–244
    clinical presentation, 244
    components, 243–244
    evaluation, 244–245
    laser devices and associated indications, 245*t*
    lasers, 244
    treatment, 245–246
Laser hair removal (LHR), 246
Latent syphilis, 82–83
LDH. *See* Lactate dehydrogenase (LDH)
Leg ulcers, 324–326
    arterial, 324
    evaluation, 324–325
    venous, 324–325
Leiomyoma/leiomyosarcoma, 18
Lentigines, 151–152, 152*f*
Lentigo maligna, 316, 318*t*–322*t*
Leser-Trelat sign, 12
Leukonychia, 196*t*–199*t*
Lice, 13, 79–80
Lichen planopilaris (LPP), 13, 190–192, 191*f*, 192*t*
Lichen sclerosus et atrophicus (LSA), 207–208, 318*t*–322*t*
Lichen scrofulosorum, 86
Lichenification, 96
Lidocaine, 218
Light amplification by stimulated emission of radiation (LASER), 243–244
Light therapy, 177
Lipodermatosclerosis, 96
Lipomas, 155–156, 155*f*
Liver diseases, 329*t*
Local heat contact urticaria, 104
Lofgren syndrome, 207
Longitudinal melanonychia, 196*t*–199*t*

Lupus, 201–203
Lupus pernio, 208
Lyme disease
  *Borrelia burgdorferi*, 87
  clinical features, 88–89, 88f
  diagnosis, 87
  differential diagnosis, 63–64
  incidence of, 88
  *Ixodes* tick vector, 88
  treatment, 90
  vector-borne disease, 87
Lyme neuroborreliosis (LNB), 89

# M

Maceration, 316, 326
Macrophages, 19
*Malassezia furfur*, 64
*Malassezia globosa*, 51
Male pattern baldness. *See* Androgenic alopecia
Malignant skin lesions, 157–182
  actinic keratosis, 318t–322t
  BCC, 318t–322t (*see also* Basal cell carcinoma (BCC))
  CTCL (*see* Cutaneous T-cell lymphomas (CTCL))
  melanoma, 318t–322t (*see also* Melanoma)
  SCC (*see* Squamous cell carcinoma (SCC))
Malnutrition, 328t
Marfan syndrome, 17
Mast cells, 19
Mastocytosis, 19
MED. *See* Minimal erythema dose (MED)
Mechlorethamine, 138
Medication-induced pruritus, 327
Meissner's corpuscles, 14
Melanocortin-1 receptor (MC1-R), 16
Melanocytes, 10, 16
Melanocyte-stimulating hormone, 16, 338
Melanocytic nevi. *See* Nevi
Melanocytosis variants
  dermal melanocytosis, 254, 256f
  oculodermal melanocytosis, 254
  scleral melanocytosis, 254, 257f
Melanoma, 165–171, 280–281, 283f, 316, 318t–322t
  ABCDEs, 2
  biopsy, 167
  clinical presentation, 165–166, 166f
  histologic reporting and classification, 166f, 167
  incidence, 165
  risk factor, 165
  staging, 167–168, 168t
  treatment, 169–171
Melanoma 5-y mortality, 252t
Melanoma late diagnosis, 252t
Melasma, 131–134, 132f, 252t, 259t–260t
Merkel cell carcinoma (MCC), 10, 14, 16, 171–174, 282, 284f

Metastatic cutaneous squamous cell carcinoma, 164
Metformin, 189
Methicillin-resistant *Staphylococcus aureus* (MRSA), 75–76
Methotrexate, 36, 50, 129, 138, 203, 206, 358
Metronidazole, 31, 77
Miconazole, 64
Microneedling, 248–249
  clinical presentation, 248
  devices, 248
  evaluation, 248–249
  treatment, 248–249
Microphthalmia-associated transcription factor (MITF), 16
Milia cysts, 154, 293
Miliaria crystallina, 293–294
Miliaria rubra, 294
Minimal erythema dose (MED), 334
Minocycline, 28, 129, 192t
Mogamulizumab, 178
Mohs micrographic surgery (MMS), 158, 224–225
Molluscum contagiosum (MC), 59–60, 311, 312f
Mongolian spot, 136, 297, 298f
Morbilliform, drug eruption, 116, 318t–322t
Morphea, 207–208
Muckle-Wells syndrome, 104–105
Mucosal pigmentation
  complexion-associated melanosis, 254
  oral mucosal melanosis, 253f, 254
Mucous membranes, 15
Muir-Torre syndrome, 14
Multiple linear melanonychia, 254, 255f
Mupirocin, 353
*Mycobacterium marinum* infection, 86
Mycophenolate mofetil, 203
Mycosis fungoides (MF), 267. *See also* Cutaneous T-cell lymphomas (CTCL)
  erythroderma, 175, 177
  patches, 175, 176f, 177
  plaques, 175, 176f, 177
  tumors, 175, 177
Myelin, 18
Myoepithelial cells, 13

# N

Nail disorders, 196–200, 196t–199t, 318t–322t
Narrow band UVB (NBUVB), 35
  dosing, 351
  indications/use, 351
  mechanism of action, 351
  therapeutic considerations, 351
Natural killer (NK) cells, 18
Necrotizing fasciitis, 76–77
Nemolizumab, 20
Neodymium-doped yttrium aluminum garnet (Nd:YAG), 244
Neonatal and infantile dermatology, 291

aplasia cutis congenita, 291–292, 292f
congenital dermal melanocytosis, 297, 298f
erythema toxicum neonatorum, 292–293
milia, 293, 293f
miliaria, 293–294
neonatal acne, 291, 292f
nevus sebaceus, 294–295, 295f
spitz nevus, 299
subcutaneous fat necrosis, 295–296, 295f
transient neonatal pustular melanosis, 296
Neoplasms, 13–14
Neurofibromas, 12, 14
Neurofibromin, 16
Neurologic diseases, 328t
Neuromas, 14
Neurosyphilis, 82
Neurotoxins
  applications, 233–234
  BoNT, 233
  botulinum toxin formulations, 235t
  clinical presentation, 233–234
  evaluation, 234–236
  neuromuscular junction, 233
  patient counselling, 236
  posttreatment care, 236–237
  treatment, 236
    frown lines/marionette linee, 238f
    glabellar complex, 234f
    glabellar frown rhytids, 236f
    lateral canthal rhytides/crow's feet, 237f
    nasal rhytides/bunny lines, 237f
    perioral rhytides, 238f
Neutrophils, 19
Nevi, 146–148
  clinical presentation
    blue nevi, 146, 147f
    compound nevi, 146, 147f
    halo nevi, 146, 147f
    intradermal nevi, 146, 147f
  evaluation, 147
  treatment, 147
Nevus of Ito, 137–138
Nevus of Ota, 137
Nevus sebaceus, 294–295, 295f
Nevus simplex, 302–303, 302f
Nickel allergic contact dermatitis, 36
Nivolumab, 21
Nodulocystic acne, 25f
Non-Hodgkin lymphomas, 174
Nonscarring alopecia, 13, 185
Normal pigmentation variants
  melanocytosis variants, 254
  mucosal pigmentation, 254
  multiple linear melanonychia, 254, 255f
  oral mucosal melanosis, 254
  pigmentary demarcation lines, 251–254
  voigt-futcher lines, 251–254, 253f
Norwegian scabies, 317, 318t–322t
Nutritional deficiencies, 211–213, 211t–212t

## O

Ocular rosacea, 29, 32
Oculocutaneous albinism, 16, 134–136
Oculodermal melanocytosis, 254
Omalizumab, 21, 36, 107
Onycholysis, 196t–199t
Onychomadesis, 196t–199t
Onychomycosis, 317, 318t–322t
Onychorrhexis, 196t–199t
Oral contraceptive pills (OCPs), 28
Oral mucosal melanosis, 253f, 254
Oral ruxolitinib, 21
Orificial TB, 86
Ota/Hori's nevus, 254

## P

Pacinian corpuscles, 14
Palmar and plantar warts, 58
Palmoplantar keratosis, 15–16
Palpable purpura
  clinical presentation, 100
  small-vessel vasculitis, 98–100, 99f
Panniculitis, 12, 18
Papillary dermis, 12
Papular sarcoidosis, 206
Papulopustular rosacea
  clinical presentation, 29
  systemic treatments, 31
  topical medications, 31
Paronychia, 196t–199t
Patched 1 homolog (PTCH1) gene, 157
PDT. *See* Photodynamic therapy (PDT)
Pediatric dermatology, 291–314
  acne vulgaris, 311–313, 313f
  dermatitis (*see* Dermatitis)
  erythema multiforme, 313–314, 314f
  infectious diseases, 308
    molluscum contagiosum, 311, 312f
    tinea, 308–309, 308f–309f
    verrucae, 309–311, 310f
  neonatal and infantile dermatology, 291
    aplasia cutis congenita, 291–292, 292f
    erythema toxicum neonatorum, 292–293
    milia, 293
    miliaria, 293–294
    neonatal acne, 291, 292f
    nevus sebaceus, 294–295
    subcutaneous fat necrosis, 295–296, 295f
    transient neonatal pustular melanosis, 296
  pigmented lesions, 296
    Cafe au lait macules, 296–297
    congenital dermal melanocytosis, 297, 298f
    congenital melanocytic nevi, 297–299
    spitz nevus, 299
  vascular lesions, 299
    capillary malformation, 299–300
    cutis marmorata telangiectatica congenita, 300
    infantile hemangioma, 300–302
    nevus simplex, 302–303, 302f

Pediculosis, 79–80
Pembrolizumab, 21, 174
Pemphigus, 15–16
Pemphigus foliaceus (PF), 209
Pemphigus vulgaris (PV), 209–210, 316, 318*t*–322*t*
Permethrin, 80
Petechiae
 abnormal platelet function, 98
 nonblanchable and nonpalpable pinpoint macules, 98, 99*f*
 nonplatelet etiologies, 98
 thrombocytopenia, 98
Photodynamic therapy (PDT), 158, 163
Phototherapy, topical therapy
 NBUVB, 351
 PUVA, 352–353
 ultraviolet (UV) radiation, 350, 351*t*
Phymatous rosacea, 29, 30*f*, 31
Physical urticarias, 103, 106
Piebaldism, 16
Pigmentary demarcation lines, 251–254
Pilar cysts, 154–155
Pilosebaceous unit, 13
Pimecrolimus, 35, 354
Pioglitazone hydrochloride, 192*t*
Pitting nail disorder, 196*t*–199*t*
Pityriasis alba, 141
Pityriasis rosea (PR), 43–44, 43*f*
Plaques, 175
Plasma cells, 20
Platelet-rich plasma (PRP), 247–248
Plexiform neurofibromas, 18
Postadolescent acne
 clinical presentation, 26
 OCPs, 28
 spironolactone, 26–27
Postinflammatory hyperpigmentation (PIH), 141–143, 256–260, 258*f*, 259*t*–260*t*
Postinflammatory hypopigmentation (PIHo), 143, 260
Potassium hydroxide mount, 2, 3*f*
Prednisone, 101
Pressure ulcers, 316
Primary neuroendocrine carcinoma, 14
Primary syphilis, 80, 81*f*, 82
Procaine penicillin G, 84
*Propionibacterium acnes,* 24, 344
Proteoglycans, 17
Pruritus, 154, 316, 327–332, 328*t*
Pseudofolliculitis barbae (PFB), 252*t*, 270–272, 272*f*
 clinical features, 270, 272*f*
 men of African descent, 270
 treatments
  community intervention, 274*t*
  intralesional energy-based devices, 274*t*
  oral, 274*t*
  surgery/procedures, 274*t*
  topicals, 274*t*

Pseudofolliculitis barbae and acne keloidalis nuchae, 259*t*–260*t*
Pseudo-Kaposi sarcoma, 96
Psoralens plus UVA (PUVA), 352–353, 352*f*
Psoriasin, 18
Psoriasis, 11
 clinical diagnosis, 47
 clinical presentation
  chronic plaque psoriasis, 45
  guttate, 45
  inverse, 46
  psoriatic arthritis, 45
  pustular, 45, 46*f*
 immune-mediated disorder, 44
 innate and adaptive immunity, 44
 prevalence, 44
 psychosocial manifestations, 44
 systemic manifestations, 44
 treatment
  phototherapy, 49
  systemic therapy, 50
  topical therapy, 48
 triggering factors, 45
Psoriatic arthritis, 45, 46*f*
Psychogenic diseases, 328*t*
Pulsed dye laser (PDL), 244
Punch biopsy technique, 3–4, 4*f*, 220–221
Pustular psoriasis, 45, 46*f*

# R

Radiation therapy
 BCC, 158
 CTCL, 177
Rapid plasma reagin (RPR), 43–44
RAS-RAF-MEK-ERK signaling pathway, 16
Reactive disorders, 95–124
 cutaneous vasculitis
  cutaneous manifestations, 97
  definition, 98
  evaluation, 100–101
  histopathologic finding, 97
  laboratory testing, 101
  treatment, 101
 petechiae
  abnormal platelet function, 98
  nonblanchable and nonpalpable pinpoint macules, 98, 99*f*
  nonplatelet etiologies, 98
  thrombocytopenia, 98
 stasis dermatitis, 95–97, 96*f*, 318*t*–322*t*
 urticaria, 101–107, 102*f*–103*f*, 318*t*–322*t*
 viral exanthems, 107–116
Relatlimab-rmbw, 21
Remicade, 357, 359
Reticular dermis, 12
Retinoids, 164–165, 266*t*, 312, 348–350
 mechanism of action, 348
 pharmacology and teratogenicity, 348–349
 systemic retinoids
  acitretin (soriatane), 350

bexarotene (targretin), 350
isotretinoin (accutane), 349
topical retinoids compounds, 349
vitamin A, 348
Rifampicin, 194
Rifampin, isoniazid, pyrazinamide, ethambutol (RIPE) therapy, 87
Risankizumab, 20
Ritlecitinib, 21, 360
Rituximab, 36, 206, 357
Rocky Mountain spotted fever (RMSF), 91–93, 92f
Roflumilast, 355
Rombo syndromes, 157
Rosacea, 29–32, 30f, 318t–322t
Ruffini corpuscles, 14
Ruxolitinib, 21, 354

## S

Sarcoidosis, 204f, 206–207, 269–270
Sarcoidosis mortality, 252t
*Sarcoptes scabiei* var. *hominis,* 77
Saucerization, 167
Scabies, 77–79, 317, 318t–322t, 328t
Scalp skin, 15, 328t
Scar sarcoidosis, 207
Scarring alopecia, 272
  central centrifugal cicatricial alopecia, 188, 189f
  discoid lupus, 13
  folliculitis decalvans, 193–194
  lichen planopilaris, 13, 190–192, 191f
  lupus erythematosus, 190
  secondary, 194
SCC. *See* Squamous cell carcinoma (SCC)
Schnitzler syndrome, 105
Schwann cells, 18
Schwannomas, 14, 18
Scleral melanocytosis, 254, 257f
Scleroderma, 207–209
Sclerotherapy, 246
  evaluation, 246
  reticular and varicose veins, 246
  treatment, 246
Scurvy, 213f
Sebaceous carcinoma (SC), 14, 282
Sebaceous glands, 14
Sebaceous hyperplasia, 14, 152–153, 153f
Seborrheic dermatitis, 262–263, 264f, 307–308, 316
  age distributions, 51
  clinical description of, 318t–322t
  clinical presentation, 52, 307–308, 307f
  cradle cap, 51
  differential diagnosis, 52
  mild eczematous process, 51
  pathogenesis, 51
  treatment, 53–54, 308
Seborrheic keratoses, 11, 148–149, 148f, 316, 318t–322t
Secondary scarring alopecias, 194

Secondary syphilis, 80, 81f, 82–83
Secukinumab, 20, 266t
SEER. *See* Surveillance, epidemiology and end results program (SEER)
Senile purpura. *See* Actinic purpura
Septisol©, 242
Sézary syndrome (SS), 174,176f. *See also* Cutaneous T-cell lymphomas (CTCL)
Shave biopsy technique, 3–4, 4f, 219–220
Shingles. *See* Herpes zoster
S100 antibody detects, 18
Silver-impregnated dressings, 325
Skin
  anatomy
    cutaneous innervation, 14
    dermis, 11–12, 11f
    epidermis, 10
    hair functions, 12
    mucous membranes, 15
    pilosebaceous unit, 13
    scalp, nails, palms and soles, 15
  cellular and molecular biology
    dermal cells, 17
    epidermal cells, 15
  conditions, 251
  examination
    biopsy, 3, 4f
    culture, 2
    history of, 1
    indications, 1–2
    patterns of dermatologic lesions, 5, 8t
    potassium hydroxide mount, 2, 3f
    primary lesions, 5t–6t
    secondary lesions, 5, 7t
  immunology
    adaptive immunity, 19
    innate immunity, 18
Skin cancer
  basal cell carcinoma, 280, 282f
  cutaneous squamous cell carcinoma, 280, 281f
  dermatofibrosarcoma protuberans, 281, 283f
  melanoma, 280–281, 283f
  Merkel cell carcinoma, 282, 284f
  sebaceous carcinoma, 282
Skin of color (SOC) dermatology
  adult and pediatric dermatology, 260–276
  Dermatologic inequities, 251
  erythema, 254–255
  frequency and impact, 252t
  goal, 251
  lasers applications, 254–256
  normal pigmentation variants, 251–254
  postinflammatory pigmentary alteration, 256–260
  scope, 251
  skin health, 251
  surgical and procedural dermatology, 276–284
  United States, 251

# Index

Skin phototypes, 350–351, 351*t*
Smooth muscle cells, 18
Soft tissue fillers, 233
   aseptic techniques, 240
   clinical presentation, 239
   dermal fillers, 238–239
   evaluation, 239
   precautions, 240
   treatment, 239–240
Solar lentigo, 318*t*–322*t*
Solar purpura. *See* Actinic purpura
Solar urticaria, 104
Soriatane, 350
Southern tick-associated rash illness (STARI), 89–90. *See also* Lyme disease
SPF. *See* Sun protection factor (SPF)
Spironolactone, 29
Spitz nevi, 147, 147*f*, 299
Spray tanning, 338
Squamous cell carcinoma (SCC), 14, 160–165, 316, 318*t*–322*t*
   actinic keratoses, 163–164
   biopsy, 161
   chemoprevention, 164–165
   clinical features, 161, 162*f*
   follow-up and prevention, 164
   incidence, 160
   localized, 164
   metastatic cutaneous, 164
   pathogenesis, 161
   prognosis, 164
   risk factor, 160–161
   staging, 161–163
*Staphylococcus aureus,* 193
Stasis dermatitis, 95–97, 96*f*, 316, 318*t*–322*t*
   chronic venous insufficiency, 95
   clinical presentation
      acroangiodermatitis/pseudo-Kaposi sarcoma, 96
      atrophie blanche, 95
      autoeczematization, 97
      complications, 96
      hyperpigmentation, 95
      lichenification, 96
      lipodermatosclerosis, 96
      superinfection, 97
   epidemiology, 95
   evaluation, 97
   risk factors, 95
   treatment, 97
   venous hypertension, 95
Stevens-Johnson syndrome (SJS), 120, 121*t*, 122
Stratum basale, 10
Stratum corneum, 10
Stratum granulosum, 10
Stratum lucidum, 10
Stratum spinosum, 10
Stress exposure, 104

Stucco keratoses, 148
Subacute cutaneous lupus erythematosus (SCLE), 201–202, 202*f*
Subcutaneous fat necrosis, 295–296, 295*f*
Subcutaneous tissue, 12
Subungual hyperkeratosis, 196*t*–199*t*
Subungual malignant melanoma, 196*t*–199*t*
Sun protection factor (SPF), 334, 336*f*
Sun safety
   counseling, 338
   melanocyte-stimulating hormone, 338
   SPF, 334, 336*f*
   sun protective clothing, 337
   sunscreens
      broad spectrum, 336–337
      outdoor activities, 337
      regulation, 336
      risks, 336
      water resistant, 336
   tanning bed use, 337–338
   UV light radiation
      chemical absorbers, 334, 335*t*
      effects, 333
      regulation, 336
      spectrum classification, 333
      uses, 334
      UVI, 333, 335*t*
      wavelength, 333
   vitamin D, 336
Sunless tanning lotions, 338
Superficial dermatophytes
   clinical features
      tinea capitis, 61*f*–62*f*, 63
      tinea corporis, 60, 61*f*–62*f*
      tinea cruris, 61
      tinea manuum, 62
      tinea pedis, 61*f*–62*f*, 63
      tinea unguium, 61*f*–62*f*, 63
   fungal infections, 60
   potassium hydroxide preparation, 63, 64*f*
   treatments, 64
Superficial skin infections, 353
Superinfection, 97
Surgical and procedural dermatology, SOC
   dermatosis papulosa nigra, 278–280, 280*f*
   keloids, 278, 279*f*
   procedural considerations, patients of color, 276–277
   skin cancer, patients of color, 280–282
Surveillance, epidemiology and end results program (SEER), 165
Syphilis, 80–84, 81*f*
Systemic antibiotics, 266*t*
Systemic disease, 318*t*–322*t*
Systemic retinoids
   acitretin (soriatane), 350
   bexarotene (targretin), 350
   isotretinoin (accutane), 349

## T

Tacrolimus, 35, 354
Tactile corpuscles, 14
Talimogene laherparepvec (TVEC), 21
Tanning bed use, 337–338
Targretin, 349
Tazarotene, 48
Tazobactam, 77
T cells, 19
Telogen effluvium (TE), 186–187, 186*t*
Terbinafine, 64
Tertiary syphilis, 47
Tetracyclines, acne, 28
Thalidomide, 203
Tick-borne illnesses, 87
Tildrakizumab, 20
Tinea capitis, 308, 308*f*
Tinea corporis, 308–309, 309*f*
Tinea pedis, 317, 318*t*–322*t*
Tinea versicolor, 64–65
TLR7 agonist. *See* Toll-like receptor 7 (TLR7) agonist
TNM. *See* Tumor, node, metastasis (TNM) system
Tofacitinib, 360
Toll-like receptor 7 (TLR7) agonist, 163–164
Toll-like receptors (TLRs), 18
Topical antibiotics, 266*t*
Topical calcineurin inhibitors (TCIs), 354
Topical immunomodulators and chemotherapeutics
    5-fluorouracil, 356–357, 356*f*–357*f*
    imiquimod, 355–356, 356*f*
    topical calcineurin inhibitors (TCIs), 354
Topical retinoids, 27
Topical steroids
    atopic dermatitis, 34
    contact dermatitis, 42
    seborrheic dermatitis, 53
Topical therapy
    application quantity, 344–345
    clinical factors, drug absorption, 341–344
    CTCL, 177
    factors, 340–341
    glucocorticosteroids, 345–348
        dosing, 344*t*, 346
        hypothalamic pituitary axis, 345
        indications/use, 345
        mechanism of action, 345
        pharmacology, 345
        systemic therapy, 347–348
        therapeutic considerations, 345–347
    immunosuppressive and immunomodulatory agents
        anti-TNF agents, 358–359
        janus kinase inhibitors (JAKI), 359–360
        methotrexate, 358
        vaccination, 360–361
    phototherapy
        NBUVB, 351
        PUVA, 352–353
        ultraviolet radiation, 350, 351*t*
    retinoids
        mechanism of action, 348
        pharmacology and teratogenicity, 348–349
    systemic retinoids
        acitretin (soriatane), 350
        bexarotene (targretin), 350
        isotretinoin (accutane), 349
        topical retinoids compounds, 349
    vitamin A, 348
    skin barrier function, 341–344
    stratum corneum, 340
    vehicles, 341, 342*t*–343*t*
Total skin electron beam therapy (TSEBT), 177
Toxic epidermal necrolysis (TEN), 120, 120*f*, 121*t*
Trachyonychia, 196*t*–199*t*
Traction alopecia, 252*t*, 276, 277*f*
Tralokinumab, 20
Trametinib, 21
Transient neonatal pustular melanosis, 296, 296*f*
Tregs, 20
*Treponema pallidum*, 80
Tretinoin (Retin-A), 27, 349
Triamcinolone, 97
Triamcinolone acetonide, 192*t*
Trichilemmal cysts, 154–155
Trichodiscoma, 13
*Trichophyton tonsurans*, 63
Trichotillomania, 187–188, 188*f*
Truncal acne, 25*f*
Tuberculosis (TB)
    clinical presentation
        cutaneous manifestations, 85, 85*f*
        endogenous spread, 85
        exogenous inoculation, 85
        hematogenous dissemination, 86
        hypersensitivity reactions, 86
    evaluation, 87
    treatment, 87
Tumor-infiltrating lymphocytes, 21
Tumor necrosis factor (TNF) inhibitors, 20, 45
Tumor, node, metastasis (TNM) system, 161–163
Tumors, mycosis fungoides, 174
Tyndall effect, 240
Tyrosinase, 16

## U

Ugly duckling sign, 147
Ultraviolet (UV) light exposure
    BCC, 157
    melanoma, 165
    SCC, 161–163
Ultraviolet (UV) light radiation. *See also* Sun safety
    chemical absorbers, 334, 335*t*
    effects, 333

Ultraviolet (UV) light radiation. *See also* Sun safety (*Continued*)
  physical blockers, 334, 335*t*
  regulation, 336
  spectrum classification, 333
  uses, 334
  UVI, 333, 335*t*
  wavelength, 333
Ultraviolet protection factor (UPF), 337
Upadacitinib, 21, 360
Urticaria, 17–19, 101–107, 316–317, 318*t*–322*t*
  acute urticaria, 106
  causes, 102
  chronic urticaria, 106
  clinical presentation, 102*f*
    delayed pressure urticaria, 104
    dermatographism, 103, 103*f*
    physical urticarias, 103, 106
    stress exposure, 104
    vibratory angioedema, 104
  comprehensive history, 106
  definition, 101–102
  differential diagnosis, 105
  epidemiology, 102
  infections, 102
  labs, 106
  mast cells, 102
  treatment, 106–107
  urticarial vasculitis, 106
Urticarial vasculitis, 105–106
U.S. Preventive Services Task Force (USPSTF), 1
Ustekinumab, 20, 51
UV index (UVI), 333, 335*t*

## V

Vancomycin, 77
Varicella-zoster virus (VZV), 68–71, 70*f*
Vascular cell adhesion molecule 1 (VCAM-1), 17
Vascular neoplasms, 17
Vascular lesions, 259*t*–260*t*
Vasculitides, 17–18
Vasculopathies, 18
Vemurafenib, 21
Venereal Disease Research Laboratory test (VDRL), 43–44
Venous ulcer, 324–325
Verrucae, 58–59, 59*f*, 309–311, 310*f*
Vibratory angioedema, 104
*Vibrio vulnificus*, 76
Viral exanthems, 107–116
  erythema infectiosum, 108*t*–109*t*, 110, 112, 114*f*, 115–116
  hand, foot, and mouth disease, 108*t*–109*t*, 111, 115
  measles, 108*t*–109*t*, 110, 112, 113*f*, 115
  pityriasis rosea, 108*t*–109*t*, 111, 114, 114*f*
  roseola infantum, 108*t*–109*t*, 111–112, 114*f*
  rubella, 108*t*–109*t*, 110, 112, 115–116
  varicella, 110–111, 114–115
Vitamin D, 48, 336, 348
Vitiligo, 125–131, 126*f*, 252*t*
Voigt-futcher lines, 251–254, 253*f*
Volar skin, 15

## W

Waardenburg syndrome, 16
World Health Organization (WHO), 338
Wound dehiscence, 230, 230*f*
Wound healing, 228

## X

Xeomin, 235*t*
Xeroderma pigmentosum (XP), 157, 161, 165
Xerosis, 316, 327–332, 328*t*